T0252183

Clinical Cases
in Critical Care

Clinical Cases in Critical Care

Alice Myers
Department of Intensive Care Medicine
East Surrey Hospital
UK

Theophilus Samuels
Department of Intensive Care Medicine
East Surrey Hospital
UK

WILEY Blackwell

This edition first published 2023
© 2023 John Wiley & Sons Ltd

All rights reserved. No part of this publication may be reproduced, stored in a retrieval system, or transmitted, in any form or by any means, electronic, mechanical, photocopying, recording or otherwise, except as permitted by law. Advice on how to obtain permission to reuse material from this title is available at http://www.wiley.com/go/permissions.

The right of Alice Myers and Theophilus Samuels to be identified as the authors of this work has been asserted in accordance with law.

Registered Offices
John Wiley & Sons, Inc., 111 River Street, Hoboken, NJ 07030, USA
John Wiley & Sons Ltd, The Atrium, Southern Gate, Chichester, West Sussex, PO19 8SQ, UK

For details of our global editorial offices, customer services, and more information about Wiley products visit us at www.wiley.com.

Wiley also publishes its books in a variety of electronic formats and by print-on-demand. Some content that appears in standard print versions of this book may not be available in other formats.

Trademarks: Wiley and the Wiley logo are trademarks or registered trademarks of John Wiley & Sons, Inc. and/or its affiliates in the United States and other countries and may not be used without written permission. All other trademarks are the property of their respective owners. John Wiley & Sons, Inc. is not associated with any product or vendor mentioned in this book.

Limit of Liability/Disclaimer of Warranty
The contents of this work are intended to further general scientific research, understanding, and discussion only and are not intended and should not be relied upon as recommending or promoting scientific method, diagnosis, or treatment by physicians for any particular patient. In view of ongoing research, equipment modifications, changes in governmental regulations, and the constant flow of information relating to the use of medicines, equipment, and devices, the reader is urged to review and evaluate the information provided in the package insert or instructions for each medicine, equipment, or device for, among other things, any changes in the instructions or indication of usage and for added warnings and precautions. While the publisher and authors have used their best efforts in preparing this work, they make no representations or warranties with respect to the accuracy or completeness of the contents of this work and specifically disclaim all warranties, including without limitation any implied warranties of merchantability or fitness for a particular purpose. No warranty may be created or extended by sales representatives, written sales materials or promotional statements for this work. The fact that an organization, website, or product is referred to in this work as a citation and/or potential source of further information does not mean that the publisher and authors endorse the information or services the organization, website, or product may provide or recommendations it may make. This work is sold with the understanding that the publisher is not engaged in rendering professional services. The advice and strategies contained herein may not be suitable for your situation. You should consult with a specialist where appropriate. Further, readers should be aware that websites listed in this work may have changed or disappeared between when this work was written and when it is read. Neither the publisher nor authors shall be liable for any loss of profit or any other commercial damages, including but not limited to special, incidental, consequential, or other damages.

Library of Congress Cataloging-in-Publication Data applied for
PB: 9781119578901

Cover Design: Wiley
Cover Images: © Tempura/Getty Images (back cover) © Chaikom/Shutterstock, © Tempura/Getty Images

Set in 11.5/13.5 STIXTwoText by Straive, Pondicherry, India
Printed and bound by CPI Group (UK) Ltd, Croydon, CR0 4YY

C9781119578901_240124

For Alex
1978 – 2018

Contents

Foreword

The authors would like to express deepest gratitude to their families for the continued support and encouragement they gave during the writing of this book.

Alice would like to thank Gordon and Auntie Margaret.

Theophilus would like to thank Kat, Joshua and Electra.

How to Use This Book

This is not intended to be an exhaustive didactic textbook of critical care medicine. The aim of this book is to try and cover a large section of core intensive care medicine (ICM) knowledge in a practical way, keeping the science relevant to your daily work in ICU. The introductory sections provide an overview of critical care medicine and include material which is often encountered in examinations.

The main body of the book consists of the clinical cases. Cases are ordered randomly to reflect the unpredictability of clinical work and, we hope, to keep things interesting. Each case is based around a fictional vignette which amalgamates various real cases managed by the authors. As many core topics as possible are explored through relevant questions and answers as each case develops. Try and answer the questions as you go. We hope this will keep you engaged during self-study. We've done our best to ensure that the cases are accurate and free from error. However, if you spot any mistakes please feel free to let us know.

The answers provided to the questions are often more detailed than you would be required to give in an examination and individual cases are longer than most viva voce examinations. If you are practising for an oral examination, we suggest you either take a section of a case with about five or six questions and drill down into the details or take a longer segment but aim for only the main bullet point answers.

At the end of the book is a Test Yourself section. Some of the answers to these questions can be found within the cases, others cover new material to further expand your knowledge.

We hope that you find this book a useful and engaging tool for revision, learning new topics and preparation for examinations.

Author Information

Dr Alice Myers MBBS BA(Hons) MRCP FRCA EDIC FFICM
Consultant in Intensive Care Medicine and Anaesthesia
Surrey and Sussex Healthcare NHS Trust
Department of Intensive Care Medicine
East Surrey Hospital
Canada Avenue
Redhill
Surrey RH1 5RH
alicemyers@nhs.net

Dr Theophilus Samuels MBBS, BSc(Hons), FRCA, FFICM, Cert Maths (Open), Dip Maths (Open), Dip Stats (Open), BA(Hons) Math Stat (Open), AMIMA, GradStat
Level 2 British Society of Echocardiography TTE accredited
Consultant in Intensive Care Medicine and Anaesthesia
Surrey and Sussex Healthcare NHS Trust
Department of Intensive Care Medicine
East Surrey Hospital
Canada Avenue
Redhill
Surrey RH1 5RH
theophilus.samuels1@nhs.net

Acknowledgements

We are very grateful to friends and colleagues who have supported us by reading and commenting on the cases whilst they were in development.

Nawaf Al-Subaie MD(Res) FRCA EDIC FICM — Consultant in Anaesthesia and Intensive Care Medicine

Giada Azzopardi BSc MBBS MRCP — ST4 Renal Medicine and Intensive Care Medicine

Gordon Bird MBBS BSc(Hons) MRCP FRCA EDIC FFICM — Consultant in Anaesthesia and Intensive Care Medicine

Joshua Burns MBBS BSc — Clinical Fellow in Critical Care

George Chater MB BChir MRCP (UK) — ST3 Anaesthetics

Muhammadawais Cheema MBBS — Clinical Fellow in Intensive Care Medicine and Critical Care Echocardiography

Terry Collingwood MBBS BSc(Hons) MRCP FFICM DipIMC — Consultant in Intensive Care Medicine

Catherine Collins RD FBDA — Critical Care Dietitian

Jamie Conti BSc MBBS MRCP — ST4 Intensive Care Medicine

Nicholas Courtenay-Evans MBBChir MA(Cantab) FRCA PGDip — Consultant Anaesthetist

Paul Crowest BMBS BSc FRCA FFICM — Consultant in Anaesthesia and Intensive Care Medicine

Alexa Curtis MBBS BSc(Hons) MRCP FRCA FFICM — ST8 Anaesthetics and Intensive Care Medicine

Jordan Durrant MBBS FRCS(Urol) — Consultant Urologist

Gareth Ennew BSc(Hons) MBBS FRCEM FFICM — Consultant in Emergency Medicine and Intensive Care Medicine

Lynn Evans BSc MBBS MRCP FFICM PG Cert Med Ed — Consultant in Acute Medicine and Intensive Care Medicine

Professor Lui Forni MB PhD — Consultant in Renal Medicine and Intensive Care Medicine

Rebecca Gray MBBS FFICM FRCP MSc — Consultant in Acute Medicine and Intensive Care Medicine

Guy Hickson MBBS BSc FRCR — Consultant Interventional Radiologist

Luke Hodgson MD MSc MRCP EDIC FFICM BSc — Consultant in Respiratory Medicine and Intensive Care Medicine

Fiona Jones PGDip RGN — Hepatology Clinical Nurse Specialist

Fiona J Lamb MBBS FRCA FFICM — Consultant in Anaesthesia and Intensive Care Medicine

Nick Lees FRCA EDIC FFICM — Consultant in Anaesthesia and Intensive Care Medicine

Donald Leith MRCP MBBS iBSc (Hons) — Clinical Research Fellow in Acute Medicine

Finnian D Lesser MBChB MRCP — Acute Medicine and Intensive Care Registrar

Robert Loveless MBChB FRCA FFICM — ST6 Anaesthetics and Intensive Care Medicine

Jennifer Macallan BSc MBBS FRCA — ST5 Anaesthetics

Claire Mearns MBChB FRCA FFICM — Consultant in Anaesthesia and Intensive Care Medicine

Patrick Morgan MBChB FRCA FFICM — Consultant in Anaesthesia and Intensive Care Medicine

Aikaterini Papadopoulou MBBS FRCA FCAI PGDip Cert Maths (Open) — ST7 Anaesthetics

Elizabeth Potter BSc (Hons) MRCP FRCA FFICM — Consultant in Anaesthesia and Intensive Care Medicine

Nicola Raeside MBBS BSc(Hons) DipABRSM — CT1 Anaesthetics

Sameer Ranjan MBBS FCARCSI EDIC — Consultant in Anaesthesia and Intensive Care Medicine

Alana Rochester MBChB BSc MRCP — IMT3 Registrar in General Medicine

Mark Salmon MBBS FRCA DipIMC — Consultant Anaesthetist

Thomas Sanderson MBBS MmedEd — Clinical Fellow in Intensive Care Medicine and Critical Care Echocardiography

Eleanor de Sausmarez BMBS BmedSci (Hons) MSc MRCEM FRCA — ST4 Anaesthetics and Intensive Care Medicine

Matthew Sinnott MB ChB (Hons) BSc (Hons) FRCA — ST6 Anaesthetics

Amybel Belladonna Taylor BSc MBChB — IMT3 in General Medicine

Patrick Thorburn MBChB BSc(Hons) PGDip FRCA FFICM — Consultant in Anaesthesia and Intensive Care Medicine

Andrew Williams BMBS MRCP MRCA — ST3 Anaesthetic Trainee

List of Abbreviations

ABG	Arterial blood gas
ACT	Activated clotting time
AF	Atrial fibrillation
AKI	Acute kidney injury
APACHE	Acute physiology and chronic health evaluation
ARDS	Acute respiratory distress syndrome
ATLS®	Advanced trauma life support
ATP	Adenosine triphosphate
BP/SBP/ NBP/IBP	Blood pressure/systolic blood pressure/non-invasive blood pressure/invasive blood pressure
bpm	Beats per minute (heart rate)
BSA	Body surface area
CABG	Coronary artery bypass graft
CAP	Community acquired pneumonia
CD4	Cluster of differentiation 4
CMV	Cytomegalovirus
CNS	Central nervous system
COPD	Chronic obstructive pulmonary disease
CPB	Cardiopulmonary bypass
CPR	Cardiopulmonary resuscitation
CRP	C-reactive protein
CSA	Cross-sectional area
CSF	Cerebrospinal fluid
CT	Computed tomography
CTA	Computed tomography angiography
CTPA	Computed tomography pulmonary angiography
CVC	Central venous catheter
DC	Direct current
DIC	Disseminated intravascular coagulation
DKA	Diabetic ketoacidosis
DNACPR	Do not attempt cardiopulmonary resuscitation
EBV	Epstein–Barr virus
ECMO	Extracorporeal membrane oxygenation
ED	Emergency department
ERCP/MRCP	Endoscopic retrograde cholangiopancreatography/magnetic retrograde cholangiopancreatography
ETT	Endotracheal tube
FBC	Full blood count

FEV1	Forced expiratory volume in 1 second
FRC	Functional residual capacity
FVC	Forced vital capacity
GABA	Gamma-aminobutyric acid
GBS	Guillain–Barré syndrome
GCS	Glasgow Coma Scale
HFNC/HFNO	High-flow nasal cannulae/oxygen
HIV	Human immunodeficiency virus
HR	Heart rate
IABP	Intra-aortic balloon pump
IBW	Ideal body weight
ICP	Intracranial pressure
INR	International normalised ratio
IV	Intravenous
LOS	Length of stay
LV	Left ventricle
LVOT	Left ventricular outflow tract
MDT	Multidisciplinary team
MRA	Magnetic resonance angiography
MRI	Magnetic resonance imaging
NG	Nasogastric
NIV	Non-invasive ventilation
PEEP	Positive end-expiratory pressure
PLAPS	Posterolateral alveolar and/or pleural syndrome
Plat	Platelets
RCUK	Resuscitation Council UK
ReSPECT	Recommended summary plan for emergency care and treatment
ROSC	Return of spontaneous circulation
RR	Respiratory rate
RV	Right ventricle
SBT	Spontaneous breathing trial
SOFA	Sequential organ failure assessment
SVV	Stroke volume variation
TEG	Thromboelastography
TOE	Transoesophageal echocardiography
TTE	Transthoracic echocardiography
U&E	Urea and electrolytes
US	Ultrasound
VTI	Velocity time integral
WBC	White blood count
WHO	World Health Organization

Part

I

Introduction

1 A Brief Introduction to Critical Care

Setting the scene

Critical care is a specialised form of healthcare, usually a department within a hospital (often called the intensive care unit or ICU), which can provide organ support and invasive monitoring for a patient while treating a reversible illness. Working in ICU can be rewarding and challenging. The aim of this introduction is to give you a brief overview of critical care with an idea of what it can and cannot offer, and its context within the hospital.

Although the life-saving possibilities are often remarkable, many of the techniques used for providing critical care support can be aggressive, with the potential to cause discomfort and psychological distress for both the patient and their family. In addition, critical care is resource heavy, has limited availability and is expensive to deliver. For these reasons, the 'reversibility' of a patient's condition is an important consideration when deciding whether or not to admit. A risk versus benefit assessment is always appropriate – risk being the degree of harm you may cause the patient through applying your organ support interventions, and benefit being the likelihood that you will be able to reverse the acute illness and return the patient to an acceptable quality of life.

Throughout the book, we will often use the terms 'critical care', 'intensive care' and 'ICU' interchangeably. Although different hospitals may draw practical distinction between areas, for the purposes of this book, HDU (high-dependency unit) or level 2 care can be assumed to be included as part of critical care unless otherwise specified.

It is worth noting that medical knowledge inevitably advances over time. Conditions which were terminal 20 years ago may well be considered reversible now. So, one must be cautious when discussing patient selection. It is not usually acceptable to refuse admission based on advanced age alone or the presence of cancer. Sometimes you may wish to admit a patient for a lower

Clinical Cases in Critical Care, First Edition. Alice Myers and Theophilus Samuels.
© 2023 John Wiley & Sons Ltd. Published 2023 by John Wiley & Sons Ltd.

level of critical care with an 'escalation plan' in place, ensuring that, should the patient's condition deteriorate, there would be no progression to more invasive and ultimately futile treatments. For instance, a physically frail 85 year old with urosepsis and hypotension might be an excellent candidate for vasopressors and antibiotics but may not benefit from intubation and ventilation in the context of multiorgan failure secondary to severe pneumococcal sepsis.

Approximately 15–20% of patients in critical care in the UK will die before leaving hospital. ICU mortality is usually higher for patients with acute medical pathologies compared with high-risk elective postoperative patients. Recognising when a patient is dying is an important skill but identifying when efforts are futile is not always easy or possible. Timely acknowledgment that the patient is in the terminal phase of life, combined with sensitive and frank communication, allows carers to consider changing the focus of care from aggressive resuscitation to prioritising comfort, dignity and time with family.

The COVID-19 pandemic (which occurred during the writing of this book!) thrust critical care into the public eye. The pandemic was a difficult period for everyone working in ICUs throughout the world. The challenges were many:

- Academic
  - Rapidly learning as much as possible about an unfamiliar disease and its management.
- Physical
  - Caring for an overwhelming number of patients while wearing restrictive personal protective equipment.
  - Increased need for manual handling due to frequent implementation of prone positioning.
  - Increased working hours for many healthcare professionals.
- Psychological
  - The emotional challenge of seeing so many patients succumb to this terrible disease while their relatives were unable to spend time with them due to quarantine.
  - Moral injury sustained through the impact of allocating limited resources in the face of overwhelming demands.
  - Many ICU staff suffered burnout or post-traumatic stress disorder (PTSD).

However, the pandemic also allowed us to learn a great deal about such things as the importance of teamwork, psychological support, mutual aid within critical care networks, video-conferencing and the use of technology to share information. Perhaps the period which follows the pandemic will be a time for post-traumatic growth with new positive developments in light of the lessons learned.

The ICU and its role within the hospital

Levels of care

The UK National Health System (NHS) uses the following definitions:

Levels of care

Level	Definition
0	Needs can be met through normal ward care in an acute hospital
1	Patients are at risk of deteriorating – care needs can be met on an acute ward with additional support from ICU or critical care outreach services
2	More detailed observation or support is needed, e.g. where there is single organ failure or where the patient has undergone major surgery, or where patients are 'stepping down' from level 3
3	Either advanced ventilation alone is required, or two or more organ systems are failing

Some hospitals have 'Level 1+' or 'Enhanced Care' units. These are able to offer specialised postanaesthetic care to surgical patients who do not require management in a level 2 or HDU area but who need more than can be delivered in a level 1 unit.

Bed capacity

In 2016–17, the NHS reported it had 5912 critical care beds (levels 1 and 2) – 68% adult, 32% children or infants. Wong et al. (SNAP-2 and EPICCS collaborators) found in 2019 that the UK had a median of 2.7 critical care beds per 100 hospital beds (compared with, for instance, 3.7 in Australia and 3.5 in New Zealand).

It is difficult to directly compare the number of critical care beds in different countries around Europe since the definitions are heterogenous. However, one study published in 2012 (Rhodes et al., Crit. Care Med.) found that, per 100 000 of the population, the number of critical care beds differed widely across Europe – 6.6 in the UK, 11 in Switzerland, 21.4 in Romania, 21.8 in Austria, 11.6 in France, 29.2 in Germany.

Bed capacity (i.e. the number of staffed beds available) affects a hospital's ability to deliver elective services since emergencies will take priority. Insufficient critical care bed capacity can lead to cancellation of high-risk surgical procedures, delays in delivering life-saving treatment and an increase in non-clinical interhospital transfers.

'Surge capacity' is a term used to describe the additional critical care beds which can be rapidly created during times of increased demand – for instance during a pandemic. The total number of critical care beds in the UK at the peak of the COVID-19 pandemic was not available at the time of writing. However, many units doubled, tripled or quadrupled their ICU capacity in response to the overwhelming number of patients. Some centres created de novo temporary ICUs in different wards within their hospitals. It should be remembered that these units will often not have had the infrastructure of a purpose-built ICU (e.g. wall-piped oxygen, store cupboards appropriately stocked, ICU regulation ventilation levels, etc.). These temporary ICUs were sometimes in distant isolated sites, staffed by non-intensivists, had a lower staff-to-patient ratio, and used non-standard equipment (e.g. anaesthetic machine ventilators). 'Surge capacity' beds are temporary and not included in the numbers otherwise quoted here.

What can be offered in critical care?

Many hospitals have a 'general' adult ICU which cares for a mixed population of medical and surgical patients aged over 16 years. These units vary in size from a handful of beds to some with more than 100 beds. In 2015, NHS Digital reported that patients aged over 50 years accounted for 77% of the 271 079 critical care episodes in its analysis. Demographics vary between units but nationally, males accounted for 56% of admissions.

Subspecialty critical care such as neurology and neurosurgery, cardiothoracic and liver can be integrated into a larger general unit or managed in a defined, ring-fenced specialist unit. Children and neonates are usually cared for in separate paediatric and neonatal critical care units.

Although some of the following techniques can be offered in other specialised areas of the hospital (e.g. operating theatres, coronary care units, acute medical units), the equipment and training required usually necessitates admission to ICU. This list is not exhaustive:

- Advanced monitoring
  - Techniques requiring invasive catheterisation
    - Intra-arterial blood pressure monitoring.
    - Central venous pressure monitoring.
    - Cardiac output monitoring, e.g. pulse contour analysis.
  - Techniques requiring specialist interpretation that may be more easily undertaken in a higher level of care area
    - Continuous electroencephalogram.
    - Frequent thromboelastography.
    - Intracranial pressure monitoring.
    - Serial echocardiography.
- Respiratory
  - Invasive and non-invasive ventilation.
  - Extracorporeal carbon dioxide extraction.
  - Extracorporeal membrane oxygenation (primarily venovenous).
  - High-frequency oscillatory ventilation.
- Cardiovascular
  - Vasopressor drugs.
  - Inotropic drugs.
  - Intra-arterial balloon pumps.
  - Extracorporeal membrane oxygenation (primarily venoarterial).
  - Mechanical assist devices, e.g. left or right ventricular assist devices.
- Renal
  - Continuous venovenous haemofiltration and haemodiafiltration.
- Other
  - Molecular adsorbent recirculating system (MARS®) for liver failure.
  - Extracorporeal cytokine adsorption devices for sepsis.

Interface with the hospital

Critical care interacts with the whole hospital, in particular supporting the work of the emergency department, operating theatres and acute medical teams. The nuances of individual departmental relationships are unique to each organisation but there are usually rules or agreements which act as a framework for these interactions. Examples include the following:

- *Referral systems* – the specific logistics may vary (e.g. verbal versus digital referrals and whether a consultant or registrar receives referrals) but the Guidelines for the Provision of Intensive Care Services (GPICS V2.1) makes the following recommendations:
    - Decisions to admit to ICU must be discussed with the ICU consultant.
    - There should be a process to review referrals and associated decision making.
- *Open and closed units* – the traditional 'open' model of ICU allowed physicians and surgeons to admit to ICU and invite review by intensivists at their own discretion. The 'closed' model has been shown to result in improved morbidity and mortality. In this model, only intensivists have admitting rights to the ICU and the critical care team is responsible for the patient's care while they remain an inpatient on the unit. Some specialist units have a modified closed system whereby, for instance, neurosurgeons may share admitting rights to a neurocritical care alongside the neurointensivists.
- *Critical care without walls* – this concept was developed to improve recognition and response to deteriorating patients in the rest of the hospital by expanding the role and influence of intensivists beyond the four walls of the ICU. Critical care outreach teams play a key role here.

The critical care team

This list is a general overview for the UK and similar countries.

- *Doctors* – by training, doctors in critical care are usually a mixture of intensivists, physicians and anaesthetists although some other specialist doctors, e.g. microbiologists, also work routinely in critical care units. The Intensive Care Society (ICS) recommends that ICU should be led by a consultant intensivist with a consultant to patient ratio of up to 1:8 to 1:15. During the COVID-19 pandemic, this was temporarily reduced to 1:30 due to the increased volume of patients. The ICU resident to patient ratio should be up to 1:8. Residents include trainees, specialty doctors and advanced critical care practitioners (ACCPs). GPICS V2.1 recommends that consultant-led ward rounds should occur twice per day and all critical care admissions should be reviewed by a consultant within 12 hours of admission.
- *Nurses* – nursing ratios differ according to the level of care. It is recommended that the nurse to patient ratio is 1:1 in level 3 and 1:2 in level 2. The nursing team should be led by a senior, experienced nurse. There should also be additional supernumerary nurses available and a clinical co-ordinator. ICU nurses are also often heavily involved in teaching and training around the hospital. Some ICU follow-up clinics are nurse led. The value and range of work done by critical care nurses is immense.
- *Critical care outreach* – GPICS V2.1 standards state that there should be a clear hospital-wide mechanism for recognising the deteriorating patient and a clearly documented escalation process. An early warning system must be in place, e.g. NEWS (National Early Warning System). An

outreach or rapid response team is recommended to be available 24 hours per day, 7 days per week. There is NICE guidance for outreach services (NG 94, chapter 27, 2018). The National Outreach Forum defined seven core elements of outreach in 2018 (PREPARE).

- **P**atient track and trigger
- **R**apid response
- **E**ducation, training and support
- **P**atient safety and clinical governance
- **A**udit, evaluation and monitoring of patient outcome and continuing quality care
- **R**ehabilitation after critical illness
- **E**nhancing service delivery

- *Pharmacists* – GPICS V2.1 recommends that each ICU should have a dedicated pharmacist and should have access to an Advanced Stage II (excellence-level) pharmacist. Pharmacy services should be available for advice 24 hours per day, 7 days per week.

- *Physiotherapists* – physiotherapists should be involved in rehabilitation of critical care patients (NG 83). They play a vital role in helping to reduce the muscle weakness and reduced mobilisation which often accompany critical illness. Chest physiotherapy, involving positioning, percussive techniques, suctioning and breathing exercises, can be extremely useful in preventing ventilator-associated pneumonias and improving weaning from mechanical ventilatory support.

- *Psychologists* – GPICS V2.1 and NG 83 are both clear in stating the value of regular psychological assessment throughout a patient's ICU admission. Psychologists are essential in the detection, assessment and management of psychological trauma and play an integral role in successful post-ICU rehabilitation. In addition, the importance of providing psychological support for critical care staff and preventing burnout is increasingly being recognised.

- *Dietitians* – provision of nutrition for critically unwell patients is often complex, with patients at high risk of malnutrition. GPICS V2.1 recommends that ICUs should have access to a dietitian during working hours and that they should form an integral part of the multidisciplinary team (MDT), being involved in critical care meetings and training.

- *Speech and language therapists* – SALT input is hugely important in the management of patients with impaired communication, e.g. due to tracheostomy, and those with swallowing difficulties. The SALT team can help with diagnosis (performing procedures such as fine endoscopic evaluation of swallowing and videofluoroscopy), rehabilitation and teaching techniques for long-term management of irreversible problems.

- *Healthcare assistants* – HCAs carry out a large range of vital clinical and non-clinical tasks within critical care. These include recording observations, undertaking personal care, ordering medical consumables and restocking clinical areas.

- *Allied support staff* – these include ward clerks, managers, porters, orderlies and domestics. Without support staff, critical care would be unable to function efficiently.

- *Advanced critical care practitioners and physician's associates* – increasingly, critical care units are encouraging development of the ACCP and physician's associate roles to supplement and complement the work done by regular critical care nurses and doctors. They may take full part in daily physical assessments of patients, contribute to management plans, perform procedures and assist with resuscitation.

■ *Other specialists* who work closely with ICU include microbiology, palliative care, transplant surgeons, specialist physicians, pain teams, specialist nurses in organ donation, chaplains, electrophysiologists, occupational therapists and perfusionists.

Psychological and psychiatric issues in the ICU

Patients in critical care are vulnerable to both pre-existing psychiatric diagnoses and acute, ICU-related problems. Approximately 50% of critically ill patients suffer serious emotional distress (Richard-Belle, BMJ Open, 2018). Underlying psychiatric issues may be directly related to the patient's admission – e.g. drug overdose, medication compliance issues leading to status epilepticus, adverse reactions to antipsychotic medications. Psychiatric diagnoses may co-exist unrelated to the admitting diagnosis but can make managing patients challenging. Patients may present to ICU while being treated under a Section of the Mental Health Act. This is discussed in Case 18.

Acutely, up to 80% of patients develop delirium while in ICU. Delirium can be hyperactive, hypoactive or mixed. Delirium is discussed further in Case 11.

The psychological sequalae following a critical care admission can include PTSD, body image issues, poor sleep, depression and psychosocial problems, including relationship difficulties and trouble returning to work. These issues, which dramatically affect a patient's long-term physical and psychological health, can sometimes be directly traced back to traumatic experiences in ICU, e.g. a period of delirium, a painful experience, a miscommunication. Although many potential sources of distress cannot be avoided, healthcare workers in ICU can make efforts to ensure good analgesia, minimise distressing noises and try to reassure and orientate patients with good communication, even when sedated. ICU follow-up clinics can provide valuable support for patients and useful insights for the healthcare team. Multidisciplinary input from psychologists, ICU nurses, physiotherapists and doctors is vital for identifying and managing long-term sequalae.

The admitting clinician should pay attention to any pre-existing psychiatric diagnoses and review medicine prescriptions. Adverse effects of antipsychotic drugs can be multisystemic and include hepatic dysfunction (e.g. chlorpromazine), sudden cardiac death (e.g. thioridazine), prolonged QTc interval (e.g. haloperidol), renal dysfunction (e.g. risperidone) and blood dyscrasias (e.g. clozapine). The admitting clinician should be aware that some antipsychotics can be administered in depot form and asenapine is available as a transdermal patch in some countries. Drug history should also include over-the-counter remedies, smoking, alcohol and illegal drugs.

Communication

Communication is key in ensuring that the patient's and relatives' experience is as good as possible. Good communication can help to mitigate some of the negative psychological impacts of an ICU admission. Discussion with the patient themselves or, if incapacitated, their next of kin should be an early priority. The clinician should try to find a safe and quiet space, take a colleague for support, avoid interruptions from phones or bleeps, and document everything thoroughly. Additional medical history should be obtained from the patient, next of kin, general practitioner, previous hospital or clinic notes, and the police/law enforcement if necessary. When providing information, you must always consider the patient's right to confidentiality. Consult the General Medical Council's guidance on using and disclosing patient information and if in doubt, discuss with the hospital legal team.

If the patient is unconscious, you will most often be communicating with the next of kin. It is usually wise to begin managing their expectations early on, given the high overall mortality in the critical care patient population.

Psychological issues amongst ICU staff

The COVID-19 pandemic highlighted the vulnerability of critical care staff to PTSD, depression, anxiety and burnout. Psychological support and resilience training should be available for staff. Hot and cold debriefing sessions can be useful (i.e. at the time of the event and after a timely delay), as can Schwartz rounds and Balint groups (group sessions where professionals gather to reflect upon the social and emotional aspects of their work). Encouraging the MDT to debrief together can improve teamwork and help build support networks. Staff should also be encouraged to take annual leave and maintain their interests outside work.

Infection control

According to the World Health Organization (WHO), approximately 30% of patients in ICUs in high-income countries are affected by healthcare-associated infection (HCAI or nosocomial infection). Critical care patients are at particular risk due to invasive procedures, relative immune suppression and exposure to broad-spectrum antimicrobials.

Scrupulous infection control is mandatory. GPICS V2.1 recommends that all staff in ICU observe the WHO 'Five Moments For Hand Hygiene'. There should be documentation and audit systems in place for infection control practices, particularly with regard to invasive procedures, antibiotic stewardship, surveillance for nosocomial infection, and environmental infection control (e.g. surface and fomite cleaning, deep cleaning). Many units observe 'gloves and aprons' and 'bare below the elbows' policies.

Cross-infection screening is advised, particularly where patients have been transferred between healthcare institutions, including care homes and rehabilitation facilities. Microbes implicated in cross-infection include methicillin-resistant *Staphylococcus aureus* (MRSA), carbapenemase-producing organisms (CPO), *Clostridium difficile* (*C. diff*) and *Acinetobacter*. There have been deadly outbreaks of these organisms in ICUs and infections are difficult to treat. There is considerable associated morbidity and mortality. 'Care bundles' have been used to reduce the incidence of certain nosocomial infections such as ventilator-associated pneumonia and catheter-related site infection (e.g. Matching Michigan).

Space between beds should be sufficient to prevent cross-infection and ICUs should have isolation areas available for patients with contagious diseases such as tuberculosis (TB) and influenza. Isolation rooms should have pressurised antechambers to offer protection from the environment for vulnerable, immunocompromised patients, or to protect the environment from contagions.

There should be clear protocols for managing incidences of staff exposure – for instance, exposure to blood-borne viruses, measles or TB.

Clinical governance and quality assurance

The UK Department of Health (DoH) stated in 1998 that clinical governance is the 'framework through which healthcare organisations are accountable for continuously improving the quality of their services and safeguarding high standards of care by creating an environment in which excellence in clinical care will flourish'.

Standards are set by organisations such as the DoH UK, WHO, Faculty of Intensive Care Medicine (FICM) and the Intensive Care Society (ICS). The ICS publishes the Guidelines for the Provision of Intensive Care Services; version 2.1 was published in 2022: GPICS V2.1.

There should be local leads (consultant and nurse) for audit and quality improvement. Local clinical governance meetings allow presentation and discussion of clinical audit, quality improvement and morbidity and mortality data. In addition to local audit meetings, there are larger organisations such as the Intensive Care National Audit and Research Centre (ICNARC) which regularly publishes reports on national data.

Most hospitals have systems in place to facilitate incident reporting (e.g. Datix). In addition, certain issues warrant root-cause analysis or After Action Review, e.g. cases of cross-infection with MRSA.

Various signals have been considered as quality-of-care indicators in the ICU, e.g. incidences of ventilator-associated pneumonia (VAP), accidental extubation or pulmonary thromboembolism. However, there is no consensus regarding this.

It can be a challenge to keep up to date with current trends in critical care medicine while working a busy job. Journal clubs are a useful way to share knowledge, encourage critical thinking and develop skills in analysis. Not all clinicians need to carry out research, but all should be able to understand the process and appraise the results.

The GRADE system can be used to assess the quality of evidence – **G**rading of **R**ecommendations, **A**ssessment, **D**evelopment and **E**valuation. GRADE reviews limitations, internal validity, inconsistency, indirectness, imprecision and publication bias. Quality will then be graded as very low, low, moderate or high.

The hierarchy of evidence can be stratified as follows:

Ia   Systematic review or meta-analysis of randomised controlled trials (RCT)

Ib   At least one RCT

IIa   At least one well-designed controlled study without randomisation

IIb   At least one well designed quasi-experimental study (e.g. cohort study)

III   Well-designed, non-experimental descriptive studies (e.g. case–control and case series)

IV   Expert opinion

Recommendations are subsequently graded as follows:

A Based on hierarchy I
B Based on hierarchy II or extrapolated from hierarchy I
C Based on hierarchy II or extrapolated from hierarchy I or II
D Based in hierarchy IV or extrapolated from hierarchy I, II or III

A full discussion of evidence-based medicine is beyond the scope of this book. However, it is worth noting that it is possible to find contradictory evidence for almost anything in medicine! While is it important to keep up to date and well apprised of current literature and recommended guidelines, every patient is unique and may not fit neatly into a management protocol. There is no substitute for making a detailed clinical assessment. Armed with your medical knowledge, your understanding of the patient's unique set of problems and an awareness of the available evidence, you can take an individualised approach to managing each critical care patient.

Key resources are often quoted in this book. Review these sources for yourself so that you can understand how to apply the evidence to your own practice.

Further reading

- The Faculty of Intensive Care Medicine and the Intensive Care Society publish *Guidelines for the Provision of Intensive Care Services*. Version 2.1 was published in 2022. GPICS V2.1 is available online at www.ficm.ac.uk and www.ics.ac.uk.
- The King's Fund publishes an especially useful overview document called *Critical Care Services in the English NHS*. This is available online at www.kingsfund.org.uk.

2 Intubation of the Critically Unwell Patient

The aim of this section is to provide an overview of the main issues to consider when approaching intubation and initial ventilation in the critically unwell patient. The following is not intended to be a comprehensive guideline – rather, it reflects the experiences of the authors. As always, clinical judgement should be used to modify techniques and individualise management strategies. There is no 'one size fits all' when it comes to critical care.

Why?

- *Airway protection* – the patient is at risk of:
  - airway obstruction, e.g. swelling secondary to anaphylaxis
  - aspiration, e.g. due to reduced GCS
  - trauma to the airway, e.g. burns or penetrating laryngeal injury.
- *Gas exchange*
  - Failure to oxygenate, e.g. pneumonia.
  - Failure to ventilate, e.g. bronchospasm.
  - Apnoea.
- *Exhaustion or weakness*
  - Neuromuscular disorders, e.g. myasthenia gravis.
  - Fatigue, e.g. respiratory compensation for metabolic acidosis.
- *Facilitate management*
  - Patients unable to comply with treatment may require sedation and airway protection to facilitate management, e.g. a uraemic patient may be encephalopathic and intolerant of vascular access and hemofiltration.
  - Patients requiring emergency bronchoscopy or isolation of one lung (e.g. pulmonary abscess).

Clinical Cases in Critical Care, First Edition. Alice Myers and Theophilus Samuels.
© 2023 John Wiley & Sons Ltd. Published 2023 by John Wiley & Sons Ltd.

Why not?

There may be occasions where it is not in the patient's best interests to intubate them, e.g. they have previously refused intubation and intensive care admission, or they have a terminal condition which means they would not survive intensive care. Talk to the patient if you can, review the clinical notes and previous escalation plans if available. Ask about Advance Decision documentation.

When?

- *Now*
  - The patient is in extremis. There is usually time to preoxygenate as a minimum (while assistants gather drugs and equipment).
  - If delay will lead to deterioration, the airway must be secured as a matter of urgency.
- *Later*
  - There is a risk of deterioration when electing to postpone intubation once the decision has been made that it is required. Clinical judgement must always be used to evaluate the risks and benefits.
  - Consider whether you have time to bring loved ones in to see the patient before you intubate. It is not always possible or practical and it should never delay emergency management. However, even a brief moment can make an enormous difference to patients and their relatives.

Reasons to delay intubation include the following:

- *Optimisation of clinical condition* – if the patient is cardiovascularly unstable, they may benefit from fluids or vasopressors and further monitoring with an arterial line prior to induction.
- *Acquiring appropriate equipment and staff* – for example, when a newborn requires intubation and the most experienced person available has limited paediatric experience. In this case, it may be safest to wait for experienced help.
- *Transferring the patient to a more appropriate location* – for example, when a patient has deteriorated on a general medical ward but the safety benefits of intubating them in critical care outweigh the risks of delaying intubation by the time it takes to transfer them there.

Where?

- *Remote location* – sometimes there is no choice but to intubate in a remote location. If the patient is unsafe to transfer, then they must be stabilised in situ.
  - Make the environment as safe as possible by asking a trained assistant to bring monitoring, drugs and equipment.
  - Position the patient as optimally as possible (may prove difficult in the angiosuite or MRI scanner).

- Ensure there is a good supply of oxygen (use cylinders in the absence of piped oxygen).
- Ask ward staff to assist or to minimise distractions.

- *Familiar environment, e.g. ICU, operating theatres or ED resuscitation* – a routine preintubation checklist is useful. It should not be assumed that monitoring is attached and equipment is available.

Who?

Roles should be allocated within the team according to skills and experience and this should be clearly communicated. Know who to call for additional help and how to contact them. Verbalise the plan before commencing.

- *First and second intubator* – usually the second person to attempt intubation should have more airway management experience than the first. If a difficult airway is anticipated or repeated instrumentation is likely to cause complications, then the most experienced person should make the first attempt.
- *Administering drugs* – ideally, an experienced doctor with an understanding of the relevant pharmacology will take this role. Once induction drugs are given, this team member should be ready to administer drugs for blood pressure augmentation and possibly additional sedation.
- *Trained assistant* – this team member assists the intubator by passing equipment and administering cricoid pressure if requested.
- *Someone on the pulse* – if invasive blood pressure monitoring is unavailable, any other health professional can be allocated this vital role. This person palpates a central pulse (usually femoral) and informs the team whether the pulse is feeling weaker or stronger, allowing the team member administering the drugs to titrate vasopressors until invasive arterial monitoring is established.
- *Runner* – this team member can fetch equipment, gas cylinders, emergency help, make telephone calls, etc.

How?

Minimising the time between loss of consciousness (administration of induction agents) and securing the airway is crucial. Critically unwell patients are often quick to desaturate, and oxygen saturations may be poor even despite preoxygenation.

The classic rapid-sequence induction (RSI) technique involving thiopentone and suxamethonium is now rarely used by intensivists due to the potential for cardiac instability, the side-effects of suxamethonium, and the availability of newer drugs. Many favour a *modified* RSI approach which may bear little resemblance to the classic technique aside from sharing an end goal of securing the airway as quickly as possible. There are a multitude of ways to achieve this safely.

■ *Assessment*
  ■ In patients who need to be emergently intubated, a full airway assessment can be impractical. However, a basic assessment of the airway by an experienced operator can be performed in only a few seconds if needed.
  ■ A MACOCHA score ≥3 predicts difficult intubation and is the only validated airway assessment tool in the critically ill (Table 1).
  ■ Pre-emptive assessment of patients on admission to critical care may help identify potentially difficult airways and allow appropriate strategies to be devised.
■ *Setting up*
  We recommend using the Difficult Airway Society's DAS ICU Intubation Guidelines preintubation checklist.
  ■ Monitoring – minimum standards include ECG, pulse oximetry, end-tidal carbon dioxide monitoring and non-invasive blood pressure. Consider establishing intra-arterial blood pressure monitoring prior to induction in patients at risk of haemodynamic instability.
  ■ Intravenous access – ensure that reliable IV access (usually at least 20 G) is available for administration of medications. Additional IV cannulae or central venous access are likely to be required once the patient is anaesthetised. Ensure cannulae are secured as they can easily be dislodged during positioning, especially if the patient is sweating.
■ *Positioning*
  ■ Usually the optimal position is approximately 30° head up, helping to reduce the risk of aspiration through passive regurgitation and improving functional residual capacity (FRC). Use pillows to facilitate the anatomic sniffing position.

Table 1: MACOCHA score used for airway assessment in critically ill patients. The score ranges from 0 (easy) to 12 (very difficult). A score ≥ 3 predicts difficult intubation in critically ill patients.

Factors	Points
Factors related to the patient	
Mallampati class III or IV	5
Obstructive sleep **A**pnoea syndrome	2
Reduced mobility of **C**ervical spine	1
Limited mouth **O**pening <3 cm	1
Factors related to pathology	
Coma	1
Severe **H**ypoxaemia (SpO$_2$ < 80%)	1
Factor related to operator	
Non-**A**naesthetist	1
Total	**12**

- During a trauma call, the patient should be kept flat with manual inline stabilisation of the cervical spine.
- There are cases where a patient's condition is improved in recumbent position, e.g. platypnoea-orthodeoxia syndrome due to atrial septal defect or hepatopulmonary syndrome.

- *Oxygen*
  - Preoxygenation aims to wash out alveolar nitrogen and replace it with oxygen. It is achieved by applying 100% oxygen for either 3 minutes or for eight maximal inspirations and expirations. This increases oxygen in the FRC. While, in health, this technique can prolong the time until desaturation occurs by up to approximately 8 minutes, it may buy only seconds in the critically unwell patient.
  - Preoxygenation can be achieved using a Waters breathing circuit (Mapleson C) with a closely applied facemask. This has the added benefit of allowing positive end-expiratory pressure (PEEP) to be applied using the adjustable pressure limiting (APL) valve.
  - When the facemask is continually applied after cessation of breathing, apnoeic oxygenation can help maintain saturations. In health, during apnoea, approximately $250\,mL/min$ O_2 diffuses from alveoli into capillaries, but only $10–20\,mL/min$ of CO_2 diffuses back into alveoli (although CO_2 production remains around $200\,mL/min$). This deficit results in a pressure difference, creating the potential for mass flow of gas from pharynx to alveoli. Movement of gases during apnoeic oxygenation can also be aided by cardiac oscillations. Consider using high-flow nasal oxygen (HFNO) throughout, particularly during intubation attempts when the facemask has been removed.
- *Call for help* – even the most experienced intensivist may appreciate skilled back-up during intubation of the critically unwell patient.
- *Drugs* – there is no set recipe. Intensivists usually develop their own techniques, and most will adjust their approach for individual patients. The following list is not exhaustive, and agents can be used in various combinations:
  - Opioids – used as co-induction agents, opioids can obtund the laryngeal response, reduce requirement for other sedative drugs, promote cardiovascular stability and minimise changes in intracranial pressure.
    - Fentanyl – around 100 times more potent than morphine. Rapid onset. Duration of action is approximately 30 minutes.
    - Alfentanil – onset of action is three times faster than fentanyl, but duration of action can be several hours.
  - Hypnotics
    - Propofol – frequently used in combination with an opioid for induction of anaesthesia in elective surgical patients. Propofol causes significant cardiovascular depression and so the standard dose should be reduced when the patient is unstable. Caution is required as even small doses in critically unwell patients can cause catastrophic hypotension.

- Ketamine – causes direct sympathetic stimulation and, in healthy patients, there may be a small transient dose-dependent increase in blood pressure on administration. It is often preferred by prehospital specialists for this reason. However, ketamine also acts as a direct negative inotrope so caution should be employed in critically unwell patients where endogenous catecholamines may be deplete. In some cases, administration can result in reduced cardiac output and even myocardial ischaemia. Ketamine has bronchodilator properties and is useful in the management of life-threatening asthma. Doses can be titrated when used in infusion for sedation, bronchodilation or analgesia. Complications include hallucinations and raised intracranial pressure.
- Thiopentone – this rapid and short-acting barbiturate has a predictable onset and rapid offset time. This made thiopentone integral to the original RSI technique. The anticonvulsant properties make it a useful option for induction of anaesthesia in cases of status epilepticus. However, it should be used with caution in critically unwell patients as it can result in significant hypotension.
- Alternative strategy – to preserve cardiovascular stability, some clinicians avoid these hypnotic agents at induction of unstable critical care patients in favour of combining a fast-acting benzodiazepine with a high-dose, fast-acting opioid.
- Neuromuscular blockers
  - Rocuronium – this non-depolarising muscle relaxant has now largely replaced suxamethonium as part of modified RSI. It has a rapid onset of action, approximately 45 seconds, when given at a dose of 1–1.5 mg/kg. It has a long duration of action but can be rapidly reversed using sugammadex, a modified gamma cyclodextrin which chelates rocuronium, thereby inactivating it. Rarely, it can cause bronchospasm or anaphylaxis.
  - Suxamethonium – rarely used in critical care now due to its side-effect profile, suxamethonium (succinylcholine) has a rapid onset of action and short duration. It is given at a dose of 1–2 mg/kg. This depolarising muscle relaxant can cause hyperkalaemia, leading to life-threatening arrhythmias and cardiac arrest.
- Others
  - Midazolam – can be given in combination with other agents to promote greater haemodynamic stability at induction. As a benzodiazepine, it is particularly useful in patients with intractable seizures. It induces anterograde amnesia.
  - Lidocaine – can be used at induction to blunt the airway responses to laryngoscopy and endotracheal intubation. It also supplements the anaesthetic effects of the induction agent.
- Vasoactive drugs
  - Metaraminol and phenylephrine – both have alpha-2 and minimal beta-adrenergic activity so are given to treat hypotension. Both

may be given by infusion. Metaraminol may cause profound reflex bradycardia in patients with normal sympathetic tone.

- Ephedrine – a synthetic, direct- and indirect-acting, non-catecholamine sympathomimetic that has activity for both alpha and beta receptors. It is rarely used as an infusion and is effective at increasing blood pressure following a bolus dose. Tachyphylaxis occurs following repeated doses, which limits its use.
- Adrenaline – dilute adrenaline can be useful when anaesthetising very unstable patients. In experienced hands, boluses of, for example, 10–20 mcg can help stabilise blood pressure while the patient is in extremis.

- *Equipment* – ensure the right equipment is available before commencing induction.
  - Preoxygenation adjuncts
    - High-flow nasal cannulae if needed.
    - Facemask.
    - Oropharyngeal airway (Guedel) – to open the airway, assist ventilation and reduce likelihood of introducing gas into the stomach.
  - Laryngoscopy – to allow visualisation of the vocal cords (can be direct or indirect). There are many different types available; these are a few examples:
    - Direct laryngoscopes – these come in different sizes. Macintosh is commonly used in adults (a curved blade is attached at 90° to a handle with a light source). The McCoy blade has a moveable distal tip segment. Magill and Miller have straight blades.
    - Video laryngoscopes – for example, the McGrath™ video laryngoscope facilitates indirect visualisation of the cords and is often used where the patient has reduced neck movement.
    - Optical laryngoscopes – for example, the AirTraq Optical Laryngoscope™ uses a set of magnifying mirrors to visualise the cords.
    - Fibreoptic scope – the endotracheal tube is mounted onto the flexible fibreoptic scope. The scope is inserted via mouth or nose and, when the cords are identified, the endotracheal tube (ETT) can be advanced into position over the scope. This is useful when anatomical issues cause reduced mouth opening and restricted neck movement. If there is airway swelling, there is a risk of causing obstruction with the scope itself.
  - Endotracheal tube (ETT) – there are many different types and sizes available. Specialised elements include the following:
    - Cuffed or uncuffed – a polyvinylchloride or polyurethane cuff, cylindrical, round or conical in shape, can be inflated with air to create a seal between the tube and the trachea. This reduces the risk of large aspiration and improves the ability to administer positive pressure ventilation.

- Subglottic secretion drainage ports – usually used where mechanical ventilation is expected to be ongoing for several days. It allows suction of secretions which gather above the cuff, so reducing the risk of microaspiration and VAP.
- Adjuncts and manoeuvres
  - Bougie – this instrument can be used where the cords are visualised but the ETT cannot be manipulated to pass through. The bougie is inserted and the ETT passed over it. It is also often used when an ETT needs to be replaced in critical care because, for example, the cuff has lost integrity.
  - Stylet – this is a malleable metal rod which is inserted into the ETT to allow it to be bent into the optimal shape for intubating the cords.
  - BURP (backward, upward, rightward, posterior) pressure – displacement of the larynx through pressure on the cricoid cartilage can improve visualisation of the cords.
  - Cricoid pressure (Sellick manoeuvre) – this aims to prevent regurgitation of stomach contents by occluding the oesophagus through pressure on the trachea. It is no longer universally practised as several studies have demonstrated that it is ineffective and can make laryngoscopy more difficult.
  - Nasogastric tube (NG) – this may be useful to decompress the stomach after intubation to improve ventilation and reduce risk of aspiration. If an NG tube is present prior to intubation, suctioning gastric contents can help prevent aspiration pneumonitis.
  - Suction – always have suction available as there may be secretions, blood or gastric contents in the airway.
  - Supraglottic airway device (SAD) – these devices sit above the glottis and aim to allow ventilation without fully securing the airway. They may be useful in the case of failed intubation. There are many different types of SAD, e.g. laryngeal mask airway (LMA Classic® or Supreme®) or iGel®.

Failed intubation

The Difficult Airway Society (DAS) has produced useful guidelines for managing the challenging situation of failed intubation. If the first attempt at laryngoscopy fails, optimise positioning and muscle relaxation before a second attempt. Consider using airway adjuncts or selecting an alternative laryngoscope. Apply oxygen via facemask or SAD if necessary. If it is impossible to intubate or ventilate, then declare a Can't Intubate Can't Ventilate emergency and prepare for a cricothyroidotomy.

- *Front of neck access* – this is rarely required but the technique should be known to all airway trained clinicians. Emergency cricothyroidotomy is performed using a scalpel to make a stab through the cricothyroid membrane, a bougie is passed into the trachea, and a size 6.0 mm ETT is inserted over the bougie.

Following intubation

- *Sedation* – usually a combination of a hypnotic agent with an analgosedative agent. Later, when weaning, this may be reduced to purely an analgosedative agent.
  - Hypnotic – propofol infusion is commonly used in adult ICU (monitor creatine phosphokinase and lactate if propofol infusion syndrome is a concern). Midazolam infusions are often used with morphine in paediatric ICU.
  - Opioids – for example, fentanyl, alfentanil or remifentanil, are often used in adult ICU. Remifentanil is a popular choice as it is rapidly metabolised by plasma and tissue esterases, giving it a short context-sensitive half-life (3 minutes after a 3-hour infusion). Morphine is more commonly used in children.
  - Alpha-2 adrenergic agonist – such as dexmedetomidine or clonidine. These agents are sedative and analgesic. Both may induce bradycardia and hypotension.
- *Consider paralysis* – non-depolarising agents can be used in infusion. Common choices are rocuronium or cisatracurium.
- *Invasive monitoring* – critical care patients are likely to require invasive arterial and central venous catheterisation (*CVC*) for pressure monitoring and blood sampling. CVCs are used for drug administration, particularly medications such as vasopressors, chemotherapy agents and parenteral nutrition. Consider whether vascular access for renal replacement will also be required at this point.
- *Tubes*
  - Nasogastric tube.
  - Urinary catheter.
  - Drains – some patients benefit from expedited drainage of pleural effusions or ascites if ventilation is impaired.
- *Imaging* – chest radiography is used to assess the position of the ETT, the CVC via internal jugular or subclavian routes, and NG tube, as well as bone and lung fields. It may be necessary to transfer for urgent CT, MRI, angiography, etc. immediately post intubation.

Setting the ventilator

An experienced clinician will program the ventilator specifically for an individual patient using their understanding of lung mechanics, flow curves and blood gases as well as knowledge of the underlying illness. Most patients will benefit from a lung-protective strategy to minimise volutrauma, barotrauma, atelectrauma and biotrauma. Patients with brain injury may require a neuroprotective strategy.

Ventilation is discussed in more detail in the cases. A reasonable default strategy is to aim for the following:

- *Lung protection*
  - Volumes – aim for approximately 6 mL/kg ideal body weight.

- Pressures – plateau pressure should be <30 cmH$_2$O. Use PEEP to maintain open alveoli and assist oxygenation.
- Gas exchange – tolerate hypercapnia if pH >7.25. To maintain low tidal volumes, respiratory rate may need to be increased.
- Driving pressure – aim to maintain lower driving pressures, ideally less than 14 cmH$_2$O.

Further reading

- Higgs, A., McGrath, B., Goddard, C. et al. (2019). Guidelines for the management of tracheal intubation in critically ill adults. *Br. J. Anaesth.* 120: 323–352. A comprehensive guideline that includes useful information and intubation strategies.
- Cook, T., Woodall, N., Harper, J. et al. (2011). Major complications of airway management in the UK: results of the fourth national audit project of the Royal College of Anaesthetists and the Difficult Airway Society. Part 2: intensive care and emergency departments. *Br. J. Anaesth.* 106: 632–642. The NAP4 report gives key insights into the difficulties faced when intubating critically ill patients.
- De Jong, A., Molinari, N., Terzi, N. et al. (2013). Early identification of patients at risk for difficult intubation in the intensive care unit. *Am. J. Respir. Crit. Care Med* 187: 832–839. Original paper that developed and validated the MACOCHA score.

Part

II

The Cases

Part

The Cases

1 The Patient with Rising Vasopressor Requirements

During your night shift, you are asked to urgently review a 65-year-old patient named David. He is day 5 post-elective right-sided hemicolectomy with primary anastomosis for a non-metastatic colorectal carcinoma. No surgical drains in situ. Earlier that day, he was started on noradrenaline (0.04 mcg/kg/min) to maintain his mean arterial blood pressure (MAP) above 65 mmHg. He is now hypotensive (80/40 mmHg) and tachycardic (120 bpm) with a noradrenaline dose of 0.35 mcg/kg/min. He is oliguric. His respiratory rate is 32 breaths per minute with SpO_2 94% on 2 L/min nasal oxygen. There are bibasal crepitations on auscultation. David is restless, sweating profusely, talking in a confused manner, and grimacing in pain when his abdomen is palpated.

What is your initial management?

- *Airway* – his speech, though confused, suggests that he is maintaining his airway and therefore does not require immediate airway manoeuvres (e.g. chin lift, jaw thrust) or adjuncts (e.g. oropharyngeal airway).
- *Breathing* – this appears laboured. He needs high-flow supplementary oxygen, an urgent portable chest radiograph and an arterial blood sample for analysis.
- *Circulation* – ensure that he has at least one large-bore peripheral IV cannula (e.g. 18 G or 16 G) in addition to his central venous access. Take blood samples for microscopy, culture and sensitivity testing, routine blood tests including amylase, a repeat group and save, and a coagulation screen. At this point, a 250–500 mL bolus of crystalloid solution should be given over a brief period (e.g. 15–20 min). Ideally, the clinician would deliver this fluid bolus personally, using a 50 mL syringe attached to the IV access. This simple technique allows the clinician to directly observe the physiological response, while also making it possible to stop giving fluid immediately if the effect is deleterious.

Clinical Cases in Critical Care, First Edition. Alice Myers and Theophilus Samuels.
© 2023 John Wiley & Sons Ltd. Published 2023 by John Wiley & Sons Ltd.

- *Disability* – his confusion is not posing an immediate danger to himself or the nursing staff. Check his blood glucose level. Treat hypoglycaemia if present. Assess pupillary reactions to light.
- *Exposure* – assess him for signs of deep vein thrombosis, rash, and bleeding per rectum.

Following exposure, reassess whether your interventions (i.e. oxygen therapy, intravenous fluid boluses) are having any impact on his physiology. Request the senior surgical on-call doctor to review him urgently.

> Following your initial management, BP increases transiently to 96/60 mmHg, SpO_2 is maintained at >98% and blood results are as follows: Hb 105 g/L, WBC 22×10^9/L, plat 560×10^9/L, CRP >350, INR 2.1, pH 7.23, PaO_2 55.6 kPa (15 L/min), $PaCO_2$ 4.1 kPa, lactate 6.4 mmol/L, amylase 183 U/L. The chest radiograph demonstrates a mild degree of bibasal atelectasis.

With these results and examination findings, what is the most likely diagnosis?

These blood test results suggest an acute inflammatory response that is probably due to sepsis. The raised lactate is most likely due to the overall haemodynamic instability leading to reduced delivery of oxygen.

Given that the patient is day 5 post elective right-sided hemicolectomy with signs of peritonism, it is very probable that he is suffering from an anastomotic leak with resultant intra-abdominal infection and septic shock.

Which factors may affect the risk of anastomotic leakage?

Non-modifiable risk factors that are associated with an increased risk include:

- Male sex
- Age over 60 years
- Previous history of radiotherapy
- ASA grades II–IV
- Underlying pulmonary disease
- Pre-existing vascular disease
- Renal disease
- Renal replacement therapy
- Immunosuppressive therapy

Modifiable risk factors include:

- Active smoking
- Obesity
- Heavy alcohol intake (>21 units per week)
- Immunosuppressants and chemotherapy

- Recent weight loss >10%
- Hypoalbuminaemia

Anastomotic leakage is associated with severe morbidity, increased length of hospital stay and mortality.

Describe how focused ultrasonography can be useful in assessing fluid responsiveness

Images must always be integrated with the rest of the clinical assessment and should not be used in isolation. Bear in mind that David is not intubated and is breathing spontaneously.

Focused ultrasonography can be used to assess the following:

Inferior vena cava (IVC) index

In spontaneously breathing patients, the IVC *collapsibility* index (i.e. the difference between the maximum diameter in *expiration* and minimum diameter in *inspiration* expressed as a percentage) is not a reliable method for determining fluid responsiveness. Clinically, being able to recognise extremes of IVC diameters is more beneficial. Therefore, in patients that are haemodynamically unstable:

- near-total collapsibility or small IVC size (<1 cm) may suggest the patient is fluid responsive
- a large, distended and non-collapsible IVC probably suggests that the patient is not fluid responsive (Figure 1.1a).

It is worth considering that in patients receiving positive pressure ventilation, standardised loading conditions to the heart must be met before any changes in IVC diameter can be interpreted. Patients should be passively ventilated (e.g. no spontaneous efforts, completely dependent on the ventilator) and receiving a tidal volume of 8–10 mL/kg. An IVC *distensibility* index (i.e. the difference between the maximum diameter in *inspiration* and minimum diameter in *expiration* expressed as a percentage) of greater than 12–18% may suggest that the patient is fluid responsive (Figure 1.1b).

However, irrespective of whether the patient is breathing spontaneously or mechanically ventilated, emphasis should not be placed on determining an IVC index (either collapsibility or distensibility). Rather, recognising extreme IVC diameters and integrating this into the clinical picture is a more robust approach to determining fluid responsiveness.

Left ventricle appearance

In the parasternal short-axis view, you can assess for the presence of end-systolic obliteration (i.e. 'kissing' ventricle). The left ventricle appears small and the papillary muscles appear to meet at the centre at end-systole. This would suggest that the LV is underfilled and hyperdynamic, indicating that the patient may be fluid responsive.

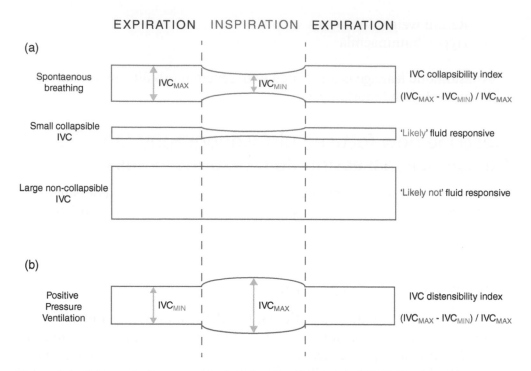

Figure 1.1: Schematic diagram representing the changes in IVC diameter. (a) In spontaneous breathing patients, the IVC collapsibility index can give an indication of the fluid responsiveness of a patient. Interpreting and recognising the extremes of IVC diameter in their clinical context is much more useful in patients who are haemodynamically unstable (see text for details). (b) In patients receiving positive pressure ventilation, the IVC diameter increases during inspiration, giving rise to an IVC distensibility index (see text for details). IVC_{MAX}, maximum diameter of IVC; IVC_{MIN}, minimum diameter of IVC.

Source: Theophilus Samuels.

Presence of A-lines and/or B-lines

A-lines are reverberation artefacts originating from the pleural line, and with adequate depth can be seen as parallel lines at regular (equidistant) intervals (Figure 1.2a). B-lines (or 'comet tails') are horizontal hyperechoic beams emanating from the inferior margin of the pleural line, which then extend through to the deep edge of the screen (Figure 1.2b). They fan out and move with the motion of the pleural line, removing the ability to visualise A-lines. Due to the lung bases possessing a greater mass of lung tissue, they will often display a B-line pattern, making examination of an upper lung field more informative for the presence of pulmonary oedema. Therefore, if lung ultrasonography demonstrates absent A-lines but abundant B-lines throughout the chest, this may suggest that pulmonary oedema has developed, and further fluid boluses may cause more harm than benefit.

Why might focused ultrasonography be difficult in this case?

It may be exceedingly difficult or near impossible to image the IVC due to the patient's intra-abdominal pathology and postsurgical abdomen, as it requires an adequate subcostal view to obtain the necessary measurements.

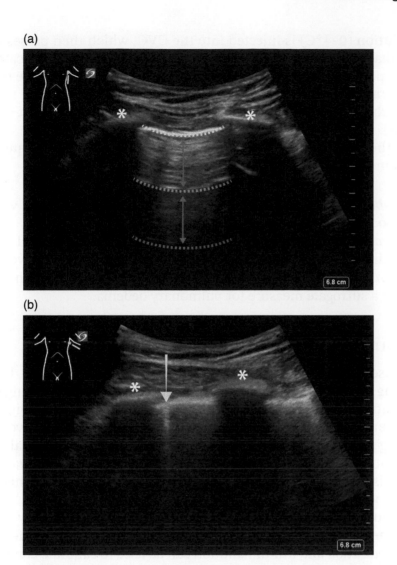

Figure 1.2: (a) A-lines are demonstrated (yellow dashed lines). (b) Single B-line is demonstrated (yellow arrow). Rib shadows are marked (*).

Source: Theophilus Samuels.

The parasternal and lung views may still be possible, but they require a co-operative patient.

His BP is maintained with a MAP >65 mmHg following further IV fluid boluses, but he is still requiring noradrenaline at 0.35 mcg/kg/min and is becoming more confused and unmanageable. You decide to start cardiac output monitoring while the surgical registrar is reviewing the patient.

Which methods can be used to measure cardiac output?

Transpulmonary thermodilution

This requires the placement of a central venous catheter (CVC) and a modified peripheral arterial catheter usually sited in the brachial or femoral artery.

Cold solution (0–4 °C) is injected into the CVC, which then passes through both cardiac and pulmonary circulations to reach the thermistor located in the modified peripheral arterial catheter. The thermistor measures the reduction in temperature over time, allowing for a thermodilution curve to be constructed from which the cardiac output is derived (using the Stewart–Hamilton equation).

Since the cold injectate passes through the entire cardiac and pulmonary circulations, other measurements can be estimated:

- *Global end-diastolic volume* (GEDV) – this represents the volume of blood in all cardiac chambers at the end of diastole.
- *Intrathoracic blood volume* (ITBV) – the volume of the blood in all four cardiac chambers plus the blood volume in the pulmonary vessels.
- *Extravascular lung water* (EVLW) – the amount of water in the lungs and a surrogate measure for pulmonary oedema.

Transpulmonary lithium dilution

This is based on a similar principle to the thermodilution method, but rather than using changes in temperature as the indicator, this uses changes in the concentration of lithium. A small dose of lithium is injected through a CVC or peripheral intravenous catheter and a concentration–time curve is generated using specialised equipment attached to the peripheral arterial line. The cardiac output is derived by measuring the area under the concentration–time curve. This technique shows good agreement with other bolus thermodilution methods.

Care must be taken when using in patients on lithium therapy and those receiving muscle relaxants as the accuracy of the results can be affected.

Thermodilution and lithium dilution can be used to calibrate commercially available pulse contour analysis devices.

Pulse contour analysis

Several commercial systems can provide almost real-time measurements of cardiac output. They use the concept that the pulsatile characteristic of an arterial waveform is considered proportional to the stroke volume. However, because stroke volume is influenced by several other factors such as arterial resistance and compliance, devices such as PiCCO™ and LiDCO™ must use the thermodilution and lithium dilution methods respectively as means of calibration.

Whilst minimally invasive and relatively easy to set up, the accuracy of these methods is affected by:

- Major changes in vascular compliance such as increasing vasopressor requirements
- Cardiac rhythm disturbances, e.g. atrial fibrillation
- Aortic regurgitation
- Over- or underdamping of the system.

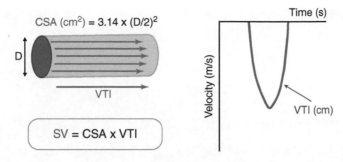

Figure 1.3: Stroke volume calculation using echocardiography. The cylinder length of the blood ejected from the LV in a single beat is the velocity–time integral (VTI) of the Doppler curve. By measuring the diameter of the left ventricle outflow tract, the cross-sectional area (CSA) can be estimated. The stroke volume can then be calculated as the product of CSA and VTI. The cardiac output can then be estimated by multiplying the SV by heart rate.

Source: Theophilus Samuels.

Echocardiography

Transthoracic or transoesophageal echocardiography can be used to determine cardiac output by estimating stroke volume using two common methods:

- measuring the difference between end-diastolic and end-systolic volumes
- using pulsed wave Doppler (PWD) techniques and 2D measurements.

Using Simpson's biplane method of disc summation, the end-systolic and end-diastolic volumes can be estimated, with the difference between the two being equal to the stroke volume. The major disadvantage to this method, particularly with a transthoracic approach, is that it relies heavily on being able to image the endocardial border, which can be notoriously difficult in critical care patients.

The second method involves measuring the velocity of red blood cells over time to create a velocity–time integral (VTI). When this velocity is measured in the left ventricular outflow tract ($LVOT_{VTI}$) along with an estimation of the cross-sectional area of the LVOT (CSA_{LVOT}), the stroke volume (SV) can be calculated from the product of these two variables, i.e. $SV = LVOT_{VTI} \times CSA_{LVOT}$ (Figure 1.3). The $LVOT_{VTI}$ can be obtained from the apical five-chamber view using PWD. The sample volume is sited within 1 cm of the aortic valve, in the LVOT (Figure 1.4). The cardiac output is easily derived by multiplying this derived SV by the heart rate. This method, although elegant, relies upon estimating the diameter of the LVOT accurately, as small errors in measurements can lead to large errors in the estimated CSA, thus over- or underestimating cardiac output.

Standard practices of echocardiography allow for these cardiac output 'snapshots' but are not continuous measurements like those described above. Real-time evaluation is possible but requires state-of-the-art equipment and appropriate training to facilitate.

Transoesophageal aortic Doppler

This semi-invasive approach uses specially designed oesophageal probes that estimate the blood velocity in the descending aorta while estimating the CSA of

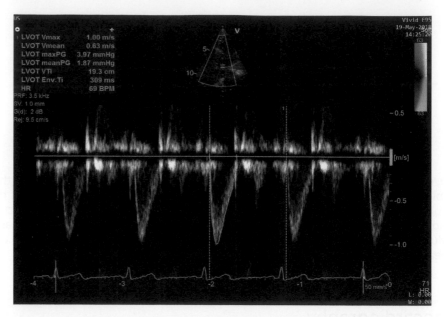

Figure 1.4: Using pulsed wave Doppler (PWD), the LVOT VTI can be measured by placing the sample volume within 1 cm of the aortic valve. By tracing around the VTI as shown, the LVOT VTI and velocity can be measured. Peak velocities of the LVOT and LVOT VTI are normally between 0.8–1.2 m/s and 18–22 cm respectively.

the descending aorta indirectly using nomograms. The probe is inserted about 30–40 cm from the teeth into the oesophagus and rotated until the Doppler signal is produced. Like the PWD approach described above, the probe measures the velocity of blood using the Doppler shift in frequency. This creates a velocity–time integral, and when multiplied with the estimated CSA and HR, the cardiac output is derived.

Thoracic electrical bioimpedance

Electrodes are placed in the neck or thorax region that continually emit and sense low-amplitude electric current. They also monitor cardiac electrical signals and changes in bioimpedance that occur with increases in intrathoracic blood volume. A pulsatile waveform is achieved by filtering out artefacts (e.g. changes in impedance due to respirations) that is then analysed to determine the cardiac output. This method is sensitive to changes in position or contact of the electrodes to the patient and may become inaccurate in the presence of acute changes in tissue water content (e.g. pulmonary oedema, pleural effusions).

The nurse looking after David sets up a pulse contour analysis device and asks you if you want to give any more fluids.

Briefly discuss how stroke volume variation (SVV) can be used to predict fluid responsiveness

Variations in stroke volume between inspiration and expiration during passive mechanical ventilation can predict which patients may be fluid responsive (i.e. 'responders') with a high degree of accuracy. The diagnostic threshold for

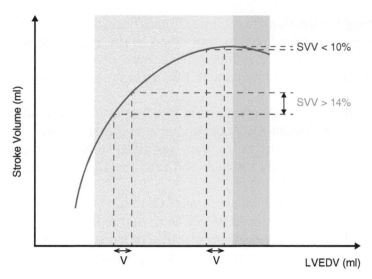

Figure 1.5: The Frank–Starling mechanism of the heart describes the relationship between stroke volume (mL) and left ventricle end-diastolic volume (LVEDV). The LVEDV is presented as a surrogate for myocardial sarcomere length. The ascending portion of the curve (green shaded area) visually depicts potential *responders*. Non-responsiveness is likely to occur after the curve begins to flatten out (orange and red shaded areas). For a given increase in volume (V), the resultant stroke volume, and therefore stroke volume variation (SVV), may suggest fluid responsiveness depending on where the patient is on the curve (green and red dashed lines).

Source: Theophilus Samuels.

SVV is reported as being between 11% and 13% with a very high sensitivity and specificity. Broadly speaking, in predicting fluid responsiveness:

- SVV less than 10% has a high *negative* predictive value (i.e. *unlikely* to require further fluid boluses and potentially need inotropic and/or vasopressor support)
- SVV greater than 14% has a very high *positive* predictive value (i.e. *likely* to require further fluid boluses).

Patients who are on the ascending portion of the Frank–Starling curve theoretically are most likely to respond to the fluid challenge by increasing stroke volume (SV) and cardiac output (CO). In contrast, patients who are on or past the flat part have little response to fluid loading, with the excess fluid potentially increasing tissue oedema and facilitating tissue dysoxia (Figure 1.5).

Describe the changes that occur in stroke volume during passive mechanical ventilation

Positive pressure ventilation (IPPV) between 8 and 10 mL/kg in a patient who is completely dependent on the ventilator (i.e. has no spontaneous breaths and therefore 'passive') induces *interpretable* cyclical changes in the loading conditions of the left and right ventricles.

- During *inspiration* (mechanical insufflation) positive intrathoracic pressure impedes the return of blood to the right ventricle (RV), thus reducing preload (i.e. reduces the venous return pressure gradient).
- RV afterload is *increased* due to the inspiratory increase in transpulmonary pressure.
- The reduction in RV preload and increase in RV afterload *decreases* RV SV, with the lowest RV SV occurring at *end-inspiration*.
- Concurrently, as the pulmonary vasculature is also compressed during inspiration, this forces blood into the LV, resulting in an initial *increase* in LV SV.
- After a delay of 2–3 cardiac cycles (due to the long blood pulmonary transit time), the reduced RV SV leads to a reduction in LV filling.
- The reduction in LV preload may lead to a decrease in LV SV, and thus CO, which is at its minimum during *expiration*.

These changes are amplified in hypovolaemic states and diminished when either ventricle is failing or the circulatory system is congested. Also, bear in mind that changes to the ventilator (increasing tidal volume to ≥ 8 mL/kg) or patient (increasing sedation and/or administering a neuromuscular blocker) may need to be performed to accurately assess fluid responsiveness. The benefit of performing these changes to determine fluid responsiveness should be assessed on a case-by-case basis.

Describe how SVV can be measured

- *Pulse contour analysis* – as described previously, variations in SV can be measured using advanced digital software. SVV can typically be displayed in real time.
- *Echocardiography* – using methods described for calculating the SV, the SVV can be calculated by taking separate measurements in inspiration and expiration (to determine the maximum and minimum values). This can be time-consuming and is not conducive to minute-to-minute monitoring unless it can be automated. Thankfully, certain ultrasound devices can automate this process by using artificial intelligence and displaying this information in real time (if the LVOT diameter is input, then SV can also be calculated). The LVOT VTI, LVOT and aortic peak velocity can be considered surrogate measures for SV (as the LVOT diameter remains constant). Some ultrasound devices can use LVOT VTI variation as a substitute for SVV. However, if the peak LVOT velocity is used, then a variation >12% suggests the patient may be fluid responsive (Figure 1.6).

The surgical registrar completes their review and requests an urgent computed tomography (CT) scan of David's abdomen and pelvis. You are tasked with taking David for his CT scan. He is now no longer obeying commands and is requiring constant nursing attention to stop him harming himself and others.

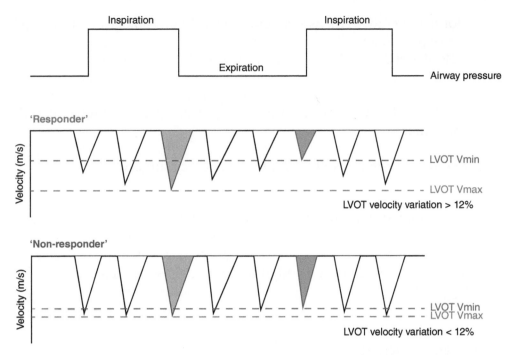

Figure 1.6: The LVOT velocity can act as a surrogate for SV (as the LVOT diameter remains constant). Therefore, the variation in maximum (LVOT V_{max}) and minimum (LVOT V_{min}) velocities can act as a measure of fluid responsiveness.

Source: Theophilus Samuels.

What are your immediate concerns regarding the transfer of David to the CT suite?

The immediate concern is David's increasing confusion and unstable clinical condition. It is also possible that once the CT is performed, the surgical team may want to proceed to surgery. The safest course of action now is to secure his airway and sedate him for transfer.

> You successfully intubate David and insert a nasogastric tube. The CT scan demonstrates multiple large collections within his abdomen and confirms an anastomotic leak. David needs to be taken back to theatres for emergency laparotomy. The anaesthetic team arrive and begin to take handover.

How would you stratify David's perioperative risk of morbidity and mortality?

Use one of the following well-recognised scoring systems:

- **P-POSSUM** – the Physiological and Operative Severity Score for the enumeration of Mortality and Morbidity (POSSUM) score was modified to the Portsmouth prediction (hence P-POSSUM) in an attempt to correct the overestimation of death in low-risk surgical patients. It has become widely accepted within the surgical community as a standard for perioperative risk assessment. It uses 12 physiological and six operative parameters.

- **CR-POSSUM** – the colorectal POSSUM score was first introduced in 2004. It provides a slightly more accurate prediction of operative mortality for patients undergoing colorectal surgery when compared to the P-POSSUM model. It uses six physiological and four operative parameters.

Both scoring systems can be used for emergency surgery.

David is returned from theatres a few hours later, following a washout and formation of a double-barrelled defunctioning stoma. He remains stable throughout the rest of your shift with a reduced noradrenaline requirement (0.10 mcg/kg/min), and you hand him over to the day team to continue his management.

Further reading

- Kobe, J., Mishra, N., Arya, V.K. et al. (2019). Cardiac output monitoring: technology and choice. *Ann. Card. Anaesth.* 22: 6–17. Informative review on the different methods of cardiac output monitoring.
- Miller, A. and Mandeville, J. (2016). Predicting and measuring fluid responsiveness with echocardiography. *Echo. Res. Pract.* 3 (2): G1–G12. Excellent review of how to use echocardiography to predict and measure fluid responsiveness.
- Zarnescu, E., Zarnescu, N., and Costea, R. (2021). Updates of risk factors for anastomotic leakage after colorectal surgery. *Diagnost.* 11: 2382. Recent informative review on risk factors for anastomotic leakage.
- Colebourn, C. and Newton, J. (2017). *Acute and Critical Care Echocardiography*. Oxford: Oxford University Press. Authoritative textbook on many aspects regarding echocardiography in critical care.

2 The Patient with Respiratory Distress I

You are asked to review 66-year-old Geoffrey in the resuscitation department. He called an ambulance earlier this evening as his breathing felt difficult and painful. He has oxygen saturations of 85% on 6 L/min oxygen via Hudson mask. He is using accessory muscles of breathing with a respiratory rate of 35–40 breaths per minute. Arterial blood gas analysis shows pH 7.14, PaO_2 7.9 kPa, $PaCO_2$ 10.6 kPa, base excess −7 mmol/L and lactate 4.3 mmol/L. He is still alert but looks tired and is unable to speak in full sentences. HR 122 bpm, BP 156/98 mmHg.

What may be the cause of the problem?

Lower respiratory tract infection

Community-acquired pneumonia (CAP) may be bacterial or viral and must be considered as a potential cause. Measure Geoffrey's temperature and inflammatory markers. Acute bronchitis occurs in 30–50 per 1000 people per year. No microbe will be identified in around a third of cases, and 90% of those cases where a pathogen is identified will be viral in origin.

Pathogens to consider include the following:

- *Viruses* – e.g. adenovirus, coronavirus, influenza, parainfluenza and respiratory syncytial virus. He may be suffering from SARS-CoV-2 infection, and he will require testing for this in the emergency department (see Case 24 for further discussion of COVID-19).
- *Bacteria* – these can be divided into the following.
  - Typical – e.g. *Streptococcus pneumoniae*, *Haemophilus influenzae*, *Moraxella catarrhalis*.
  - Atypical – e.g. *Mycoplasma pneumoniae*, *Chlamydia pneumoniae* and *Legionella pneumophila*.
- *Fungal* pneumonia can also occur but is much less common and is usually associated with immunosuppression.

Clinical Cases in Critical Care, First Edition. Alice Myers and Theophilus Samuels.
© 2023 John Wiley & Sons Ltd. Published 2023 by John Wiley & Sons Ltd.

Chronic obstructive pulmonary disease (acute exacerbation)

Geoffrey's past medical history is unknown at this point. COPD is common. The British Lung Society report that 1.2 million people, or 4.5% of the UK population over 40 years old, have a diagnosis of COPD. This episode may represent an exacerbation of COPD, whether already diagnosed or as a first presentation. It will be important to find out whether symptoms of emphysema and/or chronic bronchitis pre-exist.

Asthma

Patients with asthma suffer reversible airway obstruction through constriction of smooth muscle. This may be triggered by a variety of stimuli including smoke, dust, pollen, cold, stress, etc. The mucous hypersecretion and bronchial wall inflammation of asthma could explain Geoffrey's symptoms. However, one would also expect wheeze to feature more prominently as a symptom. More importantly, patients with asthma usually compensate for an acute attack by raising their respiratory rate, leading to hypocapnia. By the time an asthmatic's $PaCO_2$ has started to rise, they may have deteriorated to the point of exhaustion. Asthma cannot yet be fully ruled out, but it appears less likely.

Anaphylaxis

Type 1 hypersensitivity reactions are mediated by immunoglobulin E causing histamine release from degranulating mast cells and basophils. Anaphylaxis is normally accompanied by skin features (urticaria, itching or angio-oedema) and hypotension (secondary to nitric oxide-induced vasodilation and relaxation of smooth muscle). This history describes symptoms developing over time and is not consistent with anaphylaxis. This could, however, represent a different type of hypersensitivity or drug reaction so history taking should include exposure to potential allergens and their temporal relationship to the presenting symptoms.

Pneumothorax

Pneumothorax should certainly be excluded in this case. It could co-exist with several of the other possible diagnoses in this list. If present, an intercostal chest drain should be considered since Geoffrey is clearly compromised. Spontaneous pneumothorax classically presents in tall, thin men but may occur in anyone. Risk factors include smoking, genetic predisposition, bullae and connective tissue disorders.

Pulmonary oedema

Geoffrey is in respiratory distress. He may have underlying cardiac or renal failure, either of which could lead to acute pulmonary oedema presenting with shortness of breath. Examine for raised jugular venous pressure and signs of peripheral oedema.

Pulmonary embolus (PE)

Acute hypoxia of unknown cause should always alert the clinician to the possibility of PE. A massive PE is often accompanied by chest pain and may cause cardiovascular collapse when severe. Multiple small PEs may occur over time in some prothrombotic patients, leading to chronic shortness of breath. The classic ECG changes of SI, QIII, TIII (deep S wave in lead I, Q wave in lead III, inverted T wave in lead III) are much less common than sinus tachycardia or signs of right heart dysfunction, e.g. RBBB, right axis deviation, right atrial enlargement (see Case 9). Examine for signs of deep vein thrombosis (DVT).

Myocardial infarction (MI) or acute cardiac event

Myocardial infarction is usually heralded by chest pain but silent MI is possible, particularly in patients with neuropathy or poorly controlled diabetes. Cardiac chest pain may also be misinterpreted as reflux and dismissed by the patient as insignificant.

An event such as rupture of chordae tendineae would probably lead to catastrophic regurgitation and cardiogenic shock so is unlikely with a BP of 156/98 mmHg.

Renal impairment or metabolic disturbance

Metabolic acidosis due to renal impairment may lead to Kussmaul breathing ('air hunger'). Renal impairment may be present but does not alone explain the clinical picture of hypoxia unless it has also led to significant pulmonary oedema.

Underlying malignancy

Lung is the third most common type of cancer in the UK. Approximately 70% are caused by smoking. A tumour in the lung may predispose the patient to developing infection, obstruction, lobar collapse, effusions, etc. A tumour may easily be masked by consolidation on radiographic imaging. Lung malignancy can be primary or secondary.

- Primary
  - Small cell (15–20%).
  - Non-small cell (80–85%) – these include adenocarcinoma, squamous cell carcinoma, large cell and undifferentiated carcinoma.
  - Other (e.g. Pancoast).
- Secondary
  - Most cancers can metastasise to the lung but the solid tumours which commonly do this include renal, breast, colon and prostate.

While Geoffrey is *in extremis*, the priority is not to search for malignancy. If a cancer does exist, typing, grading and staging could become key in terms of assessing prognosis and treatment options later on. History should incorporate exploration of non-specific symptoms suggestive of malignancy, including anorexia and weight loss.

You are told that Geoffrey has a history of hypertension and COPD but is independent and acts as the main carer for his wife who has early dementia and severe arthritis. The chest radiograph shows hyperinflation and widespread consolidation. His temperature is 39.1 °C. His rapid test for COVID-19 is negative.

What is your analysis of the situation?

Geoffrey is extremely unwell and will not physically tolerate this degree of compromise for much longer. There is evidence of lower respiratory tract infection. This has the combined effect of impairing oxygen delivery (through reducing the available alveolar surface area) and increasing oxygen demand (through raised metabolic rate secondary to sepsis and increased work of breathing). The compensatory tachycardia and tachypnoea raise oxygen demand through increased muscle activity. Geoffrey's work of breathing is a visual reminder that oxygen demand is exceeding supply. Without intervention, Geoffrey will probably suffer cardiopulmonary arrest.

From the available information, Geoffrey is independent and so it is fair to assume he should be a good candidate for invasive organ support in critical care. He has some co-morbidities which may affect his prognosis and further information is needed once the situation is stabilised.

What is the alveolar gas equation and what is its relevance?

$$P_aO_2 = F_iO_2\left(P_{atm} - P_{H_2O}\right) - \left(P_aCO_2 / RQ\right)$$

P_aO_2 is alveolar oxygen, P_{atm} is atmospheric pressure at sea level, P_{H_2O} is partial pressure of water, F_iO_2 is the fraction of inspired oxygen, P_aCO_2 is partial pressure of carbon dioxide in the alveoli, and RQ is the respiratory quotient.

The alveolar gas equation can be used to understand how oxygenation is affected by atmospheric pressure, diet and, importantly in this case, hypercapnia. From the equation, it can be seen how, without other changes, hypoventilation can lead to decreasing alveolar oxygenation. It can also be seen that increasing the inspired fraction of oxygen should improve alveolar oxygenation.

What are the types of hypoxia and how can oxygen delivery be increased?

There are four types of hypoxia:

- Hypoxic
- Anaemic
- Stagnant or ischaemic, i.e. inadequate blood flow to tissues.
- Histotoxic or cytotoxic, i.e. inability to utilise oxygen at cellular level despite good availability.

For the bedside physician, the easiest of these to address is hypoxic hypoxia. Provide high-flow oxygen, preferably accompanied by positive end-expiratory pressure to prevent derecruitment of alveoli and therefore maintain the largest possible surface area for diffusion of oxygen across the alveolar–capillary membrane. Anaemic hypoxia may be addressed through transfusion or, in non-emergent situations, drug therapy to stimulate increased production of haemoglobin. However, the oxygen-carrying capacity of transfused blood is less than that of the patient's own blood and transfusion of blood products is not to be undertaken lightly due to the potential for complications (see Case 7). Regional hypoxia due to impaired circulation may need to be dealt with directly (e.g. intravascular stenting, thrombectomy, reperfusion techniques). Histotoxic hypoxia may or may not be treatable with specific antitoxins.

Global oxygen delivery can be improved through optimising cardiac output, haemoglobin, oxygen saturations and arterial oxygenation as reflected in the oxygen delivery equation (see Case 8).

> When you first arrived in the ED, you exchanged the Hudson mask for a non-rebreathe mask, applied 15 L/min of oxygen and gave 250 mL intravenous fluid. Now, 10 minutes later, Geoffrey is becoming drowsy. His work of breathing has not improved.

How do you proceed?

Prepare Geoffrey for intubation, call for skilled assistance and ask an appropriate person to call the patient's next of kin. There is minimal time to optimise Geoffrey's condition. He is at high risk of aspiration and is haemodynamicaly unstable. Intubate using a modified rapid sequence induction (see Introduction Section 2).

> You successfully intubate Geoffrey with a size 8.5 mm endotracheal tube. His chest feels stiff to bag, suggesting poor compliance. He now requires frequent boluses of vasopressor to maintain a MAP of 70 mmHg.

What is compliance and why may Geoffrey's lungs feel stiff, i.e. poorly compliant?

Compliance measures how volume changes with a change in pressure. Total lung compliance incorporates the compliance of both the lungs and the chest wall.

$$Transpulmonary\ pressure = Alveolar\ pressure - intrapleural\ pressure$$

$$Total\ lung\ compliance = Change\ in\ lung\ volume\ /\ transpulmonary\ pressure$$

Geoffrey has COPD which normally increases compliance. Emphysematous disease damages alveoli, resulting in a loss of elastic recoil. Decreased compliance indicates a problem in addition to his underlying COPD.

Anything which decreases the ability of the system to stretch in response to an increase in pressure will result in reduced compliance. Causes include pre-existing conditions such as pulmonary fibrosis or musculoskeletal abnormalities, acute problems such as acute respiratory distress syndrome (ARDS), bronchoconstriction, pulmonary oedema, or the rigid chest which can develop in some patients following high-dose opioids. It can also be seen from Figure 24.2 that compliance is reduced at the extremes of inflation.

What action do you take?

- *Airway* – ensure the endotracheal tube (ETT) is patent and well secured. Check chest expansion, auscultate and review a chest radiograph to assess whether the ETT is in optimal position.
- *Breathing* – set the ventilator to deliver lung protective breaths (tidal volumes approximately 6 mL/kg) at a rate sufficient to maintain $PaCO_2$ less than 8.0 kPa. Review the chest radiograph to look for CVC position, pneumothorax, consolidation, collapse and any other pathology.
- *Circulation* – insert and transduce intra-arterial and central venous catheters. Administer fluid challenges of 250 mL using a 50 mL syringe, looking for fluid responsiveness. Once Geoffrey is no longer fluid responsive, start an infusion of noradrenaline aiming to maintain a MAP sufficient to perfuse his organs (consider 70–75 mmHg given his history of hypertension).
- *Take bloods* for culture, FBC, U&Es, LFTs, CRP, coagulation, group and screen, and arterial blood gas analysis.
- Administer local protocol *antibiotics* for severe community-acquired pneumonia and oseltamivir in case of viral influenza.
- Insert a *urinary catheter* and send samples for M,C&S, urinary antigens for *Legionella* and pneumococcus.
- Request a viral influenza swab.
- Insert an NG tube.
- 12-lead ECG.
- Request ED staff to:
  - call critical care to update them regarding admission
  - obtain Geoffrey's medical records and history from the general practitioner
  - contact Geoffrey's next of kin.

You transfer Geoffrey to the critical care unit. On day 2 of admission, you discover that Geoffrey is known to have COPD, ischaemic heart disease and peripheral vascular disease. His functional capacity is poor, and he has deteriorated significantly since a prolonged admission to hospital last year for COPD. He has been increasingly short of breath at rest since then and converted to downstairs living 6 months ago. He has not left the house for some time and has been assessed for a package of care. He was deemed unsuitable for home oxygen as he is still smoking.

Does this new information affect your assessment or management of Geoffrey?

Geoffrey's premorbid state is extremely poor. Knowing that he could have been a candidate for home oxygen therapy highlights how poor his gas exchange is when he is at his best.

Although he is only 66 years old, he has significant cardiorespiratory disease which reduces his chances of surviving critical illness. His Acute Physiology and Chronic Health Evaluation score (APACHE II) is 30 points, giving him an estimated mortality of 73%. His Rockwood frailty score is 7, meaning severely frail. His Simplified Acute Physiology Score (SAPS) II is 58 points, giving him an in-hospital mortality of 64%.

Geoffrey is likely to have a poor outcome from this admission and this must be discussed with his next of kin since it cannot be discussed with him.

Do you want any further investigations or any other specialist review?

- *Echocardiography* – TTE to assess for right heart failure secondary to chronic respiratory disease and left heart function in light of ischaemic heart disease.
- *CTPA* – PE remains a potential diagnosis. PE may co-exist with other pathologies. If Geoffrey has not recently had a CT of his chest, this may also help to assess his underlying lung condition although widespread infection can limit the ability to assess lung parenchyma.
- *Respiratory physician review* – advise whether there is potential for optimising Geoffrey's COPD and perhaps to clarify his baseline respiratory function.
- *Cardiology review* – to aid in assessing the extent of Geoffrey's ischaemic heart disease and whether there is scope for optimisation.

CTPA shows widespread dense consolidation throughout both lung fields with several bullae and evidence of emphysema. Malignancy cannot be ruled out. There is no evidence of PE. TTE shows globally reduced function, right ventricle dilation and a severely impaired LV (ejection fraction 20%). The respiratory consultant tells you Geoffrey's spirometry results from last year: $FEV_1 = 25\%$ predicted, FVC = 85% predicted.

How do you interpret these lung function tests?

FVC is forced vital capacity, the volume which can be exhaled after maximal inspiration. FEV_1 is the forced expiratory volume in the first second of expiration. This measurement, recorded after administration of bronchodilators, is used to grade the severity of airway obstruction. An $FEV_1 < 30\%$ means Geoffrey's COPD is stage 4, i.e. very severe, according to the 2018 NICE guideline CG115 (>80% = stage 1, 50–79% = stage 2, 30–49% = stage 3, <30% = stage 4).

The FEV_1/FVC ratio, or Tiffeneau–Pinelli index, can be used to differentiate obstructive disease (decreased ratio <0.7) from restrictive lung disease (ratio is normal or increased).

Figure 2.1 demonstrates lung volumes and Figure 2.2 illustrates the changes in spirometry and peak flow with obstructive and restrictive lung disease.

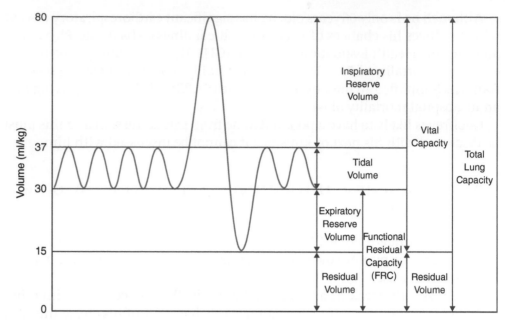

Figure 2.1: Lung volumes.

Source: Theophilus Samuels.

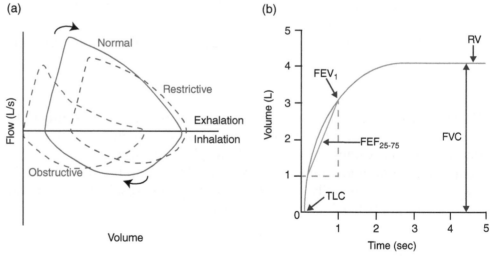

Figure 2.2: (a) Flow-volume loop demonstrating normal, obstructive and restrictive patterns. (b) A spirogram is obtained through maximal inspiration followed by rapid and forceful exhalation as maximally as possible. The FEV_1 is the volume of air exhaled in the first second (normally 70–85% depending on age). FVC is the forced vital capacity (total volume of air exhaled during a maximal forced exhalation from TLC to residual volume [RV]). The ratio of FEV_1/FVC is usually greater than 70% in healthy adults and less than 70% in obstructive pulmonary disease. FEF_{25-75} is the forced expiratory flow between 25% and 75% of vital capacity.

Source: Theophilus Samuels.

What is the pathophysiology of right ventricular dysfunction in COPD?

Hypoxaemia leads to increased pulmonary vascular resistance through hypoxic pulmonary vasoconstriction. In chronic hypoxia, this leads to remodelling of the pulmonary vascular bed, causing persistently raised right ventricle end-diastolic pressure which in turn raises right atrial pressure. Over a period of time, the right ventricle begins to decompensate, leading to right ventricular failure.

> On day 8 of admission, Geoffrey's infection has resolved. He remains intubated but is awake and appropriate with minimal sedation. He is breathing spontaneously and the pressure support has been weaned to 8 cmH$_2$O with 5 cmH$_2$O PEEP. He has a strong cough and his gas exchange is acceptable. You decide to extubate him directly onto non-invasive ventilation (NIV).

Why extubate straight to NIV?

Given Geoffrey's underlying severe COPD, his best chance of successful extubation may be with immediate non-invasive support.

There is some evidence supporting the value of immediate initiation of NIV following extubation. Ornico et al. in Crit Care 2013 showed that this approach prevents reintubation and decreases hospital mortality. Ferrer et al. in the Lancet 2009 found 90-day mortality was reduced.

> After 7 hours on NIV, Geoffrey's work of breathing increases and he looks exhausted. You reintubate him.

What is the significance of failed extubation?

Reintubation rates vary but can be as high as 25%. Reintubation is associated with increases in mortality, length of stay and risk of hospital-acquired pneumonia.

> Three days later, Geoffrey has made good progress and passes an SBT. You decide to extubate. However, he fails extubation again in a similar manner and is reintubated. You discuss the case in your critical care MDT meeting.

What is an SBT?

An SBT (spontaneous breathing trial) is a technique designed to assess a patient's suitability for extubation. When a ventilated patient is haemodynamically stable, and their pathology appears to be resolving, an SBT can be undertaken. There are methods of doing this either connected to the ventilator with minimal support or while simply on an Ayre's T-piece.

After 30–120 minutes of breathing, the patient's rapid shallow breathing index (RSBI) can be assessed:

$$RSBI = Respiratory\ rate\ /\ tidal\ volume$$

An RSBI >105 breaths/min/L has been shown to be predictive of failed extubation.

What are the main issues you would like to raise in the MDT discussion?

Geoffrey has underlying respiratory and cardiac disease. Both conditions are severe and irreversible. He has been treated for the reversible pathology which led to his admission, i.e. the lower respiratory tract infection. However, despite this, Geoffrey has failed extubation twice. He is dependent upon the ventilator.

The critical care team now consider whether Geoffrey should receive a tracheostomy or not. While he is incapacitated, the benefits and drawbacks of this should be discussed with his next of kin to find out what Geoffrey would want. It should be explained that there is a possibility, if a tracheostomy is inserted, that he may take an extremely long time to wean from the ventilator and there is a chance he may never be strong enough to breathe independently.

If it is decided not to site a tracheostomy, escalation planning and resuscitation orders need to be discussed.

Establish that safeguarding procedures have been initiated for Geoffrey's wife as she may need additional help at home. This will probably already have been raised in the ED or on admission to ICU.

Geoffrey's wife, his next of kin, is brought to the hospital by Geoffrey's best friend of 40 years. Although she has early-onset dementia, she can have a coherent conversation with you. She asks that his best friend be present as well. His wife tells you that Geoffrey does not like doctors or hospitals. She is sure that he would not want a tracheostomy. His best friend agrees.

On sedation hold the next day, Geoffrey is lucid and well enough to communicate. You discuss the issue of tracheostomy with him. He is clear that he does not want tracheostomy or reintubation again, even if it means he might die. He also does not wish to be resuscitated.

How will you document your discussions and communicate your decisions?

Document in the medical notes and in escalation planning notes that Geoffrey is for 'one-way' extubation. He should not be reintubated and his care will not be escalated should he deteriorate. He is not to be resuscitated in the case of cardiac arrest. Complete a ReSPECT form (Recommended Summary Plan for Emergency Care and Treatment) to this effect. Document all conversations in the medical notes, identifying all persons present.

With his consent, explain the situation to Geoffrey's wife. These conversations can be challenging, and it is important to tailor communication for the individual with whom you are speaking. Try to establish her baseline understanding and be aware that she may struggle to understand or retain complex concepts or large amounts of information because of both her dementia and the extreme emotion of the situation. One approach may be to explain that, if simple supportive measures fail to save Geoffrey, it is a sign that his body is too frail to survive without a ventilator. It is important to recognise when people enter the final phase of life so that medical staff can refrain from aggressive treatments designed to try and reverse what is now irreversible. Instead, understanding that this is the dying process allows the focus of care to be on comfort, prioritising dignity and time with family. Discuss Geoffrey's case with the palliative care team and offer to call the hospital chaplain.

Communicate this to the rest of the critical care team and mention the new DNACPR in the routine daily ICU team safety brief.

You extubate Geoffrey onto high-flow nasal cannulae as he finds it more comfortable than NIV. Sadly, despite your best efforts, Geoffrey dies on day 2 following extubation surrounded by his family and the hospital chaplain.

Further reading

- West, J. (2020). *West's Respiratory Physiology: The Essentials*. Philadelphia: Lippincott West's textbook of respiratory physiology is essential reading, now in its 11th edition.
- Review article about managing the end of life process in critical care
- Cook, D. and Rocker, G. (2014). Dying with dignity in the intensive care unit. *N. Engl. J. Med.* 370: 2506–2514. Review article about managing the end-of-life process in critical care.
- Weinberger, S., Cockrill, B., and Mandel, J. (2018). *Principles of Pulmonary Medicine*. St Louis: Elsevier.
- Schwartzstein, R. and Parker, M. (2012). *Respiratory Physiology: A Clinical Approach*. Philadelphia: Lippincott, Williams and Wilkins. Two excellent textbooks covering the fundamentals of respiratory medicine.

3

The Patient with Respiratory Distress II

The medical registrar calls you at the start of your night shift to inform you about a patient who has been admitted to the acute medical unit. The patient, a 46-year-old labourer called Jim, presented with double vision and lower limb weakness. His CT head was unremarkable, his inflammatory markers were not raised and he appeared otherwise relatively well. The medical team are assuming this is likely to be Guillain–Barré or myasthenia gravis but they have not made a formal diagnosis and no treatment has yet been initiated.

What is Guillain–Barré syndrome?

This is an autoimmune condition causing an acute ascending inflammatory peripheral neuropathy with areflexia and progressive motor weakness in more than one limb. Cases occur approximately 1–2 in 100 000, more commonly in Caucasians and with a bimodal incidence (teens to mid-20s, and 60–80 year olds). There are different types of Guillain–Barré which have slightly different presentations. Acute inflammatory demyelinating polyradiculoneuropathy (AIDP) is the most common subtype in Europe and North America (up to 95% of cases).

How does Guillain–Barré usually present?

Around half of cases present with glove and stocking distribution paraesthesia and a quarter present with motor weakness. The remainder present with a mixed clinical picture. In up to half of cases, cranial nerves are involved (particularly VII, IX and X) and tendon reflexes are lost.

What is myasthenia gravis (MG)?

Myasthenia gravis is also autoimmune in origin. It results in weakness characterised by fatiguability of skeletal and ocular muscles. Anti-acetylcholine antibodies develop to the alpha subunit of nicotinic receptors on the postsynaptic

Clinical Cases in Critical Care, First Edition. Alice Myers and Theophilus Samuels.
© 2023 John Wiley & Sons Ltd. Published 2023 by John Wiley & Sons Ltd.

motor endplate at the skeletal neuromuscular junction. Nerve conduction is impaired due to occupation of acetylcholine binding sites by the autoantibody. Once the number of available postsynaptic receptors decreases to 30%, patients become symptomatic. Prevalence is approximately 10 in 100000, with a female preponderance. It is often associated with thymus hyperplasia and other auto-immune diseases.

What else could cause a similar presentation?

- One of the less common variants of Guillain–Barré syndrome (GBS):
  - *Acute motor axonal neuropathy* (AMAN).
  - *Acute motor sensory axonal neuropathy* (AMSAN) – axons, rather than the myelin sheath, are affected.
  - *Miller Fisher syndrome* – the classic triad is of ophthalmoplegia, ataxia and areflexia. This disease can present as a pure oculomotor palsy. It is associated with anti-GQ1b antibodies although 1 in 10 cases is seronegative.
  - *Bickerstaff's brainstem encephalitis* – this shares similarities with the Miller Fisher variant with regard to ophthalmoplegia, ataxia and presence of anti-GQ1b antibodies. However, these patients suffer altered conscious level and may also show long tract signs (e.g. spasticity and hyper-reflexia).
  - *Pharyngeal-cervical-brachial variant* – oropharyngeal and brachiocervical weakness. There is areflexia in the upper limbs. The condition is rapidly progressive. This is an axonal neuropathy and half of cases are associated with anti-GT1a antibodies.
  - *Pan-dysautonomia* – this is an extremely rare variant which presents with autonomic symptoms alone. There is no motor involvement.
- *Lambert–Eaton myasthenic syndrome* (LEMS) – antibodies against presynaptic voltage-gated calcium channels lead to proximal limb muscle weakness, usually affecting the legs more than the arms. In contrast to MG where exercise causes worsening of symptoms, exercise can temporarily alleviate symptoms in LEMS. It is usually associated with underlying malignancy (60%) and can be the presenting feature of small cell lung cancer.
- *Toxins (especially heavy metal intoxication)* – this would usually present with abdominal symptoms and confusion, but weakness and paraesthesia are also features.
- *Botulism* – often contracted from tinned or foil-wrapped foods, *Clostridium botulinum* produces botulinum toxin which inhibits the release of acetylcholine from presynaptic nerve terminals at the neuromuscular junction. Presentation is with facial weakness, blurred or double vision, ptosis, dry mouth, postural hypotension and nausea and vomiting.
- *Lyme disease* – tick-borne Lyme borreliosis, usually *Borrelia burgdorferi*, may present in a variety of ways including facial weakness. Other symptoms include palpitations, joint pains, fever, headache and tiredness.

Erythema migrans (an erythematous bullseye rash) may be seen at the site of the tick bite.

- *Spinal cord pathology* – transverse myelitis or spinal cord compression could account for lower limb weakness but would not explain Jim's double vision.
- *Drugs* – certain drugs such as cocaine, bumetanide, amiodarone, phenytoin and vincristine can cause peripheral neuropathy.
- *Intracranial event* – this is an unlikely cause of ascending muscular weakness but is included for completeness. Jim's CT head was normal, which is reassuring. However, brainstem pathologies would be better visualised using magnetic resonance imaging (MRI). MRI imaging of the brain can require the patient to lie flat for around 45 minutes so always consider whether it is safe to do this without airway protection.

Why is the medical registrar calling you?

It is reasonable for the medical team to raise awareness of this patient who is at risk of rapid deterioration. Classically, the symptoms of GBS progress over 10–12 days. The pattern of weakness is ascending and, in some cases, can progress to involve the phrenic nerve, intercostal muscles and accessory muscles of respiration. Patients can deteriorate rapidly, leading to the requirement for invasive ventilatory support. Particularly in rapidly progressive cases, close monitoring of patients is advisable as the onset of respiratory failure can easily go unnoticed.

GBS can have profound autonomic system involvement leading to cardiac dysrhythmias, fluctuations in blood pressure, urinary retention and severe constipation leading to pseudo-obstruction.

> You decide to review Jim yourself. On examination, you find him alert and comfortable but with symmetrically reduced power in his lower limbs, more marked distally. He also has double vision at the extremes of lateral gaze. BP 127/47 mmHg lying, 93/33 mmHg sitting, HR 89 bpm, RR 14 breaths per minute with oxygen saturations of 99% on room air.

How will you assess Jim's respiratory function?

Using a combination of clinical assessment and point-of-care testing, the key is not to miss a deterioration in symptoms which could lead to Jim suffering a respiratory arrest on the ward. Assess his respiratory function and his ability to clear secretions effectively. Postural hypotension can be a manifestation of autonomic neuropathy, and approximately 30% require ventilatory support.

- *Clinical examination* – assess cough strength. Can he clear secretions? Can he sustain lifting his head off the pillow for 5 seconds? Can he raise his elbows above his head and keep them there for 5 seconds?
- *Serial lung function testing is mandatory* – 4-hourly bedside spirometry should be performed to track progress and identify deterioration. The

following parameters should raise concern and prompt admission to critical care with consideration of intubation:

- Forced vital capacity <15 mL/kg
- Maximal inspiratory pressure <30 cmH$_2$O
- Maximal expiratory pressure <40 cmH$_2$O
- Rising PaCO$_2$ on serial arterial blood gas sampling

> Jim has good respiratory function and you elect not to admit him but leave strict instructions for regular monitoring and review. Five hours later, you are called by the nurse on the ward who says that he is worried about Jim because he appears to be struggling to breathe. When you re-review him, his RR is 30–35 breaths per minute, HR 125 bpm, his cough is weak. He is too tired for spirometry.

How do you proceed?

- Admit Jim to critical care straight away. He has deteriorated rapidly which is a poor prognostic sign. Accompany him on the transfer to the ICU with monitoring in place, a skilled assistant, an emergency intubation kit and an oxygen supply.
- Ask the ward to call Jim's next of kin.
- Proceed to intubation on arrival in intensive care.
- Lung-protective ventilation.
- Insert arterial and central venous catheters, a urinary catheter and a nasogastric tube.
- Blood pressure management with fluid and vasopressors guided by clinical assessment, echocardiography and/or cardiac output monitoring.
- Prescribe thromboprophylaxis, aperients and ulcer prophylaxis.

What investigations would you like to perform now and over the next few days in addition to the standard critical care blood panel?

- *Chest radiograph* – review central venous catheter positioning and assess for development of lower respiratory tract infection, possibly secondary to aspiration.
- *Lumbar puncture* – a high protein level would be consistent with GBS. A raised white cell count could suggest an alternative cause for the presentation (e.g. Lyme disease) but could also raise the possibility of an infective or inflammatory condition leading to the development of GBS in this patient (e.g. HIV or malignancy).
- *Investigations to identify any immune activating pathogen.*
  - Stool culture for *Campylobacter jejuni*. Ask about prodromal diarrhoea, recent travel and vaccination.
  - Blood for HIV, CMV, EBV, hepatitis viruses, viral PCR (especially for arboviruses and influenza), mycoplasma antibodies.

- *Immunoglobulins and antiganglioside antibodies* (anti-GQ1b, GM1, GD3, GD1a) – high levels of anti-GM1 are associated with increased severity of GBS. Anti-GD1a is associated with acute motor axonal neuropathy.
- *MRI brain/spine* – this is sensitive but not specific. It can reveal spinal root enhancement and surface thickening.
- *Nerve conduction studies* – these may be normal in the early stages and are most useful at around 14 days. In GBS, there are low-amplitude or absent sensory nerve action potentials, an absent H reflex and an abnormal F wave. F wave abnormalities are associated with poor prognosis. Patterns of change can help identify subtypes.

What are the indications, contraindications, and complications regarding lumbar puncture?

Indications

- *Diagnostic* – sampling CSF and measuring pressure.
- *Therapeutic* – removal of CSF in certain cases of raised intracranial pressure (ICP) such as idiopathic intracranial hypertension and communicating hydrocephalus, or facilitating administration of intrathecal drugs.

Contraindications

These are mainly relative contraindications:

- Raised ICP leading to risk of brainstem herniation such as in non-communicating hydrocephalus
- Localised infection at the site of LP
- Generalised sepsis
- Coagulopathy (drug or illness induced)
- Anatomical concerns, e.g. spina bifida, trauma
- Patient refusal

Complications

- Headache
- Brainstem herniation
- Bleeding/epidural haematoma
- Infection
- Neurological injury (spinal cord or conus medullaris)

The next day, Jim is reviewed by the neurology consultant who agrees with a presumptive diagnosis of GBS.

What is the pathophysiology of GBS?

Production of auto-antibodies occurs, possibly following a trigger such as infection with *C. jejuni*. The reason why certain individuals are affected and others are not is yet to be fully elucidated. Various patterns of nerve damage can occur but demyelination is the main pathological process. Peripheral nerves (spinal and cranial) and autonomic nerves can be affected.

What are the options for management?

Immunomodulation

- High-dose intravenous immunoglobulin (IVIg) – 0.4 g/kg/day for 3–5 days.
- Plasmapheresis – five exchanges usually over 5 days.

Supportive measures

- Intubation and ventilation.
- Haemodynamic support – cardiovascular instability can result due to autonomic neuropathy.
- Pain control – opiates are useful but sedation is an unwelcome side-effect. Amitriptyline and gabapentin are often required for neuropathic pain.
- Nutrition.
- Bowel and bladder care.
- Physiotherapy.
- Venous thromboprophylaxis.

What is the evidence for plasmapheresis as compared with IVIg?

A randomised controlled trial published in the *New England Journal of Medicine* in 1992 concluded that IVIg was at least as effective as plasma exchange for GBS and may be associated with fewer complications. A similar review in the Lancet in 1997 showed similar efficacy. A Cochrane systematic review (Hughes 2004) also concluded that IVIg and plasmapheresis are similarly effective.

Cross-over therapy appears to confer no benefit. IVIg is often the more practical choice as it is easier to administer and usually more readily available.

Would your treatment plan differ if this were myasthenia gravis?

As with management of GBS, IVIg and plasmapheresis should be considered along with meticulous supportive care. There are some differences in terms of specific disease management.

- *Pyridostigmine/rivastigmine* – these drugs are acetylcholinesterase inhibitors. Therapeutic effects are achieved through delaying the breakdown of acetylcholine and hence increasing its availability to act at the reduced number of active receptors. Neostigmine and pyridostigmine act peripherally whereas rivastigmine acts centrally.

■ *Steroids and azathioprine* – steroids are not effective in GBS but are an important treatment option for modulating T cells in MG. The dose of prednisolone is gradually increased and then, as it is tapered off, it can be replaced with azathioprine to achieve longer term control through inhibition of the cell cycle.

■ *Methotrexate, mycophenolate mofetil, tacrolimus or ciclosporin* – can be considered in non-responders or those who do not tolerate steroids or azathioprine.

■ *Thymectomy* – a randomised controlled trial published by Wolfe in the *New England Journal of Medicine* (2016) found that thymectomy improved clinical outcomes over a 3-year period in myasthenia gravis.

> When you return to work after your night shifts, you find that Jim remains intubated on day 7 of his admission, having completed 5 days of IVIg. He is breathing spontaneously on the ventilator with pressure support of 18 cmH$_2$O and PEEP 5 cmH$_2$O. He has a poor cough and has marked weakness. The nurse in charge asks you whether you think this patient will need a tracheostomy.

Is there an argument to support early tracheostomy in this case?

A study published in *Neurocritical Care* by Walgaard (2017) found that patients who were unable to raise their arms from the bed or who had axonal degeneration at 1 week had a high risk of prolonged mechanical ventilation.

The TrachMan study published in *JAMA* (Young et al. 2013) compared 30-day mortality in patients receiving a tracheostomy early (day 1–4) or late (day 10 or later) in the course of their ICU admission. Although this large randomised multicentre trial found no statistical difference between the groups, it did not focus specifically on cases of neurological weakness.

Jim does not appear to be progressing quickly. He is still extremely weak. Information gathered at the multidisciplinary team meeting is particularly useful in the decision-making process.

> As a multidisciplinary team, you believe that Jim will benefit from a tracheostomy at this point due to the likely requirement for prolonged ventilatory support.

What are the indications for tracheostomy?

Some indications will be reversible and others irreversible. In some cases, reversibility may be unclear at the time of the procedure. Where possible, frank discussions should be undertaken prior to elective tracheostomy regarding reversibility and overall prognosis.

Emergency

■ Upper airway obstruction, e.g. anaphylaxis, tumour, foreign body, etc.

Elective

- Where prolonged artificial ventilation is required – reduced dead space allows for reduction in work of breathing. Tracheostomy is better tolerated than oral endotracheal tube, therefore reducing requirement for sedation.
- Airway protection – e.g. in cases of neurodegenerative disease.
- Respiratory toilet – where cough or swallow reflex is impaired.
- Surgical indications – e.g. for certain head and neck procedures.

What are the risks of tracheostomy?

Immediate or procedure related

- Haemorrhage
- Aspiration
- Airway obstruction
- Air embolus
- Pneumothorax
- Haemothorax
- Death

Medium term

- Infection
- Pneumomediastinum
- Haemorrhage (particularly from erosion into local vessels)
- Tissue necrosis
- Tracheo-arterial fistula
- Dysphagia
- Airway obstruction (tube displacement)

Long term

- Tracheomalacia
- Dysphagia
- Stricture/stenosis
- Scarring
- Fistula

How would you perform a tracheostomy?

There are various techniques for performing tracheostomy based on either the open surgical technique or percutaneous method. The following principles can be applied when performing percutaneous tracheostomy within the critical care setting.

Indications and consent

The critical care team should be satisfied that tracheostomy is indicated. Patients should be consented directly where possible and if unable to consent, then the relevant proxy consent form (Consent form 4 in the UK) should be completed (e.g. signed by two experienced medical professionals) and next of kin informed as appropriate with potential complications discussed. All decisions and discussions must be clearly documented.

Preparation

- Check coagulation.
- Group and save blood sample (two samples required in the UK).
- Aspirate NG tube.
- Position patient with neck extended.
- Ultrasound neck to check there are no blood vessels over the tracheostomy site.
- Full monitoring (including end-tidal CO_2).
- 100% oxygen.

Drugs

- Sedation.
- Muscle relaxation.
- Emergency drugs available.
- Lignocaine 1% with adrenaline 1 in 200 000 for local infiltration.

Equipment

- Drapes.
- Fibreoptic scope.
- Appropriately sized tracheostomy tube with surgical set.
- Emergency airway trolley for reintubation if needed.
- Laryngoscope (direct or video) and usually a fibreoptic scope will be required for retraction of endotracheal tube under visualisation.

Personnel

- One operator performs tracheostomy.
- One airway specialist performs bronchoscopy.
- One trained assistant helps with sedation and equipment.
- Aseptic technique with surgical scrub and personal protective equipment.

Procedure

Details of technique vary. The following description is consistent with a Seldinger method.

- Using laryngoscopy, the airway clinician deflates the ETT cuff and withdraws until the cuff can be visualised at the cords. The cuff may then be reinflated.
- Operator then inserts a 14 G cannula into the trachea (usually between the second and third or third and fourth tracheal rings).
- Positioning is verified using bronchoscopy.
- A guidewire is inserted into the trachea via the cannula.

- A series of dilators are then inserted over the guidewire until the tracheostomy tube itself can be inserted.
- Positioning can be checked via bronchoscopy.
- Once the tracheostomy tube is in place and the cuff inflated, the tube can be secured as per local protocol.

Postprocedure management

- Chest radiograph to exclude pneumothorax.
- Once the patient is no longer paralysed, sedation can be reduced or stopped.
- Full documentation in the notes.
- Reuseable equipment should be logged and returned for cleaning.
- Review ventilator settings and continue full monitoring.

> Your consultant agrees that Jim is making slow progress and will probably benefit from tracheostomy at this stage. You perform this successfully and once the effects of the paralysing agent have worn off, you stop his sedation.

What are the principles behind a respiratory weaning plan?

It is desirable to wean patients from ventilatory support as soon as possible since prolonged intubation is associated with longer length of stay, increased likelihood of ventilator-associated pneumonia and possibly increased mortality. Usually, a patient will have failed a spontaneous breathing trial before a weaning plan is created.

There are many ways to approach weaning, with some ICUs preferring to use a protocol. Some studies have shown that protocols can reduce time on mechanical ventilation.

- Weaning protocols will usually require the patient to be stable from a cardiorespiratory point of view.
- A PEEP of less than 10 cmH$_2$O is desirable.
- NAVA (neurally adjusted ventilatory assist) has been used to great effect in patients with neuromuscular disorders.
- Protocols indicate how and when to decrease pressure support and PEEP to achieve desired tidal volumes, saturations and end-tidal CO$_2$.
- Cuff deflation and use of a one-way speaking valve need to be considered.
- Weaning should challenge the patient without compromising cardiorespiratory stability.
- The aim is to reduce support as rapidly as is tolerated by the patient to expedite decannulation.
- A multidisciplinary approach involving physiotherapy, psychology and nursing is vital.

Who should be involved in Jim's ongoing care?

- Critical care physicians and nurses
- Neurologist
- Physiotherapist
- Dietician
- Occupational therapist
- Pharmacist
- Psychologist
- Pain specialist, if necessary
- And of course, Jim and his family!

Three weeks later, you are able to successfully decannulate Jim and he is discharged to a medical ward 2 days after that.

What is the likely outcome for Jim?

Approximately 85% of patients are expected to fully recover from GBS with a usual recovery period of 6–18 months. The remaining 15% have lasting disability ranging from mild paraesthesia or areflexia to severe permanent neurological damage such as ataxia, muscle wasting, foot drop, etc. Mortality is less than 5% in developed countries. Ongoing pain can be significant for some survivors. There is a recurrence rate of 7%.

Scoring systems have been devised to predict which patients will suffer worse outcomes.

- *mEGOS (modified Erasmus Guillain–Barré Outcome Score)* – patients are scored at admission or day 7 to predict a likelihood of being unable to walk independently at 6 months. This is a composite score based on age, presence of prodromal diarrhoea and Medical Research Council (MRC) muscle weakness score.
- *EGRIS (Erasmus Guillain–Barré Respiratory Insufficiency Score)* – this score predicts the probability of respiratory insufficiency within the first week of admission. The score is calculated according to days between onset and hospital admission, presence of facial or bulbar weakness, and the MRC muscle weakness score.

You invite Jim back to the ICU follow-up clinic in 6 months' time.

What post-critical care issues do patients suffer?

Specific problems related to GBS include weakness and pain. Additionally, post-intensive care syndrome (PICS) is well recognised and occurs in 25–75% of ICU survivors. The risk of developing PICS is highest in those who suffered delirium, multiorgan failure, hypoxia, severe sepsis and glucose dysregulation, or who required renal replacement therapy.

PICS comprises psychiatric and physical symptoms. Post-traumatic stress disorder, depression and anxiety are often described. Residual neuromuscular weakness can lead to reduced mobility and recurrent falls. Cognitive impairment can be a significant problem for many with PICS.

Post-intensive care syndrome can predispose patients to many other psychosocial issues including the following:

- *Personal relationships* – disturbed sleep, sexual dysfunction, fatigue and immobility can affect the patient's relationships with those close to them.
- *Social isolation* – immobility and depression may become a barrier for usual social interactions.
- *Employment* – patients may not be able to return to work in the same capacity as previously.

See Case 11 for the ICU Liberation bundle (A–F) which has been proposed as an approach to ICU management aiming to reduce the incidence of PICS.

Further reading

- Leonhard, S., Mandarakas, M., Gondim, F. et al. (2019). Diagnosis and management of Guillain–Barré syndrome in ten steps. *Nat. Rev. Neurol.* 15: 671–683. Evidence-based guidelines for dealing with GBS.
- Farrugia, M. and Goodfellow, J. (2020). A practical approach to managing patients with myasthenia gravis – opinions and review of the literature. *Front. Neurol.* 11: 604. Overview of the medical management of myasthenia gravis.
- Lee, M., Kang, J., and Jeong, Y. (2020). Risk factors for post-intensive care syndrome: a systematic review and meta analysis. *Aus. Crit. Care* 33: 287–294. Systematic review of risk factors for PICS.

4

The Patient with Abdominal Pain and Vomiting

Y ou are called to urgently review a 46-year-old named Brian in the resuscitation area of your emergency department (ED). He is a type 1 diabetic patient complaining of severe abdominal pain but with no signs of peritonism. His past medical history includes biliary colic. Observations reveal a systolic BP between 85 and 95 mmHg, sinus tachycardia 130 bpm and an SpO$_2$ 94% on 10 L/min oxygen. Brian has been vomiting profusely over the past 72 hours and has not been taking his insulin during this time. His bedside serum blood glucose is raised at 23 mmol/L and a spot urine test demonstrates the presence of ketones.

What is the likely cause of this endocrine disturbance?

Brian is most likely in diabetic ketoacidosis (DKA).

Why do you suspect DKA?

- *Absolute insulin deficiency* – Brian has not been able to take his insulin therapy. In type 1 diabetes mellitus (DM), there is a lack of circulating endogenous insulin, which requires exogenous insulin for effective management.
- *Relative insulin deficiency* – tissue insulin requirements are increased by physiological stresses such as infection, trauma and major surgery. Patients with type 1 DM can still develop DKA even if they take their regular doses of insulin. Brian appears to be critically unwell, and so probably has both an *absolute* and *relative* deficiency.
- *Ketonuria* – the presence of ketones in his urine is associated with DKA.

Describe the pathophysiology of DKA

- *Absolute or relative reduction in the effects of insulin* – this leads to altered carbohydrate metabolism. Patients with type 1 DM have virtually no functional pancreatic beta-cells (where insulin is synthesised) and can

Clinical Cases in Critical Care, First Edition. Alice Myers and Theophilus Samuels.
© 2023 John Wiley & Sons Ltd. Published 2023 by John Wiley & Sons Ltd.

neither respond to changes in blood glucose levels nor maintain a basal secretion of insulin. This absolute deficiency affects metabolism in liver, muscle and adipose tissue.

- The increased hepatic production and decreased glucose uptake by insulin-dependent glucose transporter type 4 (GLUT4) receptors located in muscle and adipose tissue result in hyperglycaemia.
- *Ketosis* – this results from the rise in the counter-regulatory hormone glucagon and other hormones such as cortisol, growth hormone and catecholamines. This leads to the mobilisation of fatty acids from adipose tissue, followed by increased hepatic beta-oxidation and synthesis of 3-hydroxybutyrate and acetoacetate. Also, in DKA, the clearance of these ketone bodies is decreased, contributing further to the rise in ketone levels.
- *Renal threshold for handling glucose is greatly exceeded* – the ensuing hyperglycaemia leads to an osmotic diuresis resulting in loss of electrolytes and water. This results in dehydration, which in turn stimulates the release of catecholamines, further exacerbating the problem.
- *Excess ketone bodies* – result in a large amount of hydrogen ions needing to be buffered. This quickly depletes the buffering capacity of the plasma, allowing the ketone anions to accumulate, which leads to a raised anion gap and contributes to the observed acidaemia.

How do you diagnose DKA?

- Anion gap metabolic acidosis (bicarbonate <15 mmol/L and/or venous pH <7.3).
- Hyperglycaemia (commonly between 19.4 and 27.8 mmol/L) or known diabetes mellitus.
- Ketonaemia (>3 mmol/L) or significant ketonuria (more than 2+ on a standard urine dipstick test).

Glucose levels typically do not exceed 44 mmol/L. However, they may be even higher in patients with DKA who are comatose.

How can the severity of DKA be classified?

Diabetic ketoacidosis can be classified as mild, moderate, or severe using various parameters including those listed here:

- *Mild* – pH 7.25–7.30, serum beta-hydroxybutyrate 3–4 mmol/L
- *Moderate* – pH 7.00–7.24, serum beta-hydroxybutyrate 4–8 mmol/L
- *Severe* – pH <7.00, serum beta-hydroxybutyrate >8 mmol/L

Can a patient develop DKA with normal serum blood glucose levels?

Yes. The class of drugs known as gliflozins (or sodium-glucose co-transporter-2 inhibitors [SGLT-2]) are a new group of oral medications used in the treatment of type 2 diabetes. By inhibiting the SGLT-2 receptors in the renal tubules, they can prevent most glucose from being reabsorbed from the glomerular filtrate to the plasma. This results in increased secretion of glucose by the urine, improving blood glucose, as well as often promoting weight loss and lowering blood pressure through the loss of sodium and water.

The DKA associated with these drugs is characterised by the usual metabolic defects such as an anion gap metabolic acidosis, ketonaemia and reduced plasma bicarbonate, but without the usual hyperglycaemia. This can occur in type 1 patients when they are started on them to promote weight loss, for example. Hence, in the absence of hyperglycaemia, the key for these individuals is to test for either urinary or serum ketones when they feel unwell.

Explain why you consider this to be DKA and not a hyperosmolar hyperglycaemic state (HHS)?

Essentially, HHS (also known as hyperosmotic hyperglycaemic non-ketotic state) is a hyperglycaemic state without ketoacidosis that occurs most often in the elderly and in those with known type 2 diabetes. It is commonly caused by acute physiological stresses, such as infection, acute abdomen, cardiac or neurological events. Drugs are also implicated, especially high-dose thiazide diuretics, corticosteroids and beta-blockers. Typically, the blood sugar level is much greater (usually 33.3 mmol/L or greater) with a markedly elevated serum osmolality of 320 mOsm/kg or greater. The mortality rates for HHS are higher than those for DKA.

The major difference between these two conditions is that HHS patients usually have enough circulating insulin to prevent ketoacidosis (prevents an increase in free fatty acids and therefore blocks ketone production in the liver), but not enough to prevent hepatic production of glucose and poor peripheral utilisation by tissues. Some urinary ketones are still present and the anion gap increases mildly, but the severe acidaemia seen in DKA is not observed. Hence, the nausea and vomiting usually seen in DKA due to the severe acidaemia is often absent. This potentially makes the onset of HHS very insidious as the osmotic diuresis and hyperglycaemia can be quite protracted (days to weeks) before medical attention is sought. This in turn can lead to severe electrolyte abnormalities and severe dehydration, particularly in the elderly and frail.

So, given that Brian is a younger patient with type 1 diabetes and has had a 72-hour history of nausea and vomiting with the presence of ketonuria, it is more likely that he is in DKA than HHS.

> You are presented with the following blood results: Na$^+$ 130 mmol/L, K$^+$ 4.5 mmol/L, urea 8 mmol/L, creatinine 121 μmol/L and arterial blood gas analysis (10 L/min oxygen therapy) – pH 7.21, PaO$_2$ 44.1 kPa, PaCO$_2$ 2.1 kPa, base excess −9 mmol/L, bicarbonate 11 mmol/L, lactate 2.1 mmol/L, chloride 101 mmol/L.

How would you calculate and interpret the anion gap for Brian?

The anion gap (AG) quantifies the difference between unmeasured cations (positively charged ions) and unmeasured anions (negatively charged ions).

$$AG = \left[Na^+\right] + \left[K^+\right] - \left(\left[Cl^-\right] + \left[HCO_3^-\right]\right)$$

The concentration of potassium is usually omitted, giving:

$$AG = \left[Na^+ \right] - \left(\left[Cl^- \right] + \left[HCO_3^- \right] \right)$$

with the typical range equal to 4–12 mmol/L in the presence of a normal albumin level (consult local laboratory reference ranges).

In healthy individuals, the anion gap mostly measures the negative charge on albumin and phosphate, but it has a low sensitivity and low specificity and is practically useless in the presence of hypoalbuminaemia.

What is the AG in this case?

The anion gap is raised at $130 - (101 + 11) = 18$ mmol/L, so Brian has a high anion gap metabolic acidosis due to severe DKA.

What are the causes for a raised AG?

Causes for a high anion gap can be outlined using the acronym *GOLDMARK*:

- **G**lycols – such as ethylene and propylene. Propylene glycol is a common diluent used for intravenous medications such as lorazepam. It is also metabolised to L-lactate and D-lactate.
- **O**xyproline (also called pyroglutaminic acid) – from chronic paracetamol ingestion, especially in malnourished women.
- **L**-lactate.
- **D**-lactate (typically seen in patients with short gut syndromes).
- **M**ethanol.
- **A**spirin.
- **R**enal failure.
- **K**etoacidosis (e.g. diabetes, starvation).

What are the main treatment goals when managing DKA?

- Commence insulin therapy and ensure that it is adequately reversing the ketogenesis (e.g. by measuring capillary beta-hydroxybutyrate using point-of-care testing).
- Ensure acidaemia is improving and returning pH to the normal physiological range.
- IV fluid therapy should adequately restore intravascular volume (typical water deficits are 100 mL/kg). Consult local guidelines on the rapidity of fluid resuscitation as these patients are prone to solute/water shifts that leave them open to severe complications. The recommended resuscitative fluid is 0.9% saline.
- Replace electrolyte losses, which can be severe (e.g. Na^+, K^+).
- Treat the underlying cause(s).
- Monitor for complications of DKA management.

How should insulin be prescribed to treat patients in DKA?

The current recommendation is to start a fixed-rate intravenous insulin infusion (FRIII) based on body weight and a serum glucose ≥14 mmol/L at a rate of 0.1 units/kg/h. As soon as serum glucose decreases to <14 mmol/L, a 10% dextrose infusion should be added. In addition, reducing the FRIII to 0.05 units/kg/h should be considered as this will reduce the risk of hypoglycaemia and hypokalaemia developing (consult your local hospital guidelines).

What are the metabolic treatment targets in DKA?

Recommended targets are:

- An increase in venous bicarbonate by 3.0 mmol/L/h
- A reduction in blood ketone concentration by 0.5 mmol/L/h
- A reduction in capillary blood glucose by 3.0 mmol/L/h
- Maintaining serum potassium concentration between 4.0 and 5.5 mmol/L.

The FRIII rate should be increased if these targets are not met (also consult your local hospital's DKA protocol and/or a specialist in the management of DKA).

What are the main complications from DKA that would concern you?

- *Hyperkalaemia and hypokalaemia* – these are potentially life-threatening complications. Due to the pre-renal acute kidney injury that may occur from severe dehydration, potassium replacement is not recommended during the initial fluid resuscitation or if the serum potassium level is greater than or equal to 5.5 mmol/L. With insulin therapy, potassium levels will almost always fall, so it is recommended that a ready-mixed bag of 0.9% saline and 40 mmol/L of potassium are prescribed if the level is less than 5.5 mmol/L and the patient is passing urine. If more concentrated solutions need to be given, this ideally should be done in a high-dependency or critical care environment where the higher concentration solutions can be given via a central vein with continuous monitoring.
- *Hypoglycaemia* – blood glucose may drop sharply once insulin therapy is commenced, and care should be taken to avoid dropping its levels to less than the normal range. This can cause cardiac arrhythmias, acute brain injury and death. In addition, it is imperative that *rebound ketosis* is avoided as this will lengthen the duration of treatment. This occurs when insulin falls to levels that create a *relative deficiency* and allow the counter-regulatory hormones to exert their ketogenic effects on metabolism once again.
- *Cerebral oedema* – symptomatic cerebral oedema is relatively uncommon in adult patients with DKA. Cerebral oedema is known to occur within the first few hours of starting treatment, suggesting that it is iatrogenic

in origin. It is more commonly associated with children who present with DKA.

- *Other* – pulmonary oedema is a very uncommon complication and usually occurs within the first few hours of commencing treatment, again suggesting an iatrogenic cause due to the rapid infusion of crystalloids over a short period of time. Those most at risk include the elderly and those with impaired cardiac function. The development of venous thromboembolic disease is also a potential complication, especially in the presence of central venous catheters.

When would you consider this episode of DKA to be resolved?

- pH *greater than* 7.3
- Bicarbonate level *greater than* 15.0 mmol/L
- Blood ketone level *less than* 0.6 mmol/L

How long would you expect it to take for Brian's DKA to resolve?

Usually, by 24 hours of appropriate treatment, the ketonaemia and acidosis should have resolved in most patients. However, should the patient fail to respond to treatment, senior and specialist input should be sought. In addition, other pathologies may be present that were difficult to identify during the initial resuscitation period. Note, relying on serum bicarbonate concentration *only* is not recommended. This is because a potential hyperchloraemic metabolic acidosis may be present due to the high volumes of 0.9% saline given.

Brian is transferred to your intensive care unit for monitoring and ongoing management. After 24 hours, he is still severely acidotic. Brian is now becoming increasingly confused and his abdominal pain is severe in the epigastric area and radiates to his back. His most recent ABG on 10 L/min of oxygen therapy demonstrates pH 7.01, base excess −17 mmol/L, bicarbonate 5 mmol/L and lactate 8 mmol/L.

With his previous history of biliary colic, what do you think may be the cause of his severe abdominal pain?

Gallstone disease is the most common cause of acute pancreatitis worldwide. Brian's history of biliary colic suggests the presence of gallstones. This would need to be confirmed using either ultrasonography or CT.

Apart from acute pancreatitis, what other conditions might cause his severe abdominal pain?

Diabetic ketoacidosis can often present with abdominal pain, but it should not be ongoing if the patient is responding to treatment. Other causes could include:

- Perforated viscus
- Bowel obstruction
- Ischaemic bowel
- Myocardial infarction
- Ruptured abdominal aortic aneurysm
- Biliary colic, acute cholecystitis or cholangitis
- Viral hepatitis and gastroenteritis
- Sickle crisis

What are the causes of acute pancreatitis?

Gallstone disease or alcohol is the cause in 80% of cases in the developed world. Alcohol-induced pancreatitis should be considered when alcohol ingestion greater than 50 g/day has occurred for at least 5 years. However, it is not always possible to obtain such an accurate history. Apart from these two causes, the others are rare and should only be considered if gallstone disease and alcohol are not implicated. These causes and others can be remembered using the mnemonic I GET SMASHED:

- **I**diopathic
- **G**allstones
- **E**thanol
- **T**rauma
- **S**teroids
- **M**umps/Malignancy
- **A**utoimmune
- **S**corpion venom
- **H**yperlipidaemia, hypothermia, hypercalcaemia
- **E**ndoscopic retrograde cholangiopancreatography (ERCP)
- **D**rugs (e.g. azathioprine, sulfonamides, OCP)

Which biochemical tests could you request for presumed acute pancreatitis?

- *Serum amylase* – due to its wide availability and sensitivity, this is commonly requested. It may be normal in 10–20% of cases (especially if the patient presents late in the course) and has low specificity.
- *Serum lipase* – this increases within 4–8 hours and remains elevated for 8–14 days and therefore is useful diagnostically in late presentations. It has a very high sensitivity for acute alcoholic pancreatitis. The combination of both serum amylase and lipase will provide sensitivity and specificity of 90–95% for detecting acute pancreatitis.
- *Serum triglyceride* – this should be requested if a lipaemic serum is suspected (e.g. triglyceride levels are above 11.3 mmol/L) or when the cause of the pancreatitis is not clear.
- *Urinary trypsinogen-2* – this a novel test, which has a reported sensitivity of 80% and specificity of 92%. It is not widely available.

Which imaging studies can be used in the diagnosis of acute pancreatitis?

- *Ultrasonography (US)* – an initial test that should ideally be performed on all patients suspected of acute pancreatitis. It can be used in unstable patients suspected of having gallstones or biliary disease. The use of contrast-enhanced ultrasound has a reported sensitivity and specificity of 82% and 89% respectively.
- *Endoscopic ultrasonography (EUS)* – this is a combination of endoscopy and ultrasound that is less invasive than ERCP and is useful in diagnosing acute pancreatitis and choledocholithiasis. When CT and US fail to show common bile duct stones, EUS may prove useful. Additionally, due to the absence of ionising radiation, it can be performed in pregnant patients and those who are too unstable to be transferred out of the critical care unit.
- *Computed tomography (CT)* – the gold standard for grading acute pancreatitis and diagnosing pancreatic necrosis and peripancreatic collections. Although CT has a high accuracy, it does not usually need to be performed before 72 hours unless the diagnosis is in doubt, or the patient fails to improve clinically.
- *Endoscopic retrograde cholangiopancreatography (ERCP)* – an effective means to treat common bile duct stones. It is, however, not indicated in the treatment of mild pancreatitis or pancreatitis not due to biliary disease.
- *Magnetic resonance cholangiopancreatography (MRCP)* – with the advantage of being non-invasive and not using ionising radiation, this modality is able to depict abnormalities of the pancreatic duct and parenchyma. Disadvantages of using MRCP include imaging artefacts (e.g. gastrointestinal air or metallic clips) and increased acquisition time compared to CT in a critically unwell patient at a remote site.

You request an ultrasound of Brian's abdomen and pelvis, which demonstrates a dilated common biliary duct. In conjunction with his signs and symptoms and a grossly elevated serum amylase, you make the diagnosis of acute pancreatitis secondary to gallstone-related disease.

Which grading systems are you aware of for acute pancreatitis?

- *Ranson's criteria* – with a reported sensitivity and specificity of 74% and 77% respectively, this scoring system uses 11 prognostic signs in total at presentation and at 48 hours later. It was originally used for alcohol-induced pancreatitis.
- *Glasgow–Imrie score* – re-evaluating the Ranson's criteria, it was found that only eight of the 11 variables were predictive for mortality. This score can be used for both biliary and non-biliary acute pancreatitis. Three or more positive variables at 48 hours following admission suggest severe pancreatitis and should prompt transfer to critical care (Table 4.1).

Table 4.1: Glasgow–Imrie score for acute pancreatitis. The variables can be remembered using the mnemonic **PANCREAS**.

PaO$_2$	<8 kPa
Age	>55 years
Neutrophils	WBC >15×10^9/L
Calcium	<2 mmol/L
Renal function	Urea >16 mmol/L
Enzymes	LDH >600 IU/L, AST >200 IU/L
Albumin	<32 g/L (serum)
Sugar	Blood glucose >10 mmol/L

AST, aspartate aminotransferase; LDH, lactate dehydrogenase.

- *APACHE II (Acute Physiology and Chronic Health Evaluation II)* – used throughout the world, this generic scoring system incorporates the worst values within the first 24 hours following admission to ICU and is therefore not entirely suitable to monitor progress during the illness. However, in predicting severe disease and hospital survival, it appears to perform similarly when compared to the Ranson or Glasgow–Imrie scores.
- *Atlanta classification* – revised in 2012, this classification system grades presentation clinically into the following categories:
  - Mild acute pancreatitis – no organ failure and no local or systemic complications.
  - Moderately severe acute pancreatitis – organ failure that resolves within 48 hours, local or systemic complications without persistent organ failure.
  - Severe acute pancreatitis – persistent organ failure.
- *Balthazar index* – this score assesses disease severity based upon CT findings. It should be noted that radiographic manifestations of acute pancreatitis tend to lag behind the clinical condition.
- *Bedside index of severity in acute pancreatitis (BISAP) score* – this can be calculated relatively quickly at the bedside, and it uses the systemic inflammatory response syndrome (*SIRS*) criteria, along with age, urea level, mental status and presence or absence of a pleural effusion to predict mortality.

Why is grading the severity of acute pancreatitis useful?

Potentially, by failing to recognise the more severe presentation of acute pancreatitis, the lack of initial aggressive management and support may lead to increased morbidity and prevent the appropriate resources being allocated. Furthermore, it is important that a patient with severe acute pancreatitis is managed in an intensive care unit.

What are the management strategies for patients presenting with acute pancreatitis?

- *Fluid resuscitation* – regardless of the severity of pancreatitis, it is well recognised that initial management should include adequate fluid resuscitation (usually at a rate of 5–10 mL/kg/h unless contraindicated), especially for severe acute pancreatitis. The rapid restoration and replacement of intravascular volume has the potential to reduce the incidence of acute renal failure in severe acute pancreatitis. In addition, adequate volume repletion can help to restore pancreatic microcirculation and prevent further cellular death. Higher rates of pancreatic necrosis are associated with inadequate intravascular volume replacement. However, care should be taken when administering excessive volumes of fluid as this may be associated with an increased need for mechanical ventilation and a greater risk for intra-abdominal compartment syndrome, sepsis and mortality.
- *Managing respiratory failure* – respiratory dysfunction is a common manifestation in acute pancreatitis and can be due to both mechanical and biochemical factors. Severe acute pancreatitis can often cause marked abdominal distension, which reduces the functional residual capacity (FRC), impairing both spontaneous and mechanical ventilation. The release of pancreatic phospholipase A2 into the circulation is also thought to degrade lung surfactant and therefore affect lung compliance. These, along with other factors, give rise to acute respiratory distress syndrome (ARDS) that may require mechanical ventilation.
- *Analgesia* – the pain associated with acute pancreatitis can be severe, often necessitating the use of opioids. In addition, adequate pain relief may improve respiratory dysfunction.
- *Nutritional support* – patients with mild pancreatitis can usually be started on oral supplements within a few days of presentation, so long as nausea, vomiting or ileus is not present. For severe acute pancreatitis, enteral nutrition when compared to parenteral nutrition has been shown to reduce the risk of death, multiple organ failure, infection, surgery and mean length of hospital stay. Moreover, total parenteral nutrition (TPN) should be avoided in patients with acute pancreatitis as higher rates of infection and line-related complications have been observed.

> Brian continues to improve for the next 10 days on your unit, but on day 11 he begins to experience pyrexia, abdominal pain and haemodynamic compromise requiring vasopressor support.

Which complication of acute pancreatitis could this be?

With evidence of systemic infection in the presence of an episode of acute pancreatitis, Brian may have developed intra-abdominal sepsis, a pseudocyst or necrotising pancreatitis.

What is necrotising pancreatitis?

Necrotising pancreatitis is a serious local complication that can either be sterile or infected. It is defined by the presence of focal or diffuse areas of non-viable pancreatic parenchyma.

How would you diagnose necrotising pancreatitis?

This can be difficult to establish since clinical manifestations of systemic inflammation and nosocomial infections are common in patients with acute pancreatitis. An increase in procalcitonin levels or air in the necrotic tissue as demonstrated by CT may suggest infection. However, the gold standard involves CT-guided fine needle aspiration that should only be performed when infection is suspected on clinical grounds.

What is the role of surgery in pancreatic necrosis?

It is now generally accepted and expected that a conservative approach is taken in managing patients with suspected pancreatic or peripancreatic infection. Discovering infection on a CT-guided fine needle aspiration is no longer a firm indication for surgery. In fact, administration of antibiotics directed by the results of culture and sensitivity and percutaneous drainage alone may be curative.

Surgical debridement or endoscopic drainage with necrosectomy is generally reserved for deteriorating patients on antibiotics who fail to respond.

What are the long-term outcomes for these patients?

Severe acute pancreatitis and necrotising pancreatitis can be difficult and challenging to manage. In patients with end-organ failure for greater than 48 hours, and/or infectious complications of pancreatic necrosis, mortality is in the range of 15–20%.

Survivors can have prolonged ICU and hospital stay and may still require other interventions once the episode has resolved (e.g. cholecystectomy or drainage of pancreatic pseudocysts). In addition, up to a third of survivors of severe necrotising pancreatitis may develop diabetes mellitus. Other long-term sequelae include pancreatic fistulae and chronic pancreatitis with chronic abdominal pain that can be debilitating and difficult to manage. Nevertheless, most survivors can return to a quality of life that is equal to age-matched controls.

> Brian responds appropriately to his course of antibiotic therapy, and is successfully discharged to the ward under the joint care of the surgical and medical teams.

Further reading

- Mehta, A., Emmett, J., and Emmett, M. (2008). GOLD MARK: an anion gap mnemonic for the 21st century. *Lancet* 372: 892. Original article detailing the use of the acronym GOLDMARK and the rationale for its use.
- Dutta, A., Goel, A., Kirubakaran, R. et al. (2020). Nasogastric versus nasojejunal tube feeding for severe acute pancreatitis. *Cochrane Database of Systematic Reviews* 3: CD010582. Highly informative Cochrane systematic review.
- Joint British Diabetes Societies Inpatient Care Group (2021) The Management of Diabetic Ketoacidosis in Adults. London: Diabetes UK. Authoritative guideline that gives excellent clinical strategies for managing DKA.

5 The Patient Involved in a Road Traffic Collision

A 25-year-old female patient named Danielle has been involved in a head-on road traffic collision travelling at approximately 50 mph. She was the driver, wearing a seatbelt, and has remained GCS 15 throughout. Extraction time was under 30 minutes. She is brought to the Major Trauma Centre (MTC) resuscitation area. You are nominated as team leader, taking an end-of-the-bed approach and delegating specific tasks.

What are the goals of the primary survey?

The primary survey is designed to detect and correct all immediate threats to life. After ensuring that there is no danger from the environment or situation (e.g. petrochemical spill, risks of electrocution), an ABCDE assessment (Airway, Breathing, Circulation, Disability and Exposure/Environmental) with cervical spine immobilisation as per Advanced Trauma and Life Support® (ATLS®) guidance should be performed. In an emergency department setting, the risk of danger to staff may still be present depending on the scenario (e.g. the rare case of organophosphate poisoning). In a team situation, roles and responsibilities would ideally be assigned prior to the patient arriving. This enables effective communication throughout and allows for concurrent interventions to be applied, such as oxygen therapy and intravenous cannulation.

During the primary survey, Danielle begins saying she 'can't breathe' and that her 'chest hurts'. The examining doctor informs you that the left side of her chest is not expanding fully and despite 15 L/min oxygen therapy, her pulse oximetry is 92%. Her respiratory rate is over 30 breaths per minute. Her GCS is 15. You are informed that her blood pressure is 90/60 mmHg, and she is tachycardic at 130 bpm.

Clinical Cases in Critical Care, First Edition. Alice Myers and Theophilus Samuels.
© 2023 John Wiley & Sons Ltd. Published 2023 by John Wiley & Sons Ltd.

What are the potentially life-threatening conditions associated with these clinical findings and how should each one be managed?

- *Tension pneumothorax* – as air progressively accumulates in the pleural space, it begins to compress the lungs and heart, which leads to respiratory and haemodynamic compromise. Tension pneumothorax should be suspected in any case of chest trauma with otherwise unexplained haemodynamic instability. Classic clinical findings (e.g. hyper-resonance, tracheal deviation, absent breath sounds) may present late and can be difficult to detect. Immediate needle decompression should be performed by inserting an appropriately sized cannula into the *fifth* intercostal space along the midclavicular line in adults. Resolution of the haemodynamic instability should occur very quickly, with the patient stabilising soon thereafter. It is important at this stage, whether needle decompression was successful or not, to insert an intercostal chest drain and attach it to an underwater seal for ongoing management.

- *Open (sucking) pneumothorax* – following penetrating chest trauma, if air enters the pleural space through this defect but is not able to exit, then pressure will increase and potentially cause mediastinal compression and cardiorespiratory compromise. This is managed by applying a non-adherent dressing to the wound by sealing it along three edges only. This allows air to escape but does not allow air to enter. It is imperative that you insert an intercostal chest drain away from the defect site.

- *Massive haemothorax* – this occurs when more than 1500 mL of blood or over one-third of the patient's blood volume rapidly accumulates within the chest cavity. With the potential to cause marked hypovolaemia and reduced venous return to the heart, this can lead to life-threatening cardiovascular collapse. Immediate drainage of >1500 mL of blood or >200 mL for 2–4 hours may indicate a need for urgent thoracotomy.

- *Flail chest* – consider a flail chest if two or more consecutive ribs are fractured in two or more places and paradoxical movement occurs during breathing. If conservative management fails (e.g. oxygen therapy or non-invasive ventilation) and respiratory failure begins to occur, then mechanical ventilation and intubation should be considered. Usually, prolonged mechanical ventilation is not required, unless associated injuries and co-morbidities are severe. Surgical stabilisation can be considered if the flail chest is severe. However, this is not routinely carried out.

- *Pericardial tamponade* – excess pericardial fluid can lead to severe disruption of myocardial dynamics. The ability of the right ventricle to fill during diastole is severely impaired. Increasing extrinsic pressure applied by the accumulation of fluid prevents the free wall from relaxing completely. With the right ventricle unable to eject blood effectively into the pulmonary circulation, it simultaneously reduces the volume of blood ejected into the systemic circulation by the left ventricle, leading to severe haemodynamic compromise. A subcostal view of the heart using ultrasound can quickly be obtained as part of a focused assessment by an experienced operator. Assuming the image quality is adequate, it can rule out significant pericardial effusion.

A useful and widely used pneumonic for ruling out life-threatening chest injuries during the primary survey is ATOM-FC:

- Airway obstruction or disruption
- Tension pneumothorax
- Open pneumothorax
- Massive haemothorax
- Flail chest
- Cardiac tamponade

While intravenous access is being established and blood withdrawn for the appropriate tests, a focused ultrasonographic assessment of Danielle's chest is performed at the same time.

What are the advantages and disadvantages of using focused assessment with sonography in trauma (FAST) versus radiographic imaging?

Advantages

- Ultrasonography can be completed much faster than radiography.
- Specific areas can be targeted for assessment.
- Higher diagnostic accuracy for pneumothorax and haemothorax.
- Avoids the use of ionising radiation (especially in women of child-bearing age).
- Can be performed at the same time as the primary survey with minimal interruption.

Disadvantages

- Requires an experienced operator.
- It does not demonstrate rib fractures or other bony injuries.
- Acquisition of images and their storage require robust clinical governance.

How might bedside focused lung ultrasonography help identify the cause of Danielle's deterioration?

- *Pneumothorax.*
  - Lung sliding – has a very high negative predictive value for diagnosing a pneumothorax (should lung sliding be observed then pneumothorax is not present at the point where the probe is applied to the chest wall). However, the absence of sliding is not enough to make the diagnosis as many other disorders are also consistent with absent lung sliding (e.g. atelectasis, acute respiratory distress syndrome).
  - B-lines – the widening of the subpleural interlobular septa due to fluid accumulation, for example, produces these characteristic

vertical ray-like artefacts. However, if a pneumothorax were present, this interface between the visceral pleura and interlobular septa would be lost and therefore the presence of a single B-line effectively rules out the diagnosis of a pneumothorax. Sadly, even the absence of both lung sliding and B-lines still does not diagnose a pneumothorax.

■ Lung point – with a partially collapsed lung that remains adherent to the parietal pleura, this lung point can be visualised as a transient appearance of a recognised ultrasonographic lung pattern (e.g. lung sliding and/or B-lines). This lung point is 100% specific for the diagnosis of pneumothorax but cannot be visualised in totally collapsed lungs.

■ Lung pulse – when lung sliding is synchronous with the heartbeat, it creates a lung pulse on ultrasound. Therefore, even in the absence of all the other described findings, if the slightest lung pulse is seen it effectively rules out a pneumothorax.

■ *Haemothorax* – fluid within the pleural space appears as an anechoic area between the two pleural layers in the most dependent chest areas (e.g. lateral-basal lung areas in the supine patient). It is important to identify the diaphragm and solid organs immediately below (e.g. liver or spleen) as normal lung will transiently move into view with breathing, obscuring these landmarks like a curtain (hence the 'curtain sign'). However, the absence of this curtain sign and presence of a large anechoic area are highly suggestive of an effusion (Figure 5.1), with the visualisation of internal echoes (e.g. filaments or mobile particles) being highly suggestive of haemothorax.

Focused lung ultrasonography confirms the presence of a large left-sided effusion. Danielle remains hypotensive and tachycardic and is becoming mildly confused (unable to give her correct date of birth when asked).

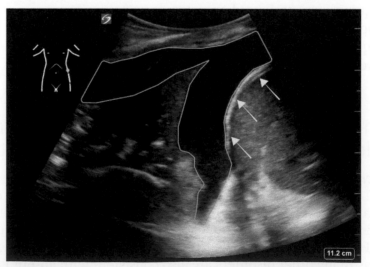

Figure 5.1: Lung ultrasound taken at the left PLAPS point demonstrating a large anechoic area (blue outline) consistent with a pleural effusion (diaphragm – yellow arrows).
Source: Theophilus Samuels.

What might the effusion suggest and what are the treatment goals?

Danielle is demonstrating signs of haemodynamic compromise from a potentially massive haemothorax. Your goals at this point would be as follows:

- *Management of the haemothorax* – your team need to insert an intercostal drain and attach it to an underwater seal. It would be appropriate to activate the hospital-wide 'major haemorrhage/code red trauma' alert to facilitate provision of emergency blood products.
- *Managing hypotension* – consider that the hypotension may in part be due to hypovolaemia from blood loss. Administering O-negative blood if type-specific or cross-matched blood is not immediately available may be indicated. Most institutions will have policies in place for emergency provision of blood products. Fluid resuscitation should be ongoing until blood products are available and being administered, but care should be taken to avoid extensive haemodilution using crystalloid solutions (as these can affect both procoagulant and anticoagulant levels, leading to a complex coagulation disorder).
- *Source/site of bleeding* – identifying an ongoing source of the bleeding, if present, is imperative as uncontrolled bleeding will make continued transfusions ultimately futile. Thoracotomy may need to be performed.
- *Tranexamic acid* – the Clinical Randomisation of an Antifibrinolytic in Significant Haemorrhage-2 trial (CRASH-2) demonstrated that if administered within the first 3 hours of presentation, tranexamic acid can safely reduce in-hospital mortality within 28 days of injury.

What are the most common blood groups?

- *Blood group A* – these are patients with surface antigen A and plasma antibodies to surface antigen B.
- *Blood group B* – these are patients with surface antigen B and plasma antibodies to surface antigen A.
- *Blood group AB* – possess no plasma antibodies to either group A or B and are known as a universal recipient.
- *Blood group O* – no surface antigens are present to react to plasma antibodies. Known as the universal donor.
- *Rhesus system* – in addition to the ABO blood grouping system, patients can be either Rhesus antigen positive or negative.

> You suspect that Danielle will need blood transfusion, but her blood type is unknown at this point.

What issues should you consider when transfusing Danielle specifically with regard to blood typing?

- In a life-threatening exsanguination, group O blood can be given if type-specific blood is not immediately available. However, type-specific uncross-matched blood can then be used as it is considered relatively safe since the benefit of transfusion outweighs the risk of a reaction. In addition to administering blood, every attempt must be made to control the source/site of bleeding.

- Universal donor blood should preferably be group O and Rhesus negative, particularly if it is to be administered to women of child-bearing age.
- Identifying type-specific blood involves ensuring the donor blood is ABO and Rhesus compatible with the recipient's blood and can be provided by most blood banks within 10 minutes.
- Fully cross-matched blood is ultimately desirable and involves comparing the donor's and recipient's blood using not only the ABO and Rhesus blood antigens, but also by directly testing for antibodies against antigens present within the blood from the recipient. This process takes longer and can be completed usually within 60 minutes.

Haemothorax is confirmed following insertion of the intercostal drain. Type-specific blood is being given and her BP and HR begin to improve. No further life-threatening injuries are found during the primary survey.

What would be your next steps in Danielle's management?

Once the primary survey has been completed with all immediate life-threatening injuries recognised and resuscitative efforts under way, consider performing diagnostic imaging as soon as possible. Usually, trauma patients would be expected to have CT imaging performed within 1 hour (or 30 minutes if in an MTC). Given that CT scanning is very rapid, it can be considered appropriate to take an unstable patient 'through the scanner' accompanied by the trauma team and with resuscitation ongoing. CT imaging of the head, neck, chest, abdomen and pelvis with intravenous contrast (e.g. for aortic angiography) is commonly requested.

Prior to transferring Danielle to the CT scanner, she becomes unresponsive. Her blood pressure is elevated at 150/80 mmHg, heart rate is 90 bpm and her pulse oximetry reads 100% on 15 L/min of oxygen.

What do you think could be causing this change in her neurological status?

You are concerned that Danielle has also suffered a traumatic brain injury (TBI). This may include the following.

- *Subdural haematoma* (SDH) – found between the delicate arachnoid mater (middle layer of dura) and the dura mater (outermost layer), this 'potential' space contains numerous bridging veins that connect the cerebral hemispheres to the superior sagittal sinus (Figure 5.2a). Shear

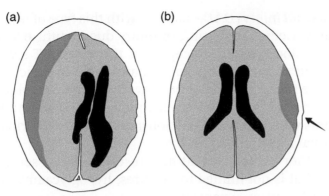

Figure 5.2: Schematic diagram representing a computed tomography (CT) scan of head demonstrating (a) subdural haematoma with midline shift (note the concave shape of the lesion), (b) epidural/extradural haematoma (note the biconvex shape that is classic) and fracture (arrow).

Source: Theophilus Samuels.

forces applied to these bridging veins by rapid acceleration and deceleration of the brain result in tearing and consequent haemorrhage; arteries can also be affected. The overall mortality is higher than EDH, usually reported as being between 40% and 60%. Prognosis is particularly poor in patients aged 60 years and over, particularly when they present with an acute SDH.

- *Epidural/extradural haematoma (EDH)* – blood may accumulate between the dura mater and the skull. Most associated with road traffic collisions, haemorrhage usually occurs from damage to the middle meningeal artery, but may also involve the middle meningeal veins, diploic veins or venous sinuses (Figure 5.2b). Typically, patients will present with a transient loss of consciousness followed by a period of lucidity where they often appear neurologically intact. However, as blood begins to accumulate, the brainstem becomes compressed, resulting in loss of consciousness.

- *Traumatic subarachnoid haemorrhage (SAH)* – the CSF-filled compartment between the subarachnoid mater and brain parenchyma contains the major cerebral blood vessels. Cerebral vasospasm may occur with traumatic SAH (though it is seen more commonly in aneurysmal SAH) and result in further parenchymal damage (e.g. ischaemia, infarction). It is important to note that traumatic SAH can be a marker of severe primary brain injury.

- *Contusions and haematomas* – these entities may be considered as two ends of a spectrum, where contusions are smaller heterogeneous areas of haemorrhage or oedema and haematomas are homogeneous demarcated collections of blood within the brain parenchyma. Contusions can potentially increase in size relatively soon after they are found, hence the use of early CT scanning. Contusions can be categorised as follows:
  - Coup – usually due to inertial forces causing injuries to brain parenchyma at the impact site (e.g. as possibly in this case, the patient's head striking the steering wheel of her car).
  - Contre-coup – these are located away from the site of impact and are usually associated with deceleration injuries resulting in areas of low pressure and increased tensile strain.

- *Diffuse axonal injury (DAI)* – patients with this type of injury will be rendered unconscious at the time of injury due to diffuse tearing of axons and small blood vessels. Deceptively, the initial CT scan may appear normal, due to the damage being mainly microscopic. Sadly, patients with severe DAI who survive may have profound neurological disability. Those with mild DAI may recover completely. DAI should be suspected in patients with impaired consciousness alongside normal CT findings and normal intracranial pressures.
- *Other* – other pathology that may result in depressed consciousness includes, but is not limited to, seizures, hypoglycaemia, toxins, drugs, hypoxaemia and/or hypercarbia.

Danielle is promptly and safely intubated by the anaesthetic team and stabilised. CT brain confirms the presence of a small left-sided subdural haematoma with no evidence of midline shift. It does not require immediate neurosurgical intervention. CT chest demonstrated a fracture of the sternum and several left-sided rib fractures with evidence of underlying pulmonary contusions.

A total of approximately 1200 mL of blood is drained from the intercostal drain, with minimal ongoing losses. Her blood pressure and tachycardia improve, and she appears to be stable. She is admitted to your neurosurgical intensive care unit for further management.

Define the role of an antifibrinolytic agent in traumatic brain injury (TBI)

CRASH-3 was an international randomised placebo-controlled trial of tranexamic acid (TXA) in adult patients with TBI. The key finding was that TXA given within 3 hours of injury reduces deaths from mild to moderate traumatic brain injuries. It is thought that those patients with mild to moderate symptoms are likely to have smaller, slower bleeds, which are more amenable to TXA treatment. Early treatment was more effective, with a 10% reduction in effectiveness for every 20 minutes from the time of injury. There was no increased risk of death or complications, or prevalence of disability in survivors.

What is the evidence for cooling in TBI?

Inducing hypothermia had been thought to be neuroprotective and consequently improve long-term neurological outcomes. However, robust evidence in the form of randomised control trials had been lacking. The POLAR-RCT trial in 2018 by the POLAR Trial Investigators and the ANZICS Clinical Trials Group demonstrated that hypothermia compared to normothermia had no significant effect on neurological recovery at 6 months. The Eurotherm group in 2015 determined that therapeutic hypothermia with standard care did not result in better outcomes compared to standard care alone.

For which complications do you need to monitor Danielle over the next 24–48 hours?

- *Pain* – if she improves neurologically, pain can often be a significant factor in delaying recovery, especially with rib fractures where conservative management is usual. Careful titration of adequate opioid analgesia can be very difficult in these types of patients. Consideration could be given to using regional techniques.
- *Pneumonia and respiratory failure* – pulmonary contusions, rib fractures and mechanical ventilation itself can predispose patients to respiratory tract infections. This may also lead to developing an acute respiratory distress syndrome (ARDS).
- *Deep vein thrombosis* – prophylactic techniques are usually divided into mechanical and pharmacological methods. Antiembolism stockings and pneumatic devices are associated with fewer complications but may not be as effective as drugs. Although pharmacological methods (i.e. low molecular weight heparins) are generally considered most effective, but their use must be weighed against the risk of bleeding in the presence of traumatic injuries.

During the secondary survey, the nurse looking after Danielle asks you about the relevance of the sternal fracture reported on the CT.

What would be your concerns regarding this finding?

- *Pain* – sternal fractures are painful and will require adequate analgesia when Danielle is awake, and when attempting to extubate. Pain control will also need to be adequate to allow deep breathing and maintain her ability to cough, to reduce the risk of a chest infection developing.
- *Blunt cardiac injury (BCI)* – this should be considered in the presence of a sternal fracture. Given the rapid deceleration mechanism associated with road traffic collisions, the myocardium can be exposed to significant shearing forces and compression between the sternum and vertebrae. BCI should be considered in the presence of other significant injuries as it may remain a clinically silent entity (the diagnosis of BCI can be particularly challenging).

How common is BCI?

A recent inspection of 15 976 patients (between 2007 and 2015) from the US National Trauma Data Bank found that BCI was reported in less than 1% of patients.

Which types of trauma-related injuries are associated with BCI?

Blunt force trauma resulting in sternal fracture or thoracic aortic injury is strongly associated with BCI. Haemopneumothorax has been demonstrated to be the strongest predictor for BCI in patients presenting with blunt force trauma. Any patient presenting with haemopneumothorax, sternal fracture, injury to the oesophagus and/or thoracic aortic injury should ideally be screened for BCI.

What are the myocardial patterns of injury associated with BCI?

The most commonly reported injury associated with BCI is contusion. Usually, as the right side of the heart lies anteriorly, it is most prone to BCI, with the reported incidences of right atrial and right ventricle injury being 17–32% and 8–65% respectively. Left-sided chamber injuries are not as commonly reported. Patients who rupture any of the four chambers of the heart are unlikely to survive to hospital. Rarely, myocardial infarction may occur following injury to the coronary arteries.

How would you diagnose and evaluate BCI in this patient?

Clinical suspicion needs to remain high in the presence of a massive haemothorax and mechanism of blunt force trauma. Sternal fracture pain may be confounded by other thoracic injuries (e.g. rib fractures) and reduced consciousness. No gold standard exists to diagnose BCI. The following investigations are suggested:

- *Electrocardiography* – a valuable screening tool, as the presence of ventricular or atrial arrhythmias, conduction abnormalities (e.g. bundle branch block) and ST segment abnormalities may suggest BCI. However, the absence or presence of abnormalities does not conclusively rule out or rule in BCI.
- *Cardiac enzymes* – being both highly specific and sensitive for myocardial cell damage, troponin T may be elevated in the presence of BCI. Following 6–8 hours from the time of injury, if the troponin levels remain within normal limits, then BCI is highly unlikely.
- *Echocardiography* – detection of abnormalities such as regional wall motion abnormalities (RMWAs) or valvular dysfunction (e.g. regurgitant jets) in patients who are unstable or have positive ECG findings and/or troponin levels may suggest BCI. Transoesophageal echocardiography is usually more sensitive than the transthoracic approach, particularly since chest wall injuries may degrade the quality of images using the latter approach. Remember that in elderly trauma patients, the presence of regurgitation or RWMAs may be pre-existing, especially in the context of known ischaemic coronary disease.

Echocardiography does not demonstrate any anatomical abnormalities and the ECG reveals sinus rhythm at a rate of 90 bpm. The troponin T level is within normal limits. You and your team do not feel that Danielle has BCI.

Danielle improves following neurosurgical intervention, making a full neurological recovery, and is successfully extubated on day 10 of admission. She is stepped down to the neurosurgical ward and discharged home 2 weeks later.

Further reading

- Advanced Trauma and Life Support®. Student Course Manual. (2018). Definitive manual for dealing with patients presenting with trauma.
- Roberts, I., Shakur, H., Coats, T. et al. (2013). The CRASH-2 trial: a randomised controlled trial and economic evaluation of the effects of tranexamic acid on death, vascular occlusive events and transfusion requirement in bleeding trauma patients. *Health Technol. Assess.* 17 (10). Original studies demonstrating the benefit of using tranexamic acid in trauma patients.
- CRASH-3 Trial Collaborators (2019). Effects of tranexamic acid on death, disability, vascular occlusive events and other morbidities in patients with acute traumatic brain injury (CRASH-3): a randomised, placebo-controlled trial. *Lancet.* 394: 1713–1723.
- Lichtenstein, D., Mezière, G., Lascols, N. et al. (2005). Ultrasound diagnosis of occult pneumothorax. *Crit. Care. Med.* 33 (6): 1231–1238. Seminal paper on the use of ultrasound to aid in diagnosing pneumothorax.

6 The Patient with a Raised Temperature

You are asked to review an 18-year-old female foreign exchange student named Jane. She has presented to your emergency department with severe agitation, profuse sweating and hypertension. A few hours before admission, she had been attending a rave party with her friends who were able to give only a partial history for that evening due to their limited English. They are unable to provide any previous medical or drug history. She is tachycardic at 140 bpm with a BP of 180/100 mmHg and is hallucinating. Her core body temperature is raised at 39 °C.

What might be the cause of her clinical presentation?

Potential causes might include:

- Drug poisoning (overdose or adverse effects)
- Neuroleptic malignant syndrome
- Serotonin syndrome
- Sepsis
- Intracerebral haemorrhage (e.g. aneurysm).

Given the history, what do you think is the most likely diagnosis?

Jane is most likely suffering from the toxic effects of recreational drug use. The most likely 'street' drug she may have taken is 'ecstasy', a colloquial term used to describe a group of illegal drugs. These include:

- 3,4-methylenedioxymethamphetamine (MDMA)
- Gammahydroxybutyrate (GHB, also known as 'liquid ecstasy')
- Benzylpiperazines.

Clinical Cases in Critical Care, First Edition. Alice Myers and Theophilus Samuels.
© 2023 John Wiley & Sons Ltd. Published 2023 by John Wiley & Sons Ltd.

The concentration of MDMA is unregulated and inconsistent across formulations so the exact ingredients may vary. This can expose individuals to excessive doses. In addition, small doses may induce a toxic-like reaction in certain individuals who are unable to metabolise MDMA.

Which resources are available in the UK for information and advice on acute intoxications and poisonings?

The National Poisons Information Service (NPIS) operates a 24-hour telephone helpline, an online database (www.toxbase.org) and a mobile app, all of which are very useful resources for clinicians treating patients with suspected/confirmed overdose.

What are the signs and symptoms usually associated with the use of MDMA?

Given that the constituents of each formulation may differ along with their concentrations, dose-dependent clinical features may vary. MDMA is a derivative of methamphetamine, which itself is derived from its parent compound amphetamine. By increasing the net release of serotonin, noradrenaline and to a lesser extent dopamine, the effects can be classified according to subjective, physiological and adverse features:

- *Subjective* effects
    - Euphoria and arousal
    - Extroversion
    - Enhanced self-awareness
    - Mental confusion and alterations to perception
- *Physiological* effects
    - Tachycardia
    - Hypertension
    - Hyperthermia
    - Increased levels of prolactin and cortisol
- *Adverse* effects
    - Nausea
    - Headache
    - Dry mouth
    - Agitation
    - Bruxism and trismus

What are the major patterns of clinical toxicity associated with MDMA overdose?

There are four serious and potentially life-threatening patterns. These are not necessarily mutually exclusive.

Hyperpyrexic type

The most dangerous form of toxicity. The hyperpyrexic adverse effects can be exacerbated when taken at raves, due to increased physical exertion and a hot environment. Increased circulating noradrenaline causes vasoconstriction which can lead to failure of redistribution of heat from the central circulation. Severe cases may develop rhabdomyolysis, myoglobinuria and renal failure, liver damage and disseminated intravascular coagulation. This type is the leading cause of death in patients with MDMA overdose.

Hepatic failure

In mild cases, the hepatitis can often resemble a viral hepatitis with spontaneous recovery occurring over weeks or months. In the most severe cases, fulminant hepatic failure ensues. In the absence of a liver transplant, this may prove fatal.

Cardiovascular toxicity

Release of noradrenaline can produce severe cardiovascular adverse effects, most notably severe hypertension. This can lead to major intracranial haemorrhage, petechial and retinal haemorrhages, and tachycardia which can lead to cardiac failure due to increasing cardiac workload.

Cerebral toxicity

Excessive fluid intake and potential release of antidiuretic hormone (ADH) can lead to the increased movement of water into tissues, including the brain. Patients can develop epileptic-type seizures and fatal compression of the brainstem and cerebellum.

> While you are assessing Jane, the ED doctor tells you she has been considering that this presentation could be caused by serotonin syndrome or neuroleptic malignant syndrome in addition to the possibility of MDMA toxicity.

What is serotonin syndrome?

Serotonin (5-HT) is a monoamine neurotransmitter that contributes to many biological processes within the human body. In the presence of increased release, reduced metabolism, reduced reuptake or stimulation of its receptors, serotonin excess may produce a syndrome that includes:

- CNS effects (e.g. agitation, confusion, delirium, coma)
- Neuromuscular excitability (e.g. clonus, tremor, bruxism)
- Autonomic instability (e.g. flushing, diarrhoea, tachycardia, hyperthermia).

Which factors may increase the risk of serotonin syndrome?

This syndrome becomes more prevalent if the patient:

- already takes prescription medications that increase or potentiate serotonin levels, e.g. tricyclic antidepressants, selective serotonin reuptake inhibitors and/or
- consumes other stimulant recreational drugs in parallel, e.g. cocaine, amphetamines, mephedrone.

What is the treatment for serotonin toxicity?

Benzodiazepines should be used as a first-line treatment. These might include:

- Oral or intravenous diazepam
- Lorazepam
- Midazolam (intramuscularly).

For severe overdoses with persistent hyperthermia, the use of cyprohepta-dine (5-HT$_{2A}$ antagonist) or chlorpromazine (5-HT$_1$ and 5-HT$_2$ antagonist) is suggested.

What is neuroleptic malignant syndrome (NMS) and how does it compare to serotonin syndrome?

Principally, NMS is associated with antipsychotic drugs such as chlorpromazine or haloperidol. It may also occur with the newer drugs olanzapine, clozapine and risperidone. It has a very low incidence amongst patients being treated with these drugs (0.01–0.02%) and generally occurs during the first 2 weeks of treatment. It can also occur with chronic use. Increasing the dose of an anti-psychotic rapidly and/or increasing its bioavailability (e.g. oral to intravenous route) may also predispose a patient to NMS.

Its clinical features can mimic those of serotonin syndrome:

- Hyperthermia
- Altered mental status
- Muscle rigidity
- Autonomic instability (e.g. hypertension, tachycardia)
- Raised creatine kinase levels

As with the serotonin syndrome, initial treatment consists of using benzodi-azepines (as described above). However, in NMS, consideration could be given to using dopamine agonists, such as bromocriptine or amantadine, following discussion with the NPIS.

> You now measure Jane's temperature to be 40 °C. She is increasingly agitated and remains tachycardic and hypertensive. The ED team have already inserted a peripheral intravenous cannula and sent blood samples for analysis of FBC, U&E, LFTs, clotting and a group and screen. They have sent blood cultures, requested paracetamol and salicylate levels and toxicology analysis of blood and urine. Someone is attempting to obtain an arterial sample for blood gas analysis, but it is proving challenging due to Jane's agitation.

What is your initial management of Jane's hyperpyrexia?

Hyperpyrexia in this context is a potentially life-threatening feature which is associated with disseminated intravascular coagulation and multiple organ failure. Jane needs urgent cooling, utilising both passive and active methods.

Active cooling measures include cold fluid lavage (e.g. bladder, gastric), ice baths and administration of cold intravenous fluids. Ice pads can be placed in the groins and armpits and forced cold air blankets can be applied. Sedation using diazepam should also be used when the temperature exceeds 38.5 °C, and high doses may be required which may place the patient at risk if airway reflexes become suppressed. It can prove extremely challenging to reduce body temperature to within the normal range.

What specific medication should you consider for muscular hyperactivity in MDMA overdose?

- *Dantrolene* – an initial dose between 2 and 3 mg/kg (maximum dose 10 mg/kg) IV can be given. This markedly reduces the ability for muscle to contract by reducing intracellular calcium. It is believed that dantrolene binds to ryanodine receptor 1 in the sarcoplasmic reticulum of skeletal muscle cells.

Which additional biochemical test should you request and what might it demonstrate?

- *Serum creatine kinase* – damage to skeletal muscle directly leads to elevated levels of this enzyme in the bloodstream. Significantly increased levels suggest considerable muscle breakdown, with subsequent release of muscle proteins such as myoglobin (which can cause myoglobin-associated renal failure). If the initial level is normal but there is ongoing concern regarding muscle damage then repeat measurements should be taken.

Jane has been in the emergency department for 30 minutes now. Despite the active and passive cooling measures that have been used so far, her core body temperature remains elevated above 38.5 °C.

How could her hyperpyrexia be further managed?

The continued presence of hyperpyrexia increases the risk of mortality associated with MDMA toxicity. It is imperative that her temperature is brought down rapidly, and the next step would be to intubate, sedate and ventilate Jane with complete muscle paralysis to reduce heat generated through muscle contraction alongside the ongoing passive and active cooling interventions.

Sedating and invasively ventilating will also help facilitate other management priorities, including obtaining a CT head to rule out an intracranial event, stabilising her cardiovascular system, managing her gas exchange and correcting any electrolyte disturbance.

The laboratory calls you to say that Jane's serum sodium is 115 mmol/L.

What might be the cause of her low serum sodium?

One might assume that hypernatraemia would be more likely due to large insensible losses secondary to increased environmental temperature and muscle activity through energetic dancing. However, individuals consume a large amount of fluid to combat dehydration, resulting in a dilutional hyponatraemic state. In addition, as described previously, increased release of antidiuretic hormone may also play a part.

> You intubate Jane and initiate mechanical ventilation. Her temperature begins to decrease below 38 °C and she appears to be stabilising physiologically. Her BP is now 120/70 mmHg and heart rate 100 bpm. CT brain is unremarkable. You safely transfer her to your ICU following discussion with your consultant. Her serum creatine kinase is found to be elevated at 20000 U/L. Serum creatinine is 200 μmol/L, and over the past 2 hours her urine output has been consistently less than 0.5 mL/kg/h.

When does rhabdomyolysis occur?

Rhabdomyolysis occurs when there is damage to muscle cells that leads to necrosis and the release of large amounts of intracellular solutes (e.g. potassium, uric acid, lactic acid and myoglobin). It has myriad causes, which include trauma, medications (e.g. statins, antimalarials), toxins (e.g. MDMA, cocaine, snake venom), hyperthermia, ischaemia, electrical injury and infection. Its main sequelae are acute kidney injury and potentially life-threatening metabolic abnormalities. The level at which a raised creatine kinase is suggestive of rhabdomyolysis is generally accepted to be around 5000 U/L, but it should be noted that myoglobin-induced renal failure can still occur below this level if other predisposing factors are present (e.g. sepsis, hypovolaemia). Jane's serum CK is 20000 U/L and she should be managed as having rhabdomyolysis.

Describe the Kidney Disease Improving Global Outcomes (KDIGO) staging of AKI

KDIGO separates AKI into three stages (Table 6.1).

How does rhabdomyolysis cause acute kidney injury?

- *Free radical toxicity* – most myoglobin that is released is normally bound to haptoglobin. However, when the level of myoglobin increases beyond the capacity for this buffering action to take place, as in rhabdomyolysis, the free myoglobin passes into the glomerular filtrate and causes damage to the renal tubular cells through overproduction of oxygen free radicals. This damage involves lipid peroxidation of fatty acids and polymerisation of protein and DNA by malondialdehyde.
- *Renal vasoconstriction* – the movement of fluid into the damaged muscle cells leads to a hypovolaemic state and therefore reduced renal blood flow, which is exacerbated further by extraneous losses (e.g. profuse sweating without increasing oral intake) and activation of the renin-aldosterone-angiotensin pathway. Additionally, it is also proposed that the ability of myoglobin to scavenge nitric oxide and release cytokines may also play a part in the observed renal vasoconstriction.

Table 6.1: KDIGO classification for acute kidney injury.

Stage	Serum creatinine	Urine output
1	1.5–1.9×baseline or ≥26.5 µmol/L increase	<0.5 mL/kg/h for 6–12 h
2	2.0–2.9×baseline	<0.5 mL/kg/h for ≥12 h
3	3.0×baseline or Increase in serum creatinine to ≥353.6 µmol/L or Initiation of renal replacement therapy or In patients <18 yr, decrease in estimated glomerular filtration rate to <35 mL/min per 1.73 m²	<0.3 mL/kg/h for ≥24 h or Anuria for ≥12 h

- *Intratubular casts* – the precipitation of myoglobin with Tamm–Horsfall protein creates intratubular casts. This is accelerated in the presence of a low pH (some practitioners induce an alkaline diuresis in these patients for this reason).

How would you manage the rhabdomyolysis that has occurred?

- *Early and aggressive fluid resuscitation* – restoring renal perfusion and thereby increasing urine output are of paramount importance. Crystalloid solutions are most commonly used. Consideration should be given to the patient who presents with severe oliguria or anuria as they may be at risk of developing pulmonary oedema with rapid fluid resuscitation (particularly if a significant cardiac history is present).
- *Bicarbonate therapy* – the theoretical advantage of urine alkalinisation in reducing the formation of casts has led to the use of intravenous 8.4% bicarbonate to increase the urine pH above 7.5. However, there is no strong evidence from randomised controlled trials to support its use. Ideally, since the drug is highly irritant to veins and can cause local necrosis from extravasation, it should be administered via a central intravenous catheter.
- *Renal replacement therapy (RRT)* – it is important to remember that starting RRT should not be guided by the creatine kinase level but instead by the status of renal impairment. In addition, as myoglobin has a molecular mass of 17 kDa, it may be poorly removed using conventional techniques. However, in critical care, the use of continuous venovenous haemofiltration (CVVH) is common and is effective at removing myoglobin from the circulation in most cases.
- *Mannitol* – this osmotic agent can effectively decrease fluid within the damaged muscle, prevent cast formation and increase renal blood flow and glomerular filtration. However, in patients with post-traumatic rhabdomyolysis and creatine kinase levels >5000 U/L, the use of mannitol does not prevent renal failure or the need for renal replacement therapy or decrease mortality.

After 12 hours of supportive management, Jane's creatinine has risen to 600 μmol/L, her potassium has increased to 6.5 mmol/L and her urine output has decreased significantly. You decide to initiate continuous renal replacement therapy (CRRT).

What are the indications for RRT in critical care?

- Metabolic acidosis (pH <7.1).
- Hyperkalaemia refractory to medical management (K^+ >6.5 mmol/L).
- Uraemic complications (e.g. encephalopathy, pericarditis, myopathy or bleeding).
- Removal of dialysable toxins (e.g. salicylate, methanol, ethylene glycol, lithium).
- Pulmonary oedema unresponsive to diuretics.
- Hyperthermia (temperature >40 °C).
- Anuria or oliguria.
- Management of fluid overload.

Has optimal timing been established for when CRRT should be initiated in the critical care patient?

There is still no consensus on the optimal timing of when to start CRRT acutely in these patients. Several trials have attempted to review this but there has been inconsistency regarding methodology and even definitions of what constitutes 'early' and 'late' initiation of therapy (notable trials include AKIKI, ELAIN and IDEAL-ICU). To date, no significant mortality benefit has been found in association with the timing of CRRT.

Where creatinine and urea were historically used in studies as substitutes for the severity of AKI, they do not necessarily determine outcome for patients requiring CRRT. Mortality associated with AKI requiring CRRT in the critically ill is usually associated with volume overload, hyperkalaemia and severe metabolic acidosis. Thus, current practice continues to include early commencement of RRT in the setting of oliguria, established volume overload, metabolic acidosis or electrolyte derangements (local guidelines should also be followed). The rapidity of initiation of RRT within an intensive care unit can depend a great deal upon the available resources and trained personnel, which can vary throughout the day.

You successfully insert a VasCath™ into the right internal jugular vein to enable commencement of CRRT.

Describe the characteristics that form the basis of RRT

- *Mode of delivery* – RRT is either continuous or intermittent. Continuous treatments result in a slow and steady clearance of solutes and permit lower average serum urea levels compared to intermittent techniques. Continuous methods also avoid the hazardous peaks of solute clearance

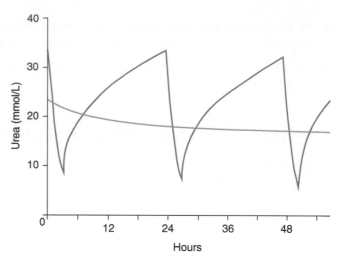

Figure 6.1: RRT patterns of urea removal using continuous (green line) versus intermittent techniques (orange line). Note the potentially hazardous peaks associated with intermittent techniques.

Source: Theophilus Samuels.

that can occur when using intermittent RRT. Compared to intermittent therapies, continuous forms of RRT (e.g. CVVH) result in a greater average mass clearance of urea (Figure 6.1) and better acid–base control.

■ *Method of removing solutes* – using diffusion, convection or a combination of both methods.

■ *Access* – this is usually via either large veins (venovenous) or arteriovenous fistulae.

Briefly describe the different methods for delivering RRT

■ *Haemofiltration (e.g. continuous venovenous haemofiltration)* – this method uses a hydrostatic pressure gradient to move large volumes of plasma water and solutes across a semipermeable membrane by *convection*. This describes *mass transfer* due to the bulk motion of a fluid (e.g. the flow of plasma water transports the molecules and ions that are located within this physiological compartment). An extracorporeal pump is used to power the movement of venous blood through a hollow-fibre cartridge. Certain solutes and plasma water pass through the semipermeable membrane, forming an ultrafiltrate. This ultrafiltrate is then removed and replaced with a physiological crystalloid solution that can be infused either prefilter or postfilter. Prefilter replacement dilutes the blood entering the filter and acts to reduce the incidence of clots forming within the haemofilter. However, it also dilutes the solute content of the blood and reduces the effective solute clearance. Postfilter replacement has no effect on clot formation or solute clearance. This is the least efficient method of RRT and is conducted continuously for 24 hours per day. However, it is efficient at removing large molecules (<60 kDa) and water (Figure 6.2a).

■ *Haemodialysis (e.g. intermittent haemodialysis)* – in this method, the solutes are removed by utilising a concentration gradient. It relies on the process of *diffusion*, a term that describes (a) the random movement

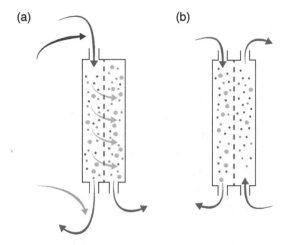

Figure 6.2: (a) In CVVH, blood (red arrows) is pumped through the circuit, creating a hydrostatic pressure gradient (yellow arrows) that moves large volumes of water and solutes across a semipermeable membrane (blue dashed line). This creates an ultrafiltrate (blue arrow) that is removed and then discarded. Replacement fluid can be infused prefilter (dark grey arrow) or postfilter (light grey arrow). It is an efficient method for removing larger molecules (green dots) and water (blue dots). (b) In IHD, blood (red arrows) and dialysate (blue arrows) move countercurrent to one another separated by a semipermeable membrane (blue dashed line). It is an efficient method for removing smaller molecules (orange dots).

Source: Theophilus Samuels.

of particles and (b) movement of particles from regions of high concentration to low concentration. Blood and dialysate run countercurrent to one another, also separated by a semipermeable membrane. Solutes that have high concentrations in the plasma will preferentially move down their concentration gradients into the dialysate (e.g. urea, creatinine). This is an intermittent procedure and is typically performed for 3–4 hours per day, 3–4 times a week. This method is avoided in critically ill patients as it causes hypotension. It is very efficient at removing small molecules, less than 20 kDa (e.g. ammonium, potassium, creatinine), but *not* at removing larger molecules and water (Figure 6.2b).

- *Haemodiafiltration (e.g. continuous venovenous haemodiafiltration)* – this method combines both diffusion and convection to remove fluid and solute.
- *Peritoneal dialysis (PD)* – this method typically makes use of an intra-peritoneal catheter. This permits a glucose-rich (hypertonic) solution to be inserted into the peritoneal cavity, which then acts as a dialysate. Following a specified period, this solution is removed and discarded. It contains the extra fluid and toxins that have crossed into this dialysate from the peritoneal blood vessels. PD is rarely used for the treatment of AKI in developed countries and is more suitable for chronic dialysis.
- *Slow low-efficiency dialysis (SLED)* – this method is performed by using dialysis machines that can deliver a slow dialysate flow for periods ranging from 8 to 12 hours per day. This technique has an excellent solute removal capability, is well tolerated haemodynamically, and does not require any additional equipment to perform if access to haemodialysis machines is readily available. SLED has similar uraemic clearance and haemodynamic stability to CVVH or CVVHD and can be used without anticoagulation. This potentially makes it less labour intensive compared to CVVH.

Your unit uses CVVH.

What dose (mL/kg/h) would you prescribe for Jane?

Evidence from two large clinical trials, the VA/NIH Acute Renal Failure Trial Network (ATN) study and Randomized Evaluation of Normal versus Augmented Level of RRT (RENAL) study, demonstrated no benefit in high doses of CRRT (e.g. >35 mL/kg/min) for critical care patients with AKI. This data suggested that the minimal dose of 20–25 mL/kg/h would be satisfactory in most cases. However, in clinical practice, higher doses can often be employed in patients with sepsis and liver failure.

Why are continuous therapies preferred over intermittent therapy in critical care?

- *Reduce risk of hypotension or cerebral oedema* – changes in plasma osmolality occur at a lower rate. This makes it the mode of choice in patients with haemodynamic instability.
- *Increase systemic vascular resistance (SVR)* – the continuous nature of filtration tends to lower body temperature despite the presence of a warming element in the system. This unintended consequence can lead to an increase in systemic vascular resistance, making it less haemodynamically unstable.
- *Safety profile* – this therapy can be safely conducted by critical care nurses.

What are the disadvantages of continuous RRT therapies in critical care?

- *Anticoagulation* – in almost all patients, the circuit needs to be anticoagulated, particularly if low flow rates are used. Heparin is most commonly used, but its anticoagulant effect may become systemic. Alternatively, citrate can be used – this possesses the best regional effect, but calcium and pH must be carefully monitored and corrected.
- *Labour intensive* – CRRT can be used safely in critical care, but it requires a one-to-one nurse-to-patient ratio as each day a large volume of effluent must be discarded and replaced with an appropriate electrolyte solution.
- *Cost* – the volume of replacement electrolyte solution required for a single patient during the length of stay can be very high.
- *Limited patient mobility* – as the therapies are continuous, patients can be literally confined to bed, especially in the presence of venous access that is 'position dependent'. As such, mental well-being should be considered in awake patients with single organ dysfunction and the use of filter-free periods is encouraged if appropriate (e.g. in between changing expired circuits), allowing the patient to mobilise if able.

Since Jane has no immediate family that can be contacted, and she has had to be intubated and ventilated without discussion or consent, one of your team suggests that deprivation of liberty has taken place.

What is a Deprivation of Liberty Safeguards (DoLS) order?

A DoLS is designed to protect vulnerable people in a hospital or care home (or even their own home) where they are deprived of their 'freedom' (i.e. the freedom to do the things they want to do and live where they want to live) and who lack the capacity to consent to the care or treatment needed. In legal terms, a person is deprived of their liberty if they are both 'under continuous supervision and control and not free to leave'.

How does DoLS apply in intensive care?

In 2017, the Court of Appeal passed judgement in R(Ferreira) v HM Senior Coroner for Inner South London & Ors and stated that in general, when life-saving medical treatment is required then there shall be no deprivation of liberty. The court affirmed that the test for deprivation of liberty as defined above requires that the patient themselves wants to leave but is being prevented by the hospital or care institution they are being held in. Therefore, when their underlying medical condition prevents them from 'leaving' then this test is not met.

Should Jane be referred for DoLS?

No. Given that her medical condition deteriorated to the point where she required intubation and mechanical ventilation to treat her persistent and life-threatening hyperpyrexia, she has not been deprived of her liberties and therefore does not require a DoLS referral.

Jane spends 48 hours on your intensive care unit and is successfully extubated on day 2, having required only 12 hours of RRT. She makes a full recovery and is discharged within 1 week of admission.

Further reading

- Toxbase. www.toxbase.org (accessed 1 February 2022). Definitive online reference for clinical toxicology for UK medical professionals.
- Tandukar, S. and Palevsky, P. (2019). Continuous renal replacement therapy. *Chest* 155: 626–638. Excellent review on who, when, why and how to use CRRT.
- KDIGO AKI Work Group (2012). KDIGO clinical practice guideline for acute kidney injury. *Kidney Int. Suppl.* 2: 1–138. Seminal work on the various aspects of AKI by world leading experts.

7 The Patient with Haematemesis

You are called urgently to your HDU to review John, a 46-year-old man who was admitted from the ward with hepatic encephalopathy. Around 4 hours into his admission, he suddenly had a single episode of haematemesis. Vital signs are HR 100 bpm, BP 110/60 mmHg and RR 20 breaths per minute. His oxygen saturations are 96% on room air despite him refusing supplementary oxygen. He is confused and agitated.

How would you initially assess John?

- *Airway* – John is confused but able to maintain his airway at present. However, his neurological status could quickly deteriorate which could necessitate emergency intubation. Haematemesis could make this a difficult airway due to potential blood in the oropharynx altering the view at laryngoscopy. Endotracheal intubation is usually required in cases of significant haematemesis where the airway is compromised or when urgent endoscopy is required.
- *Breathing* – ideally, John should receive high-flow oxygen therapy, but due to his agitation and confusion this is not possible.
- *Circulation* – ensure that two large-bore intravenous cannulae are in situ. Care needs to be taken, as attempting to site a cannula in agitated and combative patients increases the risk of a needlestick injury. Given that John is tachycardic, commence resuscitative fluids. He should have a blood group and save sample sent and ask the lab to cross-match at least four units of packed red cells (or according to your local unit policies).
- *Disability/exposure* – easily correctable factors, such as hypoglycaemia, should be identified and corrected, as well as appropriately exposing the patient to assess for other sources of bleeding (e.g. PR bleeding).

Clinical Cases in Critical Care, First Edition. Alice Myers and Theophilus Samuels.
© 2023 John Wiley & Sons Ltd. Published 2023 by John Wiley & Sons Ltd.

How might you assess bleeding severity at the bedside?

Assessment of haemodynamics and vital signs allows broad categorisation (as per ATLS*).

- *Mild bleeding* – when the approximate blood loss is between 15% and 30%, this usually produces few physiological changes. Vital signs (e.g. pulse rate, respiratory rate, blood pressure, mental status, urine output) remain relatively unchanged.
- *Moderate bleeding* – when the approximate blood loss is between 31% and 40%, this usually results in detectable changes in postural blood pressure, tachycardia, tachypnoea and oliguria. Metabolic acidaemia may be present, with attempted compensatory increases in minute ventilation (e.g. respiratory rate and tidal volumes). However, it should be noted that aspiration of blood and/or agitation and anxiety may also contribute to the increase in respiratory rate.
- *Severe bleeding* – when the degree of lost blood exceeds approximately 40%, a shocked state will most likely develop. This results in profound hypotension, marked tachycardia and tachypnoea, greatly diminished urine output and mental status, and requires a massive transfusion.

What primary prophylaxis is available for preventing upper gastrointestinal bleeding (UGIB) in acutely unwell critical care patients?

The National Institute for Health and Care Excellence (NICE) UK guidance (CG141) recommends offering these patients acid suppression therapy (H_2-receptor antagonists or proton pump inhibitors) for the prevention of UGIB, and where possible to use the oral form of the drug.

Following insertion of your second large-bore cannula, you withdraw blood samples and send them to the laboratory for urgent full blood count, cross-matching and coagulation studies. You are informed that John's haematocrit is 45%.

How useful is the haematocrit at this initial stage?

In the acute setting, it is important to understand that the patient is losing whole blood. Therefore, the loss of both plasma and red blood cells (RBCs) will result in the percentage of RBCs (the haematocrit) remaining at a similar level as before the acute bleeding occurred. As fluid from the extravascular space moves into the intravascular compartment between 24 and 72 hours after the bleeding event, and along with resuscitation using crystalloid solutions, the haematocrit will begin to decrease. Therefore, in the acute stages the haematocrit can remain nearly normal despite massive losses until resuscitative fluids are administered.

How can you differentiate clinically between an upper and lower gastrointestinal bleed?

An upper GIB may present with:

- haematemesis or coffee grounds vomiting (indicating recent but not active UGIB)
- melaena (black, tarry stools), which indicates that the blood has been present within the GI tract for at least 14 hours. However, brisk upper GI bleeding may result in rapid GI transit and present with fresh rather than transformed blood
- hyperactive bowel sounds
- raised serum urea, due to blood proteins absorbed in the small intestine.

A lower GIB typically presents with fresh blood per anus (haematochezia).

Discuss the potential sources of non-variceal upper gastrointestinal bleeding

- *Peptic ulcers* – these are the most common causes of UGIB, with an approximate incidence between 30% and 50%. Prognostic information can be obtained at endoscopy by examining these lesions. Approximately 20% of these patients will demonstrate findings of active bleeding, adherent clot or a non-bleeding viable vessel. Around one-third of this cohort will experience further bleeding and therefore benefit from endoscopic therapy with bipolar electrocoagulation, heater probe, injection therapy (e.g. absolute alcohol, 1:10000 adrenaline) and/or clips. Clean-based ulcers seen at endoscopy have nearly zero risk of rebleeding. If no measures are taken in this cohort to prevent rebleeding, then approximately 10–50% will suffer another episode. Prevention is focused on three main strategies:
  - *Helicobacter pylori* eradication decreases rebleeding rates to less than 5%.
  - Stopping non-steroidal anti-inflammatory drugs (NSAIDs) if being taken.
  - Indefinite proton pump inhibitor (PPI) therapy (42% incidence of rebleeding at 7 years if not adhered to).
- *Erosive gastritis, oesophagitis or duodenitis* – these occur in approximately 10–15% of cases and are confined to the mucosa. As there are no arteries or veins within the mucosa, these 'breaks' do not cause major bleeding. The most important precipitating factor for these erosions is the use of NSAIDs. It is estimated that 50% of patients taking long-term NSAIDs may have gastric erosions. Other causes include stress, alcohol consumption and *H. pylori* infection. Critically ill patients are most prone to stress-related gastric mucosal injury where reduced splanchnic blood flow disrupts the integrity of the mucosa. Severe bleeding should not occur unless ulceration develops. Due to their critical illness, the mortality rate is very high in these patients.
- *Mallory–Weiss tear* – accounts for approximately 2–10% of UGIB hospitalisations. The patient will usually give the classic history of vomiting,

retching or coughing followed by haematemesis. In 80–90% of patients, bleeding from these tears will stop spontaneously. They are usually found on the gastric side of the gastro-oesophageal junction. Recurrence rates are low, with estimates being up to 10%. Actively bleeding tears should be managed endoscopically.

- *Other causes* – malignancies, oesophagitis, angiodysplasia or vascular malformations (e.g. Osler–Weber–Rendu syndrome, Dieulafoy lesion), and aortoenteric fistulae are other less common causes of UGIB.

What are the options for patients who need to continue NSAIDs after they present with bleeding peptic ulcers?

- Cyclo-oxygenase-2 selective NSAID with PPI therapy.
- If taking low-dose aspirin for secondary prevention of established cardiovascular disease, then this should be restarted as soon as possible (between 1 and 7 days) after the bleeding event.
- For primary prevention of cardiovascular disease, aspirin should be discontinued in most patients who develop an UGIB.

You determine from John's clinical history that he has been recently diagnosed with cirrhosis of the liver due to alcohol.

How could cirrhosis contribute to the development of varices in John?

The hepatic venous pressure gradient (HVPG) is the difference between the portal vein pressure and free hepatic vein pressure. Portal hypertension occurs when this pressure is greater than 5 mmHg and is most associated with cirrhosis. Interestingly, if the HVPG remains less than 12 mmHg, varices do not develop and there is therefore very little risk of bleeding. When the HVPG exceeds 12 mmHg, there is little correlation between the risk of bleeding and the pressure gradient. In response to portal hypertension, portosystemic collateral venous drainage results in variceal formation, most commonly in the distal oesophagus and stomach. Varices can also occur within the small and/or large bowel and in the anorectal area.

Non-cirrhotic causes of portal hypertension include Budd–Chiari syndrome, portal vein thrombosis and constrictive pericarditis.

Describe the Child–Pugh classification of cirrhosis

This score is used to predict survival in many liver diseases and for cirrhosis can predict the likelihood of major complications, such as variceal bleeding and spontaneous bacterial peritonitis. The classification scores the patient between 5 and 15 on bilirubin, INR, albumin, ascites and encephalopathy:

- Score 5–6: class A ('compensated cirrhosis').
- Score 7–9: class B.
- Score 10–15: class C.

A score of ≥7 indicates decompensated cirrhosis. The Child–Pugh score was used to assess a candidate for liver transplantation and prognosticate in cirrhotic patients. However, for listing patients for transplantation, it has been superseded (see Case 19).

Despite the ongoing administration of IV fluid boluses, John remains tachycardic (now 120 bpm) and his BP is lower than before (95/60 mmHg).

What do you think is the source of John's bleeding?

The most likely source of bleeding in this case is ruptured oesophageal varices. This remains the most common site of portal hypertensive bleeding in these patients. In all patients with cirrhosis, approximately 50% will have oesophageal varices. However, varices will develop in most cirrhotic patients eventually.

What is the recommended haemoglobin level for transfusion in variceal bleeding?

Currently, transfusion is recommended when the haemoglobin level falls below 70 g/L. Evidence suggests that adhering to this threshold when compared to a threshold of 90 g/L decreases rebleeding, multiorgan failure and death. In addition, transfusing a patient to a haemoglobin level above 100 g/L should be avoided. However, you should consider other factors that might require transfusing at a higher threshold, such as underlying cardiac disease (e.g. peripheral vascular surgery, heart failure or ischaemic heart disease), the presence of tissue hypoxaemia (suggested by rising lactate levels) and haemodynamic status.

In rapid exsanguination, it may not be possible to use laboratory haemoglobin level as a guide to transfusion. In these circumstances, repeated clinical assessment of haemodynamics, regular estimation of overt blood loss and possibly the use of real-time thromboelastography are used to guide transfusion.

What is the role of tranexamic acid in acute UGIB?

The HALT-IT study investigated the effects of a high-dose 24-hour infusion of tranexamic acid on death and thromboembolic events in patients with acute gastrointestinal bleeding. The trial suggested that the use of tranexamic acid does not reduce death and should *not* be incorporated into management strategies to treat GI bleeding.

Describe the treatment options available for variceal bleeding

Non-endoscopic

- *Pharmacotherapy* – this aims to reduce intrahepatic resistance or decrease portal blood flow. Several agents can or have been used.
  - *Terlipressin* – a synthetic analogue of vasopressin, this has a longer duration of action and safer profile. It is the only agent that has been

shown to reduce mortality when compared to placebo. In the UK, it is licensed for bleeding from oesophageal varices.

- *Somatostatin* – this naturally occurring peptide causes splanchnic vasoconstriction without affecting systemic vasculature. It reduces portal pressure and has fewer side-effects when compared to vasopressin.
- *Octreotide* – a somatostatin analogue, it is best used in conjunction with endoscopic therapy and is used in the United States due to the unavailability of somatostatin.

Balloon tamponade – generally used in cases of exsanguinating variceal haemorrhage, this can be used to control active variceal bleeding when other forms of therapy fail or are not immediately available or while awaiting endoscopy. It is best seen as a temporising measure until definitive treatment can be given. However, as endoscopic techniques have improved, experience in the use of balloon tamponade has dramatically fallen. Nevertheless, control of bleeding can be achieved in most patients, but the risk of rebleeding is high after balloon deflation. The most commonly used balloon device is the Sengstaken–Blakemore tube, which has three ports: one for oesophageal balloon inflation, one for gastric balloon inflation and one for gastric aspiration. The tube is passed to the 50 cm mark and the gastric balloon is inflated to its full recommended volume of air, around 400–500 mL. Once correct placement is confirmed using a chest radiograph, the tube can be pulled back gently until resistance is felt (due to the diaphragm). Inflation time should be limited due to the risk of perforation, which is highest when the oesophageal balloon is also needed for haemorrhage control. Duration and timing of removal should be co-ordinated closely with the endoscopic team. In current practice, the oesophageal balloon is rarely inflated.

Transjugular intrahepatic portosystemic shunt (TIPS) – using a percutaneous approach, this technique creates a portosystemic shunt. An expandable metal stent is advanced under angiographic guidance and creates a direct portocaval shunt between the portal and hepatic vein, bypassing the liver parenchyma and significantly decreasing portal pressure. When acute variceal bleeding fails to respond to endoscopic and pharmacological therapies, this procedure should be considered. In more than 90% of patients, this technique can control active bleeding, with less than 20% experiencing a rebleeding episode. Performing a TIPS procedure within 24–48 hours in a patient with an HVPG >20 mmHg or with Child–Pugh class C disease has been shown to reduce mortality. Encephalopathy develops in up to 20% of patients undergoing this procedure and stenosis/complete occlusion of the shunt occurs in 5–15% of cases.

Endoscopic

- *Band ligation* – this technique is the preferred choice for controlling active oesophageal variceal bleeding and for subsequent eradication of oesophageal varices. Ligation involves suctioning a varix into a cap fitted on the end of the endoscope, which is then ligated by a rubber band that is released from the cap. Band ligation will control acute bleeding in up to 90% of patients. Oesophageal stenosis and postligation ulcer bleeding are uncommon complications following band ligation. In addition, this technique is less successful when oesophageal varices extend into the proximal stomach.

- *Sclerotherapy* – this involves injecting a sclerosing, thrombogenic solution into or next to the varices. This technique is generally used to control bleeding when band ligation fails but it is associated with a higher incidence of complications.
- *Stenting* – this has been demonstrated to increase 15-day survival without serious complications or further bleeding when compared to balloon tamponade. It is also associated with less need for transfusion and has a greater success at controlling bleeding

What is the role of prophylactic antibiotics in patients with variceal bleeding?

Evidence from randomised controlled trials and a meta-analysis suggests that prophylactic antibiotics in patients with variceal bleeding decreases overall mortality, death from bacterial infection, rebleeding and length of hospital stay. As bacterial infection can be present in up to 20% of these cases and up to 50% will develop a hospital-acquired infection, the use of prophylactic antibiotics appears self-fulfilling. In addition, variceal bleeding is more likely to occur in cirrhotic patients who are infected. Quinolones and cephalosporins have been used with good success, but antibiotic resistance can dramatically lower their effectiveness and local guidelines should be followed.

> About 1 hour after you began reviewing John, he has another larger episode of haematemesis. He is much quieter and only responds to pain. His oxygen saturations are now 85% on high-flow oxygen and his blood pressure is 70/50 mmHg.

How would you proceed?

This is a life-threatening situation.

- *Emergency intubation and ventilation* – the decrease in conscious level puts John at very high risk of aspiration due to the potential loss of protective airway reflexes and a stomach full of blood. Therefore, secure a definitive airway and intubate his trachea (see Introduction Section 2). Care should be taken as massive haematemesis may obscure the airway, so effective suction and experienced airway support are essential. In addition, ensure that appropriate personal protective equipment is available and used (e.g. faceshield, aprons, gloves).
- *Declare a major haemorrhage* – as part of the ongoing fluid resuscitation, John will need blood products. It should be clear that he is undergoing a massive haemorrhage and so alerting your transfusion service to this emergency will ensure that blood products are made available as rapidly as possible. Consult your local hospital policies for the major haemorrhage protocol.

- *Consider balloon tamponade* – as described previously, balloon tamponade can be considered as a bridging measure to definitive endoscopic treatment.
- *Get expert help* – alert the on-call endoscopy team to facilitate emergency endoscopy.

> With trained airway assistants, you successfully intubate John. You begin transfusing him according to your local major haemorrhage protocol (e.g. 1:1 RBC/FFP transfusion). As the on-call consultant for emergency endoscopy is mobilising their team, you are informed that the international normalised ratio (INR) is 2.3.

How can massive transfusion (MT) be defined?

The most common definitions of MT are as follows:

- Transfusion of ≥10 units within 24 hours.
- Transfusion of >4 red blood cell units in 1 hour with the anticipation of a continued need for blood product support.
- Replacement of >50% of the total blood volume by blood products within 3 hours.

However, these definitions do not direct attention to the coagulopathy that also exists in these patients and fuels the process underlying the haemorrhage.

What are the complications associated with a massive transfusion?

There are multiple ways to categorise the complications, e.g. immediate, early and delayed or immune versus non-immune. Here we divide the complications into six categories:

1. Coagulation abnormalities
   - Dilutional abnormality due to use of crystalloids or massive transfusion.
   - Dilutional thrombocytopenia.
2. Related to blood storage
   - Increased inflammatory response.
   - Immunosuppression.
   - Blood cell haemolysis.
   - Metabolic acidosis.
   - Hyperkalaemic cardiac arrest.
   - Hypocalcaemia.
   - Hypomagnesaemia.
3. Immunosuppression and infection
   - Infection (bacterial, viral, etc.).
   - Increased length of stay.
   - Increased mortality.

4. Lung-associated injury
   - Transfusion-related acute lung injury (TRALI).
   - Acute respiratory distress syndrome (ARDS).
5. Metabolic
   - Anaerobic metabolism.
   - Lactate production.
   - Hypothermia.
6. Fluid overload.

In general, non-massive transfusion can also be associated with the complications of pain, fever and anaphylaxis.

In the UK, serious adverse reactions associated with blood transfusion should be reported to SHOT (Serious Hazards Of Transfusion), the UK haemovigilance scheme.

How does this INR result affect the ability to perform endoscopy?

Endoscopy should not be delayed while treatment is ongoing to normalise the INR. It is useful to seek expert haematological advice regarding these coagulation abnormalities. Usually, coagulation defects due to liver disease or warfarin therapy can be treated using fresh frozen plasma (FFP). In patients with cirrhosis, the INR only reflects changes in procoagulant factors. However, there is often a balanced coagulopathy present with altered levels of anticoagulant factors (e.g. protein C, protein S) in addition. In this context, thromboelastography may help guide blood product administration. If patients are taking antiplatelet therapy (e.g. clopidogrel or aspirin) then platelet transfusion may be warranted. If taking warfarin, the INR may be corrected with FFP or administration of prothrombin complex concentrate (e.g. Beriplex®). In addition, platelet transfusion is also indicated when platelet levels fall below 50×10^9/L in patients with acute GIB.

Describe factors that increase the risk of death after hospital admission for acute UGIB

The mortality rate for patients presenting with UGIB ranges between 3% and 14%. The following risk factors are associated with an increased risk of death:

- Presenting in a shocked state (e.g. systolic BP <100 mmHg).
- Advanced age.
- Presence of advanced upper gastrointestinal malignancy.
- Co-morbidities such as renal or hepatic failure or disseminated cancer.
- Certain endoscopic findings such as active, spurting haemorrhage from a peptic ulcer, non-bleeding visible blood vessel.
- Rebleeding, which increases mortality 10-fold.

The endoscopy team arrive and perform emergency endoscopy. They find bleeding oesophageal varices and perform variceal band ligation successfully. With the ongoing resuscitative measures you and your team have employed, John begins to show signs of stabilising.

Further reading

- Jameson, J., Fauci, A., Kasper, D. et al. (2018). *Harrison's Principles of Internal Medicine*. New York: McGraw-Hill Education. Chapter 44. Authoritative information on gastrointestinal bleeding.
- Kamboj, A., Hoverston, P., and Leggett, C. (2019). Upper gastrointestinal bleeding: etiologies and management. *Mayo. Clin. Proc.* 94 (4): 697–703. Succinct review on the aetiologies and management of UGIB.
- García-Pagán, J., Caca, K., Bureau, C. et al. (2010). Early use of TIPS in patients with cirrhosis and variceal bleeding. *N. Engl. J. Med.* 362: 2370–2379. Formative RCT showing that early use of TIPS resulted in significant reductions in treatment failure and mortality.

8

The Patient Who Is Difficult to Ventilate

At the start of your night shift, you are asked to review 45-year-old Susan. She was admitted earlier in the day with sepsis secondary to a lower respiratory tract infection. She was agitated and severely hypoxic on arrival in ED so was intubated and brought to ICU. Throughout the day, she has been becoming increasingly difficult to ventilate. The nursing staff say that her blood gases have deteriorated, and she is now 'fighting the ventilator'.

What may be causing lack of synchrony with the ventilator?

- *Ventilator dyssynchrony due to inappropriate settings or mode of ventilation* – Susan probably received neuromuscular blockade at the time of intubation. Initially, the ventilator would need to have been set to deliver mandatory breaths. The paralysing agent is likely to have been metabolised by now, allowing Susan to initiate her own breaths.
  - Modes of ventilation can be divided into spontaneous, mandatory or a combination. There are multiple parameters which can be programmed inappropriately, e.g. inspiratory:expiratory ratio, respiratory rate, inspiratory ramp time, etc. In a spontaneous or combination mode, the ventilator can be set to detect and augment breaths initiated by the patient. Support is usually delivered as a target pressure or volume and the success of these breaths will depend upon the patient's respiratory mechanics, clinical condition and flow dynamics within the system. If augmentation is inadequate, the patient may increase their work of breathing to try and compensate.
  - If mandatory breaths are delivered out of sync with the patient's own breathing, a situation may develop where the patient wants to inspire when the ventilator is programmed for expiration, or vice versa. This results in a pattern of respiration which looks uncomfortable and is often accompanied by erratic tidal volumes and high peak pressures. Work of breathing may be increased, there is a risk of alveolar damage from shear forces within the lungs, and there may be a worsening of gas exchange.

Clinical Cases in Critical Care, First Edition. Alice Myers and Theophilus Samuels.
© 2023 John Wiley & Sons Ltd. Published 2023 by John Wiley & Sons Ltd.

- *Pain, distress, or inadequate sedation* – many patients find the presence of an endotracheal tube painful and distressing and therefore sedation is often needed for tube tolerance. There are many potential sources of distress for Susan; for example, she may have delirium and be experiencing hallucinations. She could have pleuritic pain from her infection or pain from vascular access devices, etc. Other sources of pain in critical care include chest drains, surgical wounds or pre-existing chronic and atypical pain syndromes. While Susan requires ventilatory support, she will need to be appropriately sedated, usually aiming for a RASS of 0 to −2 (see Case 11). Commonly, this is achieved using a combination of an opioid with a hypnotic agent (e.g. remifentanil and propofol).
- *Equipment problem or misplaced ETT* – search for an equipment problem systematically by assessing every element of the circuit from patient to ventilator, including all gas pipes and flow sensors. Perhaps the ETT has migrated, leading to endobronchial intubation and ventilation of one lung only. Alternatively, especially if high PEEP is being used, the cuff may have herniated above the vocal cords, causing a leak and reduction in the positive pressure generated by the ventilator. If flow-triggering is being used, a gas leak or impaired flow through ventilator tubing could mean Susan needs to work harder to compensate for the leak to trigger support from the ventilator.
- *Increased resistance in the system* – a water-logged HMEF (heat moisture exchange filter) or kinked tubing massively increases resistance to flow. Since resistance to flow is equal to the change in pressure divided by the flow rate

$$R = \frac{P}{Q}$$

(R = resistance to flow, P = pressure difference, Q = flow).
By combining this relationship with the Hagen–Poiseuille Law below

$$Q = \frac{\pi P r^4}{8 \eta l}$$

(Q = flow, P = pressure difference, r = radius, η = viscosity, π = pi, and l = length), we see that the following inverse relationship is apparent

$$R \propto \frac{1}{r^4}$$

assuming the viscosity of the gas and length of the breathing circuit remain constant. Hence, any small reduction in radius can lead to an increase in the work of breathing (use of accessory muscles, tachypnoea, tachycardia, etc.) as the patient struggles to overcome this increased resistance and decreased gas flow.
- *Worsening chest sepsis* – it is possible that Susan's apparent discomfort could be due to deterioration in her clinical condition. She was admitted recently, and the trajectory of her illness is not yet clear. Her chest sepsis may be getting worse and her initial ventilatory support might now be inadequate. Antimicrobial agents are unlikely to have made a positive impact yet. Ensure a full septic screen has been sent (including blood

cultures, a urinary antigen screen for pneumococcus and *Legionella*, nasopharyngeal aspirates, and flu swabs) and review her current anti-microbials with a microbiologist.

- *New pathology* – Susan could have developed a new problem in addition to her chest sepsis. This could be related to her lung pathology, interventions the critical care team have instigated, or something else coincidental. Keep an open mind when reviewing Susan, looking for evidence of pneumothorax, pleural effusions, lung collapse or sputum plugging. Ensure a complete assessment is performed to rule out problems with other organ systems which may have been missed by focusing on the acute problems. Don't forget to examine the skin for rashes (e.g. meningococcal septicaemia, measles etc.) and the abdomen for peritonitis, and ensure all invasive cannulae are clean and appropriately sited.

What is the likely cause of Susan's chest sepsis?

Chest sepsis can result from community- or hospital-acquired pneumonia. Susan's case is one of community-acquired pneumonia (CAP) and is probably bacterial or viral.

Bacterial causes in previously well adults include the following:

- Typical
  - *Streptococcus pneumoniae* (approximately 50% of cases).
  - *Haemophilus influenzae.*
  - *Moraxella catarrhalis.*
- Atypical
  - *Mycoplasma pneumoniae.*
  - *Legionella pneumophila* is a possibility, particularly if there has been exposure to stagnant water.
  - *Chlamydia* spp.
- *Staphylococcus aureus* and gram-negative pathogens should also be considered given the severity of Susan's condition. Secondary bacterial infection can complicate recovery from viral infection.

Viral causes include the following:

- *Influenza virus* – 'seasonal flu' due to influenza A or B. After *S. pneumoniae*, influenza A is the most common cause of CAP. Surface proteins (haemagglutinin and neuraminidase) are used in classification. Empirical treatment may be started (e.g. oseltamivir) if unable to rule this out immediately. Influenza C causes only mild infection and D mainly affects cattle.
- *Coronavirus* – consider the need to isolate the patient and wear an FFP3 mask if there is any chance of contagion, e.g. SARS-CoV (see Case 24).

Other causes include the following:

- It would be wise to explore causes of immune suppression (e.g. HIV, use of immunosuppressants) underlying lung disease (e.g. fibrotic or obstructive processes), and exposure to unusual pathogens (e.g. recent foreign travel, exposure to moulds). If none of these are present, the cause is less likely to be fungal, though this should be reviewed as a possibility if Susan fails to respond to treatment.

You review Susan and find the following on examination. Weight 82 kg, height 165 cm, BMI 30.1. The ventilator is in synchronised intermittent mandatory ventilation (SIMV) mode: FiO_2 0.85, PEEP 12 cmH$_2$O, set RR 14 per minute (actual RR 35–40 per minute), V_T 120–700 mL (ideal body weight [IBW] 57 kg).

From the end of the bed, you can see that her HR is 125–130 bpm (sinus rhythm), BP 95/50 mmHg giving a MAP 65 mmHg on noradrenaline 0.45 mcg/kg/min. Her chest is moving asynchronously with the ventilator (Figure 8.1), and she is using accessory muscles of respiration. You can hear the peak pressure alarm intermittently.

Her temperature is 38.4 °C. She is prescribed co-amoxiclav and clarithromycin. She is sedated with propofol 150 mg/h and fentanyl 100 mcg/h with a RASS -2.

You also note that her urine output has dropped to 0–10 mL/h for the last 6 hours.

The remainder of the examination is unremarkable.

Initial blood results – Hb 104 g/L, WBC 14.2 × 10^9/L, CRP 256, platelets 92 × 10^9/L, urea 9 mmol/L, creatinine 157 μmol/L.

ABG – pH 7.10, PaO$_2$ 7.2 kPa, PaCO$_2$ 9.3 kPa, base excess −6.4 mmol/L. Lactate is now 3.6 mmol/L (3.1 mmol/L on admission).

Plain chest radiograph shows widespread pulmonary infiltrates.

What is your assessment of the clinical situation?

From examination and review of the flow and pressure curves, Susan is dyssynchronous with the ventilator, leaving her at risk of barotrauma and atelectrauma. She appears to be deteriorating with increasing vasopressor requirements and poor urine output. She has reduced oxygen delivery and increased oxygen requirements with increased work of breathing and pyrexia. Intervention is required at this point to prevent further deterioration.

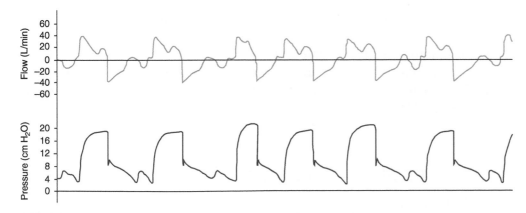

Figure 8.1: Pressure and flow curves for the patient.

Source: Theophilus Samuels.

What is synchronised intermittent mandatory ventilation?

Synchronised intermittent mandatory ventilation is a volume control mode where the ventilator is set to deliver mandatory breaths at a programmed respiratory rate while also allowing spontaneous breathing. For example, a set respiratory rate of 14 breaths per minute means the ventilator would deliver 14 breaths spread evenly throughout the 60-second time period (time-cycled). All 14 breaths would be mandatory in the way they are delivered (i.e. cycling from inspiration to expiration). The ventilator will attempt to synchronise the mandatory breaths with the patient's own breathing up to the maximum set rate. If the patient takes a breath during that time-window, the ventilator will synchronise that breath with the patient. If they do not, then a preprogrammed mandatory breath will be delivered. The patient can breathe additionally, but unless pressure support is set for those breaths (i.e. pressure-SIMV [P-SIMV]), they will be unaugmented.

Categorise the available modes of mechanical ventilation

There are several ways to categorise modes of ventilation. With huge numbers of ventilator manufacturers creating increasing numbers of new modes, many modern modes may cross several categories and nomenclature is variable.

This is one approach to answering the question:

- Conventional modes
    - Pressure – pressure assist control, pressure SIMV, pressure support.
    - Volume – volume assist control, volume SIMV.
- Adaptive modes
    - Simple – adaptive assist control, adaptive SIMV, adaptive volume support.
    - Advanced – adaptive support ventilation.
- Biphasic modes
    - BIPAP (biphasic positive airway pressure).
    - APRV (airway pressure release ventilation).

Other ways to approach categorisation could include:

- Mandatory versus spontaneous
- Control (ventilator triggered) versus support (patient triggered)
- Triggering modes – time, pressure, volume, flow, shape-signal, neural assist (NAVA)
- Cycling modes – time, volume, flow.

What types of ventilator asynchrony do you know?

- Trigger asynchronies
    - Delayed triggering – there is a delay between the patient's effort and delivery of supported breath.

- Ineffective effort – patient effort fails to trigger a breath.
- Autotriggering – mechanical breath is delivered without any spontaneous patient effort, sometimes seen with cardiac oscillations or water droplets in flow sensor tubing.
- Flow asynchrony – the delivered flow is insufficient for the patient's demands.
- Termination asynchrony
  - Double triggering – a single patient effort results in two delivered breaths without expiration in between.
  - Early cycling – the programmed breath is too short for the patient, leading to spontaneous effort during ventilator expiration.
  - Delayed cycling – duration of the mechanical breath is longer than the patient's own spontaneous effort.

What is peak pressure and how is it different from plateau pressure?

Peak pressure is the pressure generated by the ventilator to overcome the total airflow resistance (upper airways and alveolar)

$$PIP = QR + \frac{\dot{V_t}}{C} + PEEP$$

(PIP = peak inspiratory pressure, Q = flow, R = resistance, V_t = tidal volume, C = compliance, $PEEP$ = peak end-expiratory pressure).

It is measured during inspiration and sudden isolated increases may be due to obstructed ventilator tubing, kinked endotracheal tube or bronchospasm, for example.

Plateau pressure is more reflective of smaller airways and pulmonary compliance and should be measured during the inspiratory pause

$$P_{plat} = \frac{V_t}{C}$$

(P_{plat} = plateau pressure, V_t = tidal volume, C = compliance).

When both plateau and peak pressures are high, this is suggestive of low pulmonary compliance due to, for example, atelectasis, pulmonary oedema, acute respiratory distress syndrome (ARDS), pneumothorax, etc. See Case 24 for further discussion.

What are your options to combat Susan's ventilator dyssynchrony?

- *Change the mode of ventilation* – in an unparalysed patient, particularly one with a high CO_2 and light sedation, SIMV may be poorly tolerated, even with pressure-augmented spontaneous breaths. The fact that her respiratory rate is so much higher than the set rate, together with the erratic ventilator curves, reveals that Susan is initiating many additional breaths. Her tidal volumes are variable, ranging from 2 to 12 mL/kg. Ideally, aim to achieve consistent low tidal volume ventilation for Susan, approximately 340 mL, i.e. 6–8 mL/kg of IBW.

- *Adjust ventilator settings* – assess the ventilator flow curves and adjust according to Susan's individual requirements. This requires alteration of advanced ventilator settings (e.g. pressure ramp time, trigger sensitivities, etc.). When carefully considered, even small adjustments can dramatically improve tolerance of mechanical ventilation.
- *Increase sedation* – aiming to increase tolerance of mechanical ventilation.
- *Consider neuromuscular blockade* – if her drive to breathe cannot be overcome with appropriate sedation, neuromuscular blockade may need to be added.

If Susan's condition were improving and she were in the process of weaning from the ventilator, it may be appropriate to change her to a fully spontaneous mode with pressure support set to achieve appropriate volumes. However, in a deteriorating patient, it is usually more appropriate to increase the support from the ventilator and facilitate tolerance of mechanical ventilation by increasing sedation.

Susan has severe chest sepsis with associated multiple organ failure. You decide to deepen her sedation to improve synchrony with the ventilator. You increase her propofol infusion rate to 200 mg/h and her fentanyl infusion rate to 200 mcg/h. Once she is well sedated, you give her a 50 mg bolus of rocuronium and set the ventilator to a pressure-controlled, volume-guaranteed mode with a PEEP of 10 cmH$_2$O.

One of the senior ICU nurses suggests that the chest radiograph taken before admission shows ARDS (Figure 8.2).

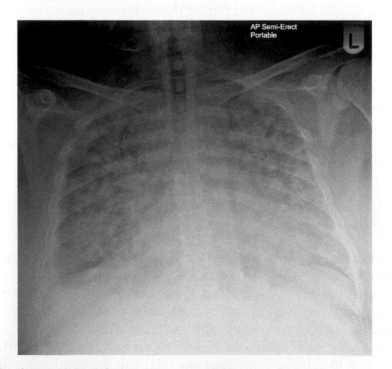

Figure 8.2: Chest radiograph demonstrating ARDS.

What is acute respiratory distress syndrome?

Acute respiratory distress syndrome is an acute diffuse inflammatory lung injury, leading to increased vascular permeability, increased lung weight and loss of aerated tissue (Ranieri et al., JAMA 2012). There is increased physiological dead space and reduced lung compliance. Diagnosis, according to the Berlin definition, requires hypoxaemia with bilateral infiltrates on chest radiograph (not explained by cardiac failure or fluid overload) with a PEEP of at least $5\,cmH_2O$. There are three categories of severity:

Category	PaO$_2$:FiO$_2$ (P:F) ratio	Mortality at 30 days
Mild	200–300 mmHg or 26.6–40 kPa	27%
Moderate	100–200 mmHg or 13.3–26.6 kPa	32%
Severe	<100 mmHg or <13.3 kPa	45%

What is the Murray score?

The Lung Injury Severity Score (LISS or Murray score) was proposed by Murray et al. in 1988. This score is used to grade severity of lung injury and can be used to aid decisions regarding whether patients with ARDS require extracorporeal membrane oxygenation (ECMO). It was not designed to prognosticate outcomes.

This composite scoring system awards points for degree of derangement within four parameters:

- Extent of consolidation on chest radiograph
- P:F ratio
- PEEP level
- Respiratory compliance

In those with a total score greater than 3, consider discussion with an ECMO centre.

Is there evidence to support the use of neuromuscular blockade in cases of ARDS?

The evidence is controversial. The ACURASYS trial in 2010 showed a 90-day mortality benefit with the use of a continuous infusion of cisatracurium early in ARDS.

The ROSE Trial in 2019 (Re-evaluation Of Systemic Early neuromuscular blockade) challenged previous trial results and showed no evidence of mortality benefit.

As with all evidence-based medicine, these published studies can be criticised, and overextrapolation is fraught with potential problems. Several other studies report an association between increased asynchrony and worse outcomes (e.g. Zhou et al., Sci Rep, 2021). A reasonable approach would seem to be to try and optimise all ventilator settings, sedation, analgesia, etc., and if the patient remains dyssynchronous with potentially harmful pressures and volumes, consider introducing a paralysing agent.

> Susan looks more settled after your interventions and she is easily achieving tidal volumes of 340 mL with pressures consistently less than 30 cmH₂O. Her HR has reduced to around 105 bpm, but her BP has also fallen. Her noradrenaline has risen to 0.65 mcg/kg/min aiming for a MAP of 65 mmHg. Her temperature is 38.6 °C. In the 60 minutes that you have been assessing and managing Susan's recent deterioration, she has passed no urine.

Why does Susan need so much noradrenaline and what can you do to improve her cardiovascular status?

Susan is in septic shock. Although the pathophysiology of sepsis is not fully elucidated, it is likely that bacterial infection induces release of proinflammatory cytokines like interleukins (IL) (particularly IL-1 and IL-6), and tumour necrosis factor (TNF-α) leading to a generalised inflammatory response. Vascular dilation occurs and total peripheral resistance decreases. This is compounded by capillary leakage. Her chest radiograph changes would be consistent with excess interstitial fluid. Susan's reduced urine output may reflect reduced renal perfusion.

Susan will be prone to losing fluid into third spaces, including the interstitial areas of the lungs, yet she is probably intravascularly depleted. While fluid accumulation in the lungs (further impairing her gas exchange) should be avoided, her circulating volume requires optimisation to reduce vasopressor requirements and preserve end-organ perfusion.

Aim to augment the cardiac output element of the oxygen delivery equation (Figure 8.3).

Stroke volume depends upon preload, inotropy and afterload, so consider fluids, vasopressors and inotropic agents at this stage, depending upon the clinical assessment of Susan's needs. Ideally, clinical assessment and fluid management will incorporate bedside echocardiography (see Case 1).

$$DO_2 = CO \times CaO_2 \times 10$$

$$HR \times SV \qquad ((Hb \times SpO_2 \times 1.39) + (0.003 \times PaO_2))$$

Figure 8.3: Oxygen delivery equation. DO_2, delivery of oxygen (mL/min); CO, cardiac output (L/min); HR, heart rate; SV, stroke volume (mL); CaO_2, oxygen-carrying capacity of the blood (mL/dL; multiplication by 10 adjusts this to mL/L); Hb, haemoglobin (g/L); SpO_2, oxygen saturations (%); PaO_2, partial pressure of oxygen (kPa); 1.39, oxygen-binding capacity of Hb per gram; 0.003, amount of dissolved oxygen in the blood (0.003 mL of oxygen gas is dissolved in 100 mL of blood).

Source: Theophilus Samuels.

You decide to establish cardiac output monitoring. Standing at the bedside and using a 50 mL syringe connected to the central venous catheter, you administer a warmed 250 mL crystalloid fluid bolus while observing the monitors. Susan's stroke volume variation (SVV) decreases from 24% to 18% and her systolic blood pressure increases from 92 to 96 mmHg. You administer three further fluid boluses. The SVV is now 11% and you reduce the noradrenaline to 0.47 mcg/kg/min. The next arterial blood gas shows gas exchange is unchanged, but the metabolic acidosis is ongoing with a base deficit of −7.5 mmol/L (lactate 2.9 mmol/L). Her saturations are holding despite the fluid challenge, but you leave instructions to maintain a PEEP of at least 10 cmH$_2$O until gas exchange has improved.

Should you instigate renal replacement therapy? What is the evidence for 'early' vs 'late' renal replacement therapy?

Susan has been in intensive care for a relatively short period of time. On arrival, assuming her previous renal function was normal, there was blood panel evidence of an acute kidney injury. She has now had decreased urine output for the last few hours.

There is no strong evidence to support early renal replacement therapy and no real consensus on what constitutes 'early' or 'late' in this context. The AKIKI, ELAIN and IDEAL-ICU trials gave conflicting results. However, they asked subtly different questions, with substantial differences in study design making meta-analysis difficult. As with many clinical problems in critical care, the best guidance remains to assess the individual patient and use clinical judgement as to how to proceed.

You decide to insert a VasCath™ now and review Susan's progress over the next few hours. If her urine output remains poor despite optimising fluids and vasopressor support, you will commence continuous venovenous haemofiltration tonight considering the likelihood that she will continue to deteriorate. Significant acidosis may impair cardiac contractility, shift the oxyhaemoglobin dissociation curve, increase pulmonary vascular resistance and impair enzyme function. Although her acidosis has a significant respiratory component, by correcting the metabolic component you will be better able to tolerate hypercapnia and continue lung protective ventilation.

What is the evidence for starting steroids?

In contrast to several earlier studies, one meta-analysis (Wu WF et al., Am J Emerg Med, 2018) suggests that use of glucocorticoids in severe CAP may reduce both the risk of in-hospital mortality and the length of hospital stay.

Steroids have also been used in critical care for a presumed positive impact on haemodynamic instability, reducing dose and duration of vasopressor requirement. However, steroids continue to be a contentious topic within critical care, with conflicting evidence regarding their use in ARDS, sepsis and in conjunction with high-dose vasopressors. It also remains unclear as to whether glucocorticoids should be given as bolus doses or as an infusion.

Surviving Sepsis guidelines (2021) suggest commencing treatment with hydrocortisone in septic shock requiring noradrenaline ≥0.25 mcg/kg/min for at least 4 hours.

> In your department, steroids tend be used when there is refractory septic shock. You prescribe 50 mg intravenous hydrocortisone QDS.
>
> You return an hour later to review the effects of your interventions. The arterial blood gas is as follows: pH 7.12, PaO_2 6.5 kPa, $PaCO_2$ 10.5 kPa, base excess −7.2 mmol/L, lactate 4.7 mmol/L.

What are the rescue methods for critical hypoxaemia in severe ARDS?

In addition to manipulating the relevant ventilator settings to optimise oxygenation (i.e. PEEP, FiO_2 and inspiratory:expiratory ratio), and considering neuromuscular blockade, the following techniques may be used:

- *Prone positioning* – this technique has more supporting evidence than the others listed below. Some of the trial data is conflicting but the weight of evidence is in favour of prone positioning being beneficial in ARDS. Of note, the PROSEVA Trial (Geurin et al., NEJM 2013) showed a significant mortality benefit in severe ARDS.
- *Airway Pressure Release Ventilation (APRV)* – APRV has some small supporting trial evidence but is yet to be evaluated in a large multicentre trial.
- *Extracorporeal membrane oxygenation* – there is some evidence to support the use of ECMO in ARDS, but this is an extremely invasive technique. The large intravascular cannulae and need for aggressive anticoagulation can lead to complications. In addition, there is limited availability of ECMO as it is only performed in a small number of centres throughout the UK.
- *High-frequency oscillatory ventilation (HFOV)* – two trials examining HFOV were published in the *New England Journal of Medicine* in 2013 (OSCAR and OSCILLATE). One showed no difference in mortality and one showed increased mortality. Since then, HFOV is less commonly used in adult patients.
- *Inhaled pulmonary vasodilators* – inhaled nitric oxide and aerosolised prostacyclin are sometimes used in rescue therapy. Study data is limited and equivocal.
- *Recruitment manoeuvres* – various methods have been proposed (e.g. staircase recruitment manoeuvre) to deliver this 'open lung' strategy. There is no strong supporting evidence. In fact, the ART trial (2017) found an increase in mortality associated with the use of recruitment manoeuvres. Recruitment manoeuvres should be used with caution and only performed in selected patients by experienced clinicians.

You decide to place Susan in the prone position and ask the nurses to prepare for haemofiltration.

How do you achieve prone positioning?

- *Assemble the team* – one airway trained doctor at the head and six other trained members of staff to assist (depending upon local protocol).
- *Staff should wear appropriate personal protective equipment (PPE)* including eye protection.
- *Ensure all lines and tubes are secured* and gathered towards either Susan's head or her feet.
- *Ensure there is plenty of padding* ready which will support and cushion potential pressure areas and allow the abdomen to remain free.
- *Stop NG feed and aspirate the NG tube.*
- *Give a bolus dose of paralysing agent and use the 'Cornish pasty' method to prone Susan* – a sheet beneath the patient and another over the top are rolled tightly together to allow the patient to be turned prone in a controlled manner. Multiple pillows are used to ensure the abdomen is free and pressure points are protected.

How does prone positioning improve oxygenation?

- Improved ventilation/perfusion matching with increased blood flow to the dependant lung.
- Increased functional residual capacity (FRC).
- Reduced atelectasis.
- More uniform distribution of plateau pressure.
- Redistribution of transpulmonary pressure with a possible reduction of right ventricle afterload.
- Increased secretion drainage.

Once Susan is safely in the prone position, what is your plan for her ongoing management at this stage (in addition to haemofiltration)?

- Prone position management should include setting ventilator parameters and instructions on how long the patient should remain prone.
  - If patient is stable, remain prone for 16 hours.
  - Check ABG after 1 hour, looking for improvement in oxygenation.
  - Regular pressure point assessment and 4 hourly alternating movement of arms and head in the 'swimmer's position'.
  - Regular suctioning.
  - Aim for lung protective ventilation with high PEEP. Use neuromuscular blockade if necessary. Consider using APRV in conjunction with prone position.

- Call the ICU consultant to discuss potential referral for ECMO.
- Ensure critical care 'housekeeping' is maintained, e.g. consider NG tube position and feed, thromboprophylaxis, glucose control and stress ulcer prophylaxis.
- Further imaging could include CT chest, but Susan is not stable enough.
- Request a formal echocardiogram when she is in the supine position.
- Call Susan's family to update them regarding a change in her condition. She is married with two small children and is very close to her three siblings.

Your consultant has just arrived in the hospital and performs bedside cardiac and lung ultrasound (limited by position). The consultant calls the regional ECMO referral centre who would like to take Susan but unfortunately, they do not have any beds available right now. They will call you in the morning but advise to keep Susan in the prone position in the meantime. The APACHE II score is 23 and the SOFA score is 10.

What is the likely outcome in this case?

Susan has a severe community-acquired pneumonia. Her CURB-65 (Confusion, Uraemia, Respiratory rate, Blood pressure and Age >65) score was 4 on admission, placing her in the highest risk group with a 30-day mortality predicted risk of 27.8%. Her APACHE II score gives her an approximate mortality of 40%. Her SOFA score gives her a mortality of 40–50%. Whichever scoring system is used, Susan has a significant chance of dying in critical care. This should be communicated to the next of kin with support for the family and safeguarding for the children offered if necessary.

Besides sepsis and multiorgan failure, what are some possible complications of pneumonia?

- Pleural effusion
- Empyema
- Lung abscess
- Pulmonary fibrosis

After 4 days in your ICU, Susan starts to show significant improvement. She is extubated on her fifth day of admission. She is discharged to a general medical ward 2 days later and goes home after 3 weeks in hospital. Her follow-up chest radiograph at 6 weeks is clear and she plans to return to work. She is invited for respiratory outpatient review and seen in the ICU follow-up clinic.

Further reading

■ Arnal, J. (2018). *Monitoring Mechanical Ventilation using Ventilator Waveforms*. Cham: Springer. Useful textbook exploring the details of ventilator waveforms.

■ Kallet, R. (2015). A comprehensive review of prone position in ARDS. *Respir. Care* 60 (11): 1660–1687. A useful review article looking at prone position prior to COVID-19.

■ Cilloniz, C., Torres, A., and Niederman, M. (2021). Management of pneumonia in critically ill patients. *BMJ* 375: e065871. State-of-the-art review (from the USA).

■ Slutsky, A. and Villar, J. (2019). Early paralytic agents for ARDS? Yes, no and sometimes. *N. Engl. J. Med.* 380: 2061–2063. Editorial on neuromuscular blockade in ARDS.

9 The Patient with Chest Pain

You attend an emergency call in your hospital's acute medical unit during daytime hours. On arrival, a 34-year-old female patient named Grace appears tachypnoeic (respiratory rate 30 breaths per minute) with oxygen saturations of 96% on 15 L/min oxygen therapy. She is tachycardic at 110 bpm with a blood pressure of 120/70 mmHg. She is pyrexial with a temperature of 38 °C. Grace is alert and able to answer questions appropriately but finds it difficult to complete sentences due to breathing difficulties. She complains of left-sided chest pain that came on abruptly (which is affecting her ability to take deep breaths) and a swollen left calf that is painful on palpation. Measures to stabilise Grace have already been initiated.

What could be the most likely causes of deterioration in this case?

Possible causes using a system-based approach include the following:

- *Respiratory* – pneumonia, pulmonary embolism, acute asthma exacerbation, spontaneous pneumothorax.
- *Cardiovascular* – acute myocardial infarction, aortic dissection, anaphylaxis, sickle chest crisis.
- *Musculoskeletal* – trauma (e.g. rib fractures).
- *Gastrointestinal* – perforated viscus, acute pancreatitis.

Given that Grace is presenting with dyspnoea, pleuritic chest pain of sudden onset, tender calf on palpation, tachypnoea, tachycardia and pyrexia, you have a high clinical suspicion that this is an acute pulmonary embolism (PE).

What are the principles of management of acute PE?

The key components of managing an acute PE involve making sure that stabilising measures are occurring at the same time as clinical evaluation

Clinical Cases in Critical Care, First Edition. Alice Myers and Theophilus Samuels.
© 2023 John Wiley & Sons Ltd. Published 2023 by John Wiley & Sons Ltd.

and diagnostic tests. It is recommended that these patients are stratified into two categories:

- Haemodynamically *stable*.
- Haemodynamically *unstable*.

How do we define haemodynamic instability in acute high-risk pulmonary embolism?

- *Cardiac arrest.*
- *Obstructive shock* – SBP <90 mmHg or vasopressors required to achieve a SBP ≥90 mmHg despite adequate fluid resuscitation and evidence of end-organ perfusion.
- *Persistent hypotension* – SBP <90 mmHg or SBP decrease ≥40 mmHg that lasts longer than 15 minutes and is not caused by new-onset arrhythmia, hypovolaemia or sepsis.

At present, Grace appears haemodynamically *stable*, so you continue with your assessment. She tells you that she has recently been confirmed antiphospholipid antibody positive after being investigated for three miscarriages over the past 12 months. Her urine pregnancy test is confirmed as negative.

How might the presence of antiphospholipid antibodies be relevant to her presentation?

The development of venous and/or arterial thromboses together with pregnancy morbidity (e.g. recurrent foetal losses) are in keeping with an antiphospholipid syndrome (APS). APS is an acquired risk factor for venous thromboembolism (VTE). This therefore supports your suspicion that PE is the most likely cause for her current clinical presentation. Of note, the Euro-Phospholipid Project (2002) described the baseline characteristics of 1000 patients with APS and found that 38.9% presented with DVT and 14.1% with PE.

What other risk factors increase your risk for VTE?

- *Genetic risk factors* – protein C and S deficiency, antithrombin III deficiency, factor V Leiden mutation.
- *Acquired risk factors* – age, obesity, previous VTE, malignancy, vasculitis, pregnancy, hormone replacement therapy, oral contraceptives.
- *ICU-related risk factors* – prolonged immobility (e.g. mechanical ventilation, paralysis, sedative drugs), femoral venous catheters, and inappropriate dosage or lack of thromboprophylaxis.

Which blood tests could aid in diagnosing PE?

- *Arterial blood gas* – hypoxaemia in the presence of a normal chest radiograph should prompt consideration for PE. However, PaO_2 is normal in approximately 14–24% of patients. An increased alveolar-arterial (A-a) gradient is present in at least 60% of patients and decreased carbon dioxide levels with respiratory alkalosis in approximately 40%. Increased arterial carbon dioxide levels can occur with large PEs due to increased dead space.

- *Serum D-dimer levels* – this is a measure of degradation products from cross-linked fibrin. Where levels are measured as normal in patients with low probability of PE, additional diagnostic testing is not necessary as it is recognised that the frequency of VTE is not increased in the subsequent 3 months.
- *Troponin I or T* – levels are elevated in 30–60% of patients with acute PE. Elevated troponin concentration is associated with an increased risk of mortality in both unselected patients and haemodynamically stable patients at presentation. High-sensitivity troponin T assays have a high negative predictive value for excluding an adverse in-hospital clinical outcome.
- *B-type natriuretic peptide (BNP) and N-terminal (NT)-proBNP* – released in response to increased myocardial stretch, plasma levels of BNP and NT-proBNP reflect the severity of RV dysfunction and haemodynamic compromise in acute PE. These biomarkers are useful for excluding an unfavourable early clinical outcome, with high sensitivity and a negative predictive value.

Which electrocardiogram (ECG) abnormalities might be found in PE?

Patients presenting with PE tend to have non-specific findings and up to 70% will present with tachycardia and non-specific ST segment and T-wave changes. The classic S1Q3T3 pattern (S wave lead I, Q wave and inverted T wave in lead III) and new incomplete right bundle branch block occur in less than 10% of patients.

Which ECG abnormalities are associated with a poor prognosis in patients diagnosed with PE?

- Tachycardia (>100 bpm).
- New and complete right bundle branch block.
- Atrial arrhythmias (e.g. atrial fibrillation).
- ST elevation in aVR.
- S1Q3T3 pattern.
- Anterior ST segment changes and T-wave inversion.

What is the rationale for ordering a chest radiograph?

The main indication is to investigate other causes for this presentation. The most common findings are non-specific, such as pleural effusion and atelectasis. Chest radiograph may appear normal in up to one-fifth of patients.

Which imaging modality is considered the 'gold standard' for diagnosing PE?

Computed tomography pulmonary angiography (CTPA) is the most sensitive and specific diagnostic imaging modality for detecting PE, especially when utilised as part of PE diagnostic protocols.

What are the advantages and disadvantages of performing a CTPA in patients with suspected PE?

Advantages

- High diagnostic accuracy for suspected PE.
- The ability to diagnose other diseases that may be present.
- Widely available technology in developed countries.

Disadvantages

- Potentially dangerous intrahospital transfer in very unwell patients.
- No immediate access to patient during scan.
- Potential for anaphylaxis to occur with the use of IV contrast agents.
- Large amount of ionising radiation used.
- Potential to worsen renal impairment through use of IV contrast.

In which circumstances might a CTPA result be indeterminate?

- Artefact (e.g. from patient movement, metallic foreign bodies, equipment leads).
- Abnormal cardiac output leading to suboptimal enhancement of the pulmonary artery and its branches.
- Morbid obesity/body habitus.

Which pretest probability scores are used for PE?

The most accepted and widely used systems are the Wells criteria and modified Wells criteria. These are calculated by adding the clinical risk variables together to determine the pretest probability (Table 9.1). It is best validated for use in an outpatient setting in patients presenting with suspected PE and may not be as accurate in older patients. However, the concomitant use of a D-dimer assay, particularly in hospitalised patients, improves its specificity and sensitivity for diagnosing PE. This effectively rules out PE if the D-dimer is negative where the patient is considered low probability.

Table 9.1: The criteria and scoring systems for the Wells and modified Wells clinical probability assessments.

Criteria	Score (points)
Clinical symptoms of DVT (e.g. leg swelling, pain on palpation)	3.0
Other diagnoses less likely than PE	3.0
Tachycardia (>100)	1.5
Immobilisation (>3 d) or surgery in the previous 4 weeks	1.5
Previous DVT/PE	1.5
Haemoptysis	1.0
Malignancy	1.0
Wells criteria – clinical probability assessment	*Total score*
High	>6.0
Moderate	2.0–6.0
Low	<2.0
Modified Wells criteria – simplified clinical probability assessment	*Total score*
PE likely	>4.0
PE unlikely	<4.0

DVT, deep vein thrombosis; PE, pulmonary embolism.

Using the Wells criteria, what would be the probability that Grace has developed a PE?

You suspect that PE is the most plausible diagnosis in your list of differentials, giving her a score of 3.0. Her clinical symptoms (e.g. pain on calf palpation with leg swelling) give her a score of 3.0. The tachycardia greater than 100 bpm scores 1.5, giving her a total score of 7.5. This suggests Grace has a high probability of having an acute PE using the standard Wells criteria and 'likely' using the modified version.

What role does echocardiography have in the work-up for diagnosing PE?

In suspected high-risk PE patients with haemodynamic instability, should echocardiography fail to demonstrate RV overload or dysfunction then this practically excludes PE as the cause. Instead, in these cases, echocardiography can further aid in diagnosing other pathologies such as acute valvular dysfunction or severe left ventricle systolic impairment. However, RV overload and dysfunction can still be found in the absence of acute PE.

The interpretation of transthoracic echocardiography (TTE) can be hindered by poor-quality images, especially when focusing on the right side of the heart. Nevertheless, the extent of RV dysfunction is directly correlated with the degree of perfusion defects on lung scans.

Echocardiography findings include the following (Figure 9.1):

- Decreased RV regional and longitudinal function.
- Increased RV chamber size – found in ≥25% patients.
- Tricuspid regurgitation.
- Abnormal septal wall motion – may indicate RV pressure overload.
- McConnell's sign – this is where the RV mid free wall becomes dyskinetic, with relative sparing of the apex and the base.
- Mobile thrombus located within the right heart cavities – associated with high mortality.
- Distended non-collapsible inferior vena cava.
- '60/60' sign describes the simultaneous finding of a right ventricular outflow tract (RVOT) acceleration time <60 ms with a midsystolic notch and an estimated pulmonary artery systolic pressure <60 mmHg (which is estimated from the tricuspid regurgitant jet velocity).

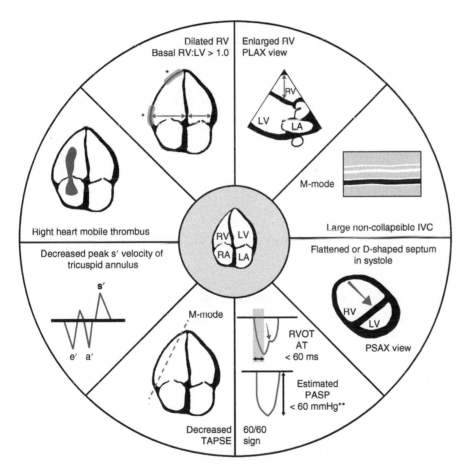

Figure 9.1: Potential echocardiography findings in acute PE. RV = right ventricle, LV = left ventricle, LA = left atrium, RA = right atrium, PLAX = parasternal longitudinal axis view, s' = peak systolic velocity of tricuspid annulus (normal 9–17 cm/s in females), e' = peak early diastolic velocity of tricuspid annulus, a' = peak late diastolic velocity of tricuspid annulus, TAPSE = tricuspid annulus plane systolic excursion (normal≥17 mm), RVOT AT = right ventricular outflow tract acceleration time (orange shaded area; normal>130 ms), PASP = pulmonary artery systolic pressure, PSAX = parasternal short axis view, IVC = inferior vena cava, midsystolic notch (red arrow), * McConnell's sign – RV mid free wall becomes dyskinetic, with relative sparing of the apex and the base (green shaded areas), ** estimated from peak tricuspid regurgitant jet velocity (normal <2.8 m/s).

Source: Theophilus Samuels.

What is the association between right ventricle dysfunction and prognosis in PE?

When right ventricle dysfunction (RVD) is present, mortality and embolic-related adverse events are increased. The mortality rates for patients presenting with shock and severe RVD approach 65%. In haemodynamically stable patients with PE and evidence of RVD, mortality rates are between 8% and 14%. Mortality rates are less than 3% for patients with PE and no evidence of RVD.

What other factors are associated with poor outcome in patients with PE?

The ICOPER study demonstrated that the following clinical features were significant independent predictors of 3-month mortality:

- Age over 70 years.
- Malignancy.
- Congestive heart failure.
- Chronic obstructive pulmonary disease.
- Hypotension.
- Tachypnoea.
- RV hypokinesis.

Which presenting clinical feature is considered the most influential predictor of outcome?

In the same ICOPER study, the investigators found that hypotension (systolic blood pressure <90 mmHg) was identified as the most influential predictor of outcome at 3 months.

Grace's condition begins to deteriorate, and she appears drowsy. She now has a sustained hypotension (80/40 mmHg) despite receiving fluid boluses over the past 20 minutes. Focused echocardiography confirms the presence of a dilated right ventricle with impaired systolic function. Her arterial blood gas demonstrates a pH of 7.0, PaO_2 6 kPa, $PaCO_2$ 11 kPa, HCO_3 11 mmol/L, lactate 7.4 mmol/L, K^+ 5.1 mmol/L. The D-dimer assay is positive. The chest radiograph appears normal.

What are your immediate concerns?

Grace's condition has now deteriorated considerably, and she is clearly haemodynamically unstable. She requires mechanical ventilation with vasopressor support (it is important to remember that mechanical ventilation may only minimally improve oxygenation due to V/Q mismatch).

Given her deterioration, following discussion with your consultant, you decide to intubate and mechanically ventilate Grace with support from your anaesthetic colleagues.

Briefly outline the steps you should consider before, during and after you perform intubation of her trachea

Before

- Explain to the next of kin why this intervention is needed, ideally prior to induction or as soon as possible. Inform them that it is not without risk given how unwell Grace has become and could potentially result in death.
- As this is an emergency, it is not possible to transfer her to a 'safer' environment (e.g. theatres) and so this will effectively be a 'remote site' induction. Ensure thorough preparation as per Introduction Section 2.
- Consider obtaining intra-arterial blood pressure monitoring prior to induction. This should not delay intubation and if it is not possible then you should allocate a member of your team to manually palpate a central pulse continuously (e.g. femoral artery).

During

- Expect further haemodynamic instability, so adjust induction agents and doses accordingly.

After

- Once Grace is intubated, ensure that the respiratory plateau pressures are not high as this may worsen right-sided cardiac impairment leading to deleterious hypotension.

> Following uneventful intubation, Grace is placed on mechanical ventilation with the aim of avoiding high plateau pressures. A central line is sited, and a noradrenaline infusion rapidly rises to 0.6 mcg/kg/min. After 30 minutes following induction, her BP remains low at 85/40 mmHg, SpO_2 is between 90% and 92% (FiO_2 1.0), and she is now more tachycardic at 130 bpm. She is receiving minimal sedation to tolerate the endotracheal tube. On clinical examination and bedside lung ultrasound, there is no evidence of a pneumothorax.

What do you think is most probably going on at this point?

Grace remains haemodynamically unstable despite resuscitative efforts and has most likely suffered a *massive PE* given the hypotension, hypoxaemia and right ventricular dysfunction. The initial cardiac depressant effects of your induction agents may also play a part in any postintubation hypotension. However, she was already persistently hypotensive prior to induction, and adequate time has now passed since they were administered, so the induction agents and ongoing sedation are unlikely to be a significant contributing factor at this point.

Do you think it is safe to transfer Grace for a CTPA at this point?

At present, she is intubated, ventilated and requires vasopressor support to improve tissue perfusion. She most likely has a life-threatening massive PE. Her condition may deteriorate even further despite your interventions, so in these circumstances intrahospital transfer is not without risk. Ultimately, obtaining a CTPA is a risk-versus-benefit decision and requires senior input and discussion. Although CTPA would not be entirely necessary to confirm the diagnosis, it would be useful for ongoing management decisions (e.g. to rule out other causes such as acute aortic dissection).

> Following discussion with your consultant, you and your anaesthetic colleagues take Grace to the CT scanner on the way to ICU. Scan confirms a massive PE with evidence of RV dysfunction.

What are your main treatment priorities at this point?

The administration of potentially life-saving therapies should be instigated:

- *Thrombolysis* – the use of thrombolytic agents is a widely accepted treatment for patients with PE presenting with or developing haemodynamic instability. The greatest benefit is seen when thrombolysis is given within 48 hours of symptom onset. Thrombolysis can still be beneficial in patients who have had symptoms for 6–14 days if deemed appropriate. In patients who have a high risk of bleeding, or who have had one failed attempt at thrombolysis, or who will probably die before thrombolysis can effectively lyse the clot, the use of catheter-directed thrombus removal with or without thrombolysis can be considered if this service is available on site. Thrombolysis is deemed unsuccessful if clinical instability persists and after 36 hours RV dysfunction remains unchanged on echocardiography.
- *Embolectomy* – in patients who have clear contraindications to thrombolysis, the emboli can be removed surgically or using a catheter. However, not all centres can offer this intervention so an interhospital transfer may be required (particularly if a surgical option is warranted as this requires an experienced surgeon and cardiopulmonary bypass). Surgery allows both diagnostic and therapeutic interventions to be applied simultaneously and it remains an option for those patients where thrombolysis has failed. Surgical embolectomy carries high mortality, particularly in elderly patients, and evidence suggests that there may be no difference in 30-day mortality between surgical embolectomy and thrombolytic therapy.

Describe the absolute and relative contraindications to thrombolysis

Absolute

- Ischaemic CVA within 3 months.
- Known malignant intracranial neoplasm.
- Known structural intracranial cerebrovascular disease.
- Prior intracranial haemorrhage.

- Suspected aortic dissection.
- Active bleeding.
- Recent spinal or neurosurgery.
- Recent significant closed head or facial trauma.

Relative

- Age greater than 75 years.
- Anticoagulant therapy.
- Pregnancy.
- Recent internal bleeding.
- CPR > 10 minutes.
- Dementia.
- Major surgery within 3 weeks.
- History of CVA within 3 months.

The decision is made to administer a thrombolytic agent.

Which thrombolytic agent(s) can be used in PE?

Drugs used in the treatment of PE include the following (https://bnf.nice.org.uk accessed 1 October 2022):

- *Recombinant tissue-type plasminogen activator or rtPA (alteplase)* – an initial 10 mg bolus over 1–2 minutes is given, followed by a 90 mg intravenous infusion over 2 hours. It is recommended for patients under 65 kg that the maximum dose does not exceed 1.5 mg/kg.
- *Streptokinase* – a dose of 250 000 units is given over 30 minutes, then 100 000 units every 1 hour for 24 hours. Alternatively, a dose of 1 500 000 units can be given over 1–2 hours.
- *Urokinase* – a loading dose of 4400 units/kg is given over 10–20 minutes, followed by 4400 units/kg/h for 12 hours.

Ensure that you check with your local hospital formulary regarding drugs, doses and administration protocols.

Describe the major advantages and disadvantages of thrombolytic therapy in acute PE

Advantages

- *Haemodynamics* – short-term improvements occur in pulmonary arterial blood pressure, RV function (e.g. reduced RV afterload) and pulmonary perfusion. It is not yet established if these short-term improvements persist beyond the initial stages, as the current evidence is equivocal.
- *Accessibility* – this treatment is widely available and easy to administer.

Disadvantages

- *Bleeding* – compared to anticoagulant therapy (e.g. heparin), systemic thrombolytic therapy increases the risk of major bleeding and intracranial haemorrhage. However, in high-risk patients (i.e. with cardiogenic shock), the benefit of thrombolysis in reducing the combined outcome of mortality and recurrent PE appears to outweigh the risk of bleeding (9.9% rate of severe bleeding and 1.7% rate of intracranial haemorrhage).

> Thrombolytic therapy is administered to Grace. She is fully ventilated and on vasopressor support (noradrenaline 0.1 mcg/kg/min) to maintain a mean arterial pressure between 60 and 65 mmHg.

Is there any role for pulmonary vasodilators in the treatment of PE?

The theoretical advantage of dilating the pulmonary vasculature to reduce RV afterload is enticing. However, at present, there are no large randomised controlled trials involving pulmonary vasodilators (e.g. nitric oxide, epoprostenol) in the management of PE and so their use is not currently recommended.

> Grace continues to improve over the next 72 hours, and formal echocardiography demonstrates a marked improvement in her right ventricular function.

What are the early and late complications associated with PE?

Early complications that can occur within 3 months include the following:

- *Haemodynamic collapse/cardiogenic shock* – the greatest risk of death from hypotension is within the first 2 hours of presentation and therefore early consideration of thrombolytic therapy as opposed to anticoagulation only is essential. Patients who present with hypotension, or develop hypotension subsequently, remain at high risk of death for up to 72 hours and are therefore best cared for within a high-dependency or intensive care setting (particularly if RV dysfunction is present).
- *Recurrence* – patients remain at risk of recurrence for at least 2 weeks after the initial presentation. The risk gradually decreases to around 6% at 3 months. Recurrence is more likely if the patient is concurrently diagnosed with malignancy and is unable to maintain anticoagulation at therapeutic levels.
- *Stroke* – the presence of a patent foramen ovale (PFO) in a patient with acute PE is thought to increase their risk of stroke. If neurological symptoms consistent with stroke develop then appropriate investigations for a PFO should be undertaken if feasible.

Late complications include the following:

- *Recurrence* – the risk of further PE events is lowered with the effective use of anticoagulation but remains increased in the presence of risk factors such as malignancy.

- *Death* – current evidence suggests that when patients with PE are compared to matched controls, there is a threefold increase in mortality at 30 years. It is important to note that most of these deaths may be due to other causes such as malignancy, sepsis, myocardial infarction, heart failure and stroke.
- *Chronic thromboembolic pulmonary hypertension (CTEPH)* – this unusual complication presents with shortness of breath and reduced exercise tolerance within 2 years after the initial event. Additionally, patients may present with symptoms of RV dysfunction such as peripheral oedema or exertional chest pain.
- *Cardiovascular* – there is an associated increase in subsequent development of atrial fibrillation and cardiovascular events.

Grace is successfully extubated on day 5 and subsequently discharged to the ward under the care of the respiratory team.

Further reading

- Konstantinides, S., Meyer, G., Becattini, C. et al. (2020). 2019 ESC guidelines for the diagnosis and management of acute pulmonary embolism developed in collaboration with the European Respiratory Society (ERS). The task force for the diagnosis and Management of Acute Pulmonary Embolism of the European Society of Cardiology (ESC). *Eur. Heart J.* 41: 543–603. Comprehensive guideline on several key aspects associated with managing patients with acute pulmonary embolism and includes excellent descriptions of right ventricle pathology.

10 The Out-of-Hospital Cardiac Arrest Patient

You are called to the emergency department during your nightshift. You find the ED team preparing for the arrival of a 68-year-old male patient named Gary. He has suffered an out-of-hospital cardiac arrest (OHCA). Gary was found collapsed on the toilet by his wife at approximately 01:00 am. She managed to provide 10 minutes of basic life support whilst waiting for the paramedic team to arrive. The paramedics have intubated his trachea and have provided 30 minutes of continuous CPR prior to return of spontaneous circulation (ROSC). The initial rhythm was shockable (ventricular fibrillation), and Gary received 6 DC shocks. He is en route to the ED.

How can we define cardiac arrest?

Cardiac arrest is defined as the sudden loss of cardiac function resulting in the cessation of effective circulation (confirmed by an absent palpable pulse) which may be reversible by rapid medical intervention. Delayed or inadequate intervention significantly lowers the chances of survival and increases the risk of permanent neurological/psychological damage. The absence of medical intervention will result in death.

What is the chain of survival?

The UK Resuscitation Council describes the chain of survival as a sequence of events, or 'links', that when performed equally well maximises the chances of survival for cardiac arrest patients:

- Immediate recognition of cardiac arrest and calling for help (first link).
- Prompt initiation of effective CPR (second link).
- Performing defibrillation as early as possible (third link).
- Optimising postresuscitation care (fourth link).

Clinical Cases in Critical Care, First Edition. Alice Myers and Theophilus Samuels.
© 2023 John Wiley & Sons Ltd. Published 2023 by John Wiley & Sons Ltd.

What are the approximate survival rates for OHCA in the UK?

It is estimated that fewer than 1 in 10 cases of OHCA in the UK survive to return home. Neurological and functional recovery varies considerably amongst survivors (e.g. ranging from being able to lead a normal life to permanent coma or vegetative state).

How could you classify the causes of OHCA?

Classifying OHCA into cardiac and non-cardiac events (NCEs), one population-based observational case series demonstrated that NCEs were the cause of 62.5% of deaths. Causes could be categorised using the acronym OOHCAS as follows:

- **O**bstructive – pulmonary embolism (PE), cardiac tamponade.
- **O**xygen ('hypoxia') – asthma, acute worsening of chronic obstructive pulmonary disease (COPD), airway obstruction and submersion.
- **H**ypovolaemia – major haemorrhage (trauma, gastrointestinal bleeding, acute aortic dissection).
- **C**erebrovascular disease – stroke, acute intracranial haemorrhage.
- **A**naphylaxis ('distributive').
- **S**epsis.

For identifying and treating reversible causes during a cardiac arrest scenario, the UK Resuscitation Council advises using the 4Hs and 4Ts aide-mémoire:

- **Hypovolaemia**
- **Hypoxia**
- **Hypo/hyperthermia**
- **Hypo/hyperkalaemia**
- **Tension pneumothorax**
- **Tamponade** – cardiac
- **Thrombosis** – cardiac or pulmonary
- **Toxins**

While you are waiting for the ambulance to arrive, the ED registrar suggests you should prepare to thrombolyse the patient.

What is the evidence surrounding thrombolysis in cardiac arrest?

For thrombolysis

- A meta-analysis in 2006, which examined one prospective and seven retrospective cohort studies, found that thrombolysis during CPR can significantly increase the chances of ROSC as it can improve/re-establish blood flow in occluded coronary arteries. Seven of the studies used tissue plasminogen activator (tPA) and one used recombinant tPA, along with either heparin, aspirin or heparin/aspirin for anticoagulation. As expected, the risk of severe bleeding (defined as life-threatening or bleeding that requires transfusion) was higher in the thrombolysis group. However, there was no clear evidence that a secondary bleed could result in death. The risk of bleeding may also have been theoretically lower due to the inherent survival bias in this cohort of patients (e.g. increased bleeding risk in those receiving thrombolysis because of their increased survival rate).

Against thrombolysis

■ In the double-blind, multicentre Thrombolysis in Cardiac Arrest trial (TROICA, 2008), the use of tenecteplase did not result in an improvement in outcome when compared with placebo. The trial was prematurely terminated for futility after enrolling 1050 patients and the incidence of intracranial haemorrhage was higher in the treatment group. This trial did not conclusively answer this question due to limitations regarding its selection criteria and was criticised for the deliberate avoidance of using aspirin and/or heparin for anticoagulation.

Should we perform immediate coronary angiography in all patients after cardiac arrest?

Coronary angiography (CA) is recommended in survivors of OHCA with ST segment elevation, with the potential for percutaneous coronary intervention. However, the benefit of CA in non-ST segment elevation remains unclear. It is important not to delay other postresuscitative modalities if these facilities are not immediately available or will take an inappropriate time to put in place.

The paramedics hand over and state that Gary is an active and generally fit individual. His past medical history includes treated hypertension and hypercholesterolaemia. He is intubated and being ventilated with a tidal volume of 500 mL at a respiratory rate of 12 breaths per minute. He is making no spontaneous respiratory efforts. Monitoring shows a HR of 100 bpm, pulse oximetry 99% on 100% oxygen and a BP of 100/50 mmHg.

While you are examining Gary, the ECG trace and invasive blood pressure flatline and the capnography trace falls to zero. You immediately perform a central pulse check and declare he is in cardiac arrest. Your team commences standard adult ALS measures according to the UK Resuscitation Council guidelines.

Describe how echocardiography can help in the management of cardiac arrest

The 10-second pulse check provides an opportunity for focused echocardiography to be performed by an experienced practitioner. It can help to determine the following:

■ *Ventricular fibrillation* (VF) – fine VF can, on occasion, be mistaken for asystole and can be detected by focused echocardiography. This can potentially avoid delays in defibrillation.

- *Hypovolaemia* – generally, the presence of a small, underfilled left ventricle with a totally collapsed inferior vena cava suggests the need for aggressive fluid resuscitation and a search for the cause.
- *Tamponade* – demonstrating a pericardial effusion should lead to the consideration of immediate drainage as the characteristic findings of tamponade may not be present during cardiac arrest. Current evidence (class I) suggests that pericardiocentesis should be performed under ultrasound guidance, as this significantly reduces the risk of complications with experienced operators.
- *Pulmonary embolism* – right ventricular dysfunction (in the absence of left ventricular disease or known pulmonary disease) suggests PE is possible. On rare occasions, demonstrating thrombus in the right atrium or ventricle, pulmonary arteries or both can confirm the diagnosis.

Can you use focused echocardiography to prognosticate in cardiac arrest?

The complete absence of cardiac activity, 'cardiac standstill', as demonstrated on the focused subcostal echocardiography view, heralds an extremely poor prognosis. M-mode can be utilised in this instance to demonstrate zero movement of the myocardium and will resemble a 'barcode' appearance.

> Gary achieves ROSC after a further three cycles and three shocks for VF. He requires inotropic support to maintain his blood pressure. After a further period of stability, you safely transfer Gary to your critical care unit to establish postresuscitation management. You successfully insert a central venous catheter and arterial line. The arterial blood gas (FiO_2 1.0) demonstrates pH 6.9, PaO_2 55 kPa, $PaCO_2$ 7.1 kPa, HCO_3 8 mmol/L, base excess −20 mmol/L and lactate 15 mmol/L.

How would you interpret the ABG result?

The ABG clearly demonstrates a severe mixed metabolic and respiratory acidaemia – a common finding in patients presenting with OHCA. With effective mechanical ventilation, the initial severe hypercarbia associated with respiratory arrest, the $PaCO_2$, can be reduced (assuming adequate cardiac output). The decreased bicarbonate and large base deficit reflect the physiological buffer present in the patient's blood that aims to neutralise the increased hydrogen ions (acid) being produced. The increased lactate is mostly due to the increased anaerobic metabolism occurring in peripheral tissues. The high PaO_2 reflects hyperoxaemia, especially given the inspired oxygen fraction is 1.0.

What is the potential association between hyperoxaemia and cardiac arrest?

One systematic review and meta-analysis in 2018 examined 16 observational studies published between 2008 and 2017, which included a total of 40 573 adult patients. Six of these studies included patients with OHCA only, eight studies included patients with both OHCA and in-hospital cardiac arrest (IHCA) and the remaining two studies included IHCA patients only. The authors managed to quantitatively analyse 10 of these studies and determined that:

- Intra-arrest hyperoxaemia was associated with significantly *lower* mortality
- Postarrest hyperoxaemia was associated with a *higher* mortality.

Some of the studies in another systematic review on the effects of hyperoxaemia in acutely ill patients suffering cardiac arrest revealed no association between poor outcome and hyperoxaemia during CPR or in the first 24 hours after cardiac arrest. However, they also found that severe hyperoxaemia (defined as $PaO_2 > 39.9\,kPa$) appeared to be independently associated with increased in-hospital mortality.

Currently there is a low level of evidence describing the effect of hyperoxaemia on clinically relevant outcomes in OHCA. Hyperoxaemia during postresuscitation care may be associated with lower survival rates and poorer neurological outcomes.

Discuss the role of targeting hypothermia at 33 °C in OHCA comatose survivors?

The Targeted Temperature Management 2 (TTM 2) trial investigated 1850 comatose OHCA survivors from any initial rhythm. In short, they found that targeted hypothermia at 33 °C did *not* lead to a lower incidence of death compared to targeted normothermia (preventing body temperature >37.7 °C) at 6 months. The only intervention that is now recommended is the active treatment of pyrexia (>37.7 °C) during the initial 72 hours in OHCA patients who remain comatose.

What is the role of targeting MAP in OHCA comatose survivors?

Part of the Carbon dioxide, Oxygen and Mean arterial pressure After Cardiac Arrest and REsuscitation trial (COMACARE) looked at low-normal (65–75 mmHg) and high-normal (80–100 mmHg) groups. Researchers used neuron-specific enolase (NSE; discussed later) at 48 hours as the primary outcome. Neurological outcome at 6 months was one of the secondary outcomes. Targeting a specified level of blood pressure was possible once admitted to the ICU. They found that there was no difference between the two groups in terms of serum concentration of NSE or any of the secondary outcomes.

You decide to target a MAP of 75 mmHg for Gary. By day 3 of admission, Gary has not demonstrated any neurological signs of recovery despite being off sedation for over 24 hours. You meet with his wife and daughter to discuss his prognosis.

Which tests can we use to predict poor neurological outcome in OHCA survivors?

Prognostication should ideally be deferred until 72 hours after the arrest and when the patient is sedation free, normothermic and other causes of coma or paralysis have been corrected, where possible.

- *Pupillary light reflex (PLR)* – the absence of this reflex at ≥72 hours is a strong predictor of poor neurological outcome following cardiac arrest. It has a high specificity but low sensitivity. However, this test can be operator dependent and qualitative, which has led to some reservation about its reproducibility in neuroprognostication. One novel method using the PLR involves automated infrared pupillometry, which provides a quantitative measure of pupil size, PLR and constriction velocity. Recent studies suggest that this technique has both a higher specificity and sensitivity when compared to standard PLR measurement by clinicians.
- *Corneal reflex* – when the corneal reflex is bilaterally absent, this suggests a probably poor neurological outcome. However, due to this reflex being more prone than PLR to the residual effects of sedatives and muscle relaxants, it has a lower specificity and similarly low sensitivity.
- *Myoclonus* – poor neurological outcome is almost invariably associated with the development of status myoclonus (defined as continuous and generalised myoclonus >30 minutes) that occurs within the first 48 hours post cardiac arrest. Myoclonus should only be used in conjunction with other indices, and it is a less robust predictor than PLR. When present, it is recommended that an electroencephalogram (EEG) is performed to exclude other more benign forms of postanoxic myoclonus (e.g. Lance-Adams syndrome).
- *EEG* – in comatose patients, the identification of burst suppression and suppressed background (with or without periodic discharges) at a median time of 77 hours after ROSC predicted poor neurological outcome with 100% specificity and 50% sensitivity. Recent evidence suggests that when continuous EEG is performed within the first 24 hours following cardiac arrest, the presence of isoelectric, low-voltage or burst suppression with identical bursts can predict poor neurological outcome at 6 months. However, the sensitivity of these findings is low. EEG will also aid in ruling out postanoxic seizure activity in the comatose patient.
- *Bispectral index (BIS)* – this form of automated EEG analysis is used to monitor depth of anaesthesia. It has a maximum value of 100 in an awake patient to a minimal value of 0, which is equivalent to a flat EEG with no signal. It was recently demonstrated that if a total duration of BIS 0 was recorded for over 30 minutes, this predicted a poor neurological outcome with 100% specificity and >60% sensitivity.
- *Short-latency somatosensory evoked potentials (SSEPs)* – the bilateral absence of N20 (negative peak at 20 ms) SSEPs is among the most robust predictors to be tested at 72 hours post ROSC. It predicts poor

neurological outcome with high accuracy and precision. Like the other modalities, SSEPs suffer from having a low sensitivity (rarely above 50%). SSEPs are less affected by sedation than an EEG, but they are prone to electrical interference.

■ *Neuron specific enolase (NSE)* – this is a cell-specific isozyme of the glycolytic enzyme enolase and is highly specific for neurons and peripheral neuroendocrine cells. There are three isozymes of enolase, with enolase-gamma being neuron specific. NSE has been shown to provide quantitative measures of brain damage and/or improve the diagnosis and outcome of OHCA comatose survivors. NSE is not affected by hypothermia or sedation but is affected by haemolysis. High levels are necessary (>97 ng/mL) to give a 100% positive prediction value of poor outcome. This test is not routinely available, and it should be used in conjunction with other tests that can predict poor neurological outcome. Sampling at multiple time points (e.g. 24, 48 and 72 hours) is currently recommended to reduce the risk of a false-positive result, which can occur in the presence of neuroendocrine tumours and small cell carcinoma.

■ *Neurofilament light chain (NFL)* – at 24 hours, this novel biomarker was found to be a highly specific predictor of poor neurological outcome at 6 months. It has been shown to possess greater predictive value than NSE, brain CT, SSEPs, EEG and clinical examination.

■ *CT brain* – attenuation of the grey/white matter interface on CT suggests cerebral oedema and is one of the main findings for hypoxic-ischaemic brain injury. The ratio of grey to white matter densities (GWR) is used to prognosticate in these individuals. When performed within 24 hours following the event, a GWR <1.22 was found to predict in-hospital mortality with a 98% specificity but was not able to differentiate survivors with poor versus good outcome. Currently, there is no consensus on when to perform CT in survivors following cardiac arrest for neuroprognostication. The presence of generalised oedema without formal GWR measurement predicts poor neurological outcome (CPC 3–5) with very high specificity and low sensitivity within 24 hours from ROSC. Both the specificity and sensitivity increase further if these findings are also present from 24 hours to 7 days following ROSC.

■ *Magnetic resonance imaging (MRI)* – current guidelines suggest that MRI can be used for prognostication between 2 and 5 days after ROSC. Modern evidence suggests that it can even predict neurological outcome when performed within 3 hours after ROSC. However, the evidence for using MRI is prone to selection bias in prognostic studies as its use is limited in unstable patients post cardiac arrest. In addition, it is only recommended in combination with other predictive measures and in specialist centres.

It is important to remember that a multifaceted approach involving these investigations and clinical findings (e.g. organ failure) will allow for robust neuroprognostication in these potentially challenging situations.

Which findings, if any, might suggest a good neurological outcome?

Despite most of the work done to identify markers of poor neurological outcome, predictors of good neurological outcome have recently been recognised (they have yet to be included in any international guidelines).

- Presence of early EEG reactivity.
- Improvement of auditory discrimination (through analysis of EEG responses to auditory stimuli) from the first to the second day after ROSC.
- Absence of diffusion weighted imaging abnormalities on MRI within 1 week of ROSC.

Describe the Cerebral Performance Category Scale

The Cerebral Performance Category (CPC) Scale is used to assess neurological outcome in cardiac arrest survivors (Table 10.1).

Table 10.1: Cerebral performance categories (CPC).

Category	Comments
1	Good cerebral performance, is alert, able to work and lead a normal life, but may have a mild psychological or neurological deficit
2	Moderate cerebral disability but enough cerebral function for independent activities of daily life (e.g. use public transport). May be able to work in a sheltered environment
3	Severe cerebral disability, depends on others for daily support and may range from being ambulatory to paralysed, usually in an institution
4	Permanent coma or vegetative state
5	Certified brain dead or death

How does the CPC relate to long-term prognosis following cardiac arrest?

A review of over 300 patients treated at Columbia University Medical between 2008 and 2015 suggested that CPC at discharge was not predictive of clinical outcome. Approximately 50% of patients with mild to no neurological or psychological defect still had a poor outcome at 1 year.

Describe the modified Rankin Scale (mRS)

This aims to incorporate both quality of life and survival and is another widely used tool in OHCA research. It uses a seven-point scale, with better recovery associated with lower scores, and has been shown to have consistent inter-rater reliability. A patient with no symptoms at all is given a score of 0 and those who die a score of 6. A good outcome is generally considered to be between a score of 0 and 3.

What are the disadvantages of using measures such as the CPC and mRS for classifying outcomes following OHCA?

It is important to understand that these scores use strictly objective measures to describe outcomes that are, in their very essence, completely subjective. These reductionist measures clearly do not consider the state of neurodisability perceived or experienced by the patient or their next of kin.

> On day 5, Gary begins to show signs of neurological recovery and is successfully extubated 8 days after the cardiac arrest and subsequently discharged from your unit. At 6 months, he can function relatively independently from others, but has mild problems with memory and recall.

Further reading

- *Advanced Life Support*, 8e. London: Resuscitation Council UK. Definitive guide to resuscitation practices in the UK.
- Sandroni, C., Nolan, J., Andersen, L. et al. (2022). ERC-ESICM guidelines on temperature control after cardiac arrest in adults. *Intensive Care Med.* 48: 261–269. Informative rapid practice guideline regarding temperature control.

11 The Patient with Hyponatraemia

At morning handover, you are informed about Gladys. She is an 80-year-old patient who has just arrived at your HDU for management of severe hyponatraemia. She had been prescribed furosemide 7 days prior to admission for symptoms of heart failure, including pedal oedema. She lives with her husband and can walk around her bungalow with the aid of a Zimmer frame, but rarely leaves her home for fear of falling. She is mildly confused, and the laboratory has called to confirm that her serum sodium concentration is 105 mmol/L.

Define hyponatraemia

Hyponatraemia is defined as a serum sodium concentration less than 135 mmol/L. It is the most common disorder of electrolytes seen in hospitalised patients.

Classify hyponatraemia according to serum sodium concentration, time of development, symptoms, serum osmolality and volume status

See Table 11.1.

Discuss and describe hyponatraemia according to severity of symptoms

See Table 11.2.

Some patients with *profound* biochemical hyponatraemia may have clinically mild symptoms, while others with *moderate* biochemical hyponatraemia may present with significant neurological symptoms. Elderly patients are prone to non-specific symptoms (e.g. nausea, malaise, anorexia), and it is worth

Clinical Cases in Critical Care, First Edition. Alice Myers and Theophilus Samuels.
© 2023 John Wiley & Sons Ltd. Published 2023 by John Wiley & Sons Ltd.

Table 11.1: Classification of hyponatraemia. Classifying hyponatraemia using volume status can be considered ambiguous. It is often not clear in this context whether volume status refers to extracellular fluid volume (ECF), to the effective circulating volume (ECV) or to the total body water. A potential workaround to reduce ambiguity is to use the terms ECV and ECF.

Classification based on	Categories	Parameters/cut-off values
Serum sodium concentration	Mild	130–135 mmol/L
	Moderate	125–129 mmol/L
	Profound	<125 mmol/L
Time of development	Acute	<48 h
	Chronic	>48 h
Symptoms	'Moderately symptomatic'	Any biochemical degree of hyponatraemia in the presence of moderately severe symptoms of hyponatraemia
	'Severely symptomatic'	Any biochemical degree of hyponatraemia in the presence of severe symptoms of hyponatraemia
Serum osmolality	Hypotonic	<275 mOsm/kg
	Non-hypotonic	≥275 mOsm/kg
Volume status	Hypervolaemic	Clinical assessment
	Euvolaemic	
	Hypovalaemic	

Table 11.2: Hyponatraemia classified according to the severity of symptoms.

Severity	Symptoms
Mild	Non-specific or may be absent
Moderately severe	Nausea without vomiting
	Headache
	Confusion
Severe (unlikely with serum sodium >130 mmol/L)	Cardiorespiratory arrest
	Vomiting
	Reduced consciousness (Glasgow Coma Score ≤8)
	Seizures
	Abnormal and deep somnolence

considering hyponatraemia if they are present. It is recommended that the management of hyponatraemia is guided by the presenting clinical symptoms and signs rather than the degree of hyponatraemia. The clinician should consider all symptoms that can be associated with cerebral oedema as symptoms that can occur with moderately severe or severe symptomatic hyponatraemia.

What is the pathophysiology behind disturbances in sodium homeostasis and what is the likely cause in this case?

The underlying principle that explains most sodium disorders centres around the imbalance that occurs between water intake and water excretion. Serum osmolality is maintained at a near-constant level through the tightly regulated homeostatic mechanisms involving water intake and the excretion of water (e.g. via increased or decreased antidiuretic hormone [ADH] release).

In this case, the profound hyponatraemia is most probably due to her furosemide therapy for hypertension (although thiazide diuretics are more commonly the culprit). Furosemide acts by blocking the sodium-potassium-chloride co-transport mechanisms in the luminal membrane of the loop of Henle (thick ascending limb). By blocking this receptor, furosemide increases urine output of water, sodium, potassium, chloride and other electrolytes by two mechanisms:

- Greater delivery of solutes to the distal nephrons. These solutes then act as osmotic agents which prevent the reabsorption of water.
- An increase in the osmolality of the medullary interstitial fluid reduces the absorption of ions from the loop of Henle into the medullary interstitium. This in turn disrupts the countercurrent multiplier system.

Both effects also reduce the ability of the kidney to dilute or concentrate the urine.

Before reviewing Gladys, you review her medical clerking and results of the blood tests that have been ordered.

What is normal serum osmolality?

A standard reference range for serum osmolality is 280–296 mOsm/kg. Normal serum osmolality is tightly controlled, and it varies less than 0.5% throughout the day in healthy individuals. Serum osmolality (P_{osm}) can be estimated by the following formula:

$$\text{Estimated } P_{osm} = (2 \times \text{serum sodium}) + \text{serum glucose} + \text{serum urea}$$

From this relationship, it becomes apparent that in health, the major determinant for serum osmolality is serum sodium concentration (representing approximately 94% of the extracellular osmoles). However, in the presence of renal disease, the contributions of urea and glucose should be considered.

Define osmolality and osmolarity. What is the difference?

Osmolarity refers to the number of dissolved particles per 1 L of solvent and is expressed as Osm/L. *Osmolality* is the number of dissolved particles in 1 kg of solvent and is expressed as Osm/kg.

The difference between the two is insignificant for dilute solutions such as when considering the physiology of body fluids. However, as the volume of a solvent changes with temperature, osmolarity is considered temperature *dependent*. Therefore, since osmolality is temperature *independent* as it is based on the mass of the solvent, it is the preferred term in biological systems.

Why is it important to establish whether hyponatraemia is hypotonic?

Hypotonic hyponatraemia is managed differently from non-hypotonic hyponatraemia. Cerebral oedema does *not* occur with non-hypotonic hyponatraemia.

Excluding hyperglycaemic hyponatraemia is also important in these patients. Several formulae can be used to correct the measured serum sodium concentration in the presence of a raised measured serum glucose concentration.

Hyponatraemia can be hypotonic, isotonic or hypertonic when *estimating* the serum osmolality. This is because the estimate depends upon which osmotically active agents are present *and* whether they are incorporated into the calculation. Conversely, a *measured* serum osmolality <275 mOsm/kg always confirms that the hyponatraemia is hypotonic.

How is normal serum osmolality physiologically maintained?

There are two basic principles for maintaining serum osmolality that should be borne in mind when considering how changes in intracellular and extracellular fluid volumes are handled by the body.

- The number of osmoles (the amount of a substance that is fully dissociated and dissolved in water) in the intracellular and extracellular compartments remains relatively constant due to cell membranes possessing almost complete impermeability to many solutes (e.g. sodium and chloride).
- The osmotic equilibrium between the two compartments remains almost exactly equal due to water being able to rapidly move across cell membranes, so no osmotic gradients exist among the body's fluid compartments. The exception to this is the renal medulla due to its need to concentrate urine, hence the osmolality is much larger than in other parts of the body.

Bearing these principles in mind, the physiological changes that occur to maintain normal serum osmolality can be summarised as follows:

- Changes in plasma osmolality are sensed by specialised cells called osmoreceptors located in the anterior hypothalamus near the supra-optic nuclei (increased osmolality causes them to shrink). These hypo-thalamic osmoreceptors then proportionately stimulate cells located in the supraoptic and paraventricular nuclei.
- Both the supraoptic and paraventricular nuclei have axonal extensions that project into the posterior pituitary. Membrane permeability to calcium ions increases following stimulation. This results in an increase in the release of stored ADH into the circulation.
- Circulating levels of ADH then affect the proportion of aquaporins (water channels) that are inserted into the collecting duct of the kidney, thus altering its permeability to free water resulting in the ability of the kidney to excrete concentrated/low-volume or dilute/high-volume urine.

Osmoreceptors can detect changes in osmolality rapidly, which results in a significant increase in ADH within minutes. In addition, they induce thirst in response to an increased extracellular fluid osmolality.

Describe how ADH works

Antidiuretic hormone (also known as arginine vasopressin) binds to type 2 vasopressin receptors (V2R), resulting in an increase in intracellular cyclic adenosine monophosphate (cAMP) levels and protein kinase A activity through a stimulatory G-protein-coupled mechanism. This then increases water permeability of the collecting ducts in the kidney through the actions of aquaporin-2 water channels (Figure 11.1).

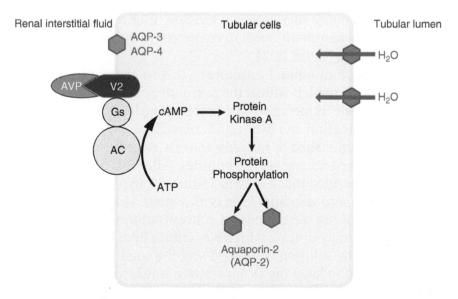

Figure 11.1: Effect of antidiuretic hormone on renal tubular cells. Aquaporin 3 and 4 channels allow passage of water out of the cell. Regulation of these aquaporins appears to be independent of AVP. AC, adenylate cyclase; AQP-3/AQP-4, aquaporin 3 and 4 channels; AVP, arginine vasopressin or ADH; cAMP, cyclic adenosine triphosphate; Gs, G stimulatory protein; V2, vasopressin-2 receptors.

Source: Theophilus Samuels.

In the absence of disease, the kidney can vary urine concentration dramatically, ranging from an osmolality of 1200 mOsm/kg at maximal activity to as low as 50 mOsm/kg. However, in a diseased state, as in critically unwell patients, this range can be considerably smaller. This is important as when daily solute load is increased or decreased, the ability of the kidneys to react to these changes to maintain serum sodium concentration within normal limits is diminished.

What other factors influence the synthesis and release of ADH?

While plasma osmolality plays an important role as described above, an equally if not more powerful stimulation of ADH release occurs in the setting of low arterial blood pressure and low effective arterial volume. It is therefore plausible for a hypotensive patient to have low plasma osmolality but high circulating levels of ADH. Other factors that can increase ADH levels include pain, stress, hypoxia, hypercapnia, nausea and medications (e.g. adrenaline).

Following review of the notes and results, you go to review Gladys. Her measured serum osmolality is 233 mOsm/kg. She is now drowsy, and her GCS has reduced to 11 (E3, V3, M5) so you assess her to be severely symptomatic from the hypotonic hyponatraemia.

Describe the management of severe symptomatic hyponatraemia

Irrespective of the cause or whether it is acute or chronic, severe symptomatic hyponatraemia requires *immediate treatment* with the appropriate clinical monitoring in place (Figure 11.2).

The current recommended guidance aims to increase serum sodium concentration by 5 mmol/L within the *first hour of treatment*. This threshold ideally minimises the immediate risk of cerebral oedema and reduces the risk of osmotic demyelination and over-rapid correction.

This can be accomplished by infusing 150 mL 3% hypertonic saline solution (or equivalent) intravenously over 20 minutes. After this first infusion has finished, it is recommended that a second 150 mL 3% hypertonic saline infusion is started while the serum sodium level is measured. This entire process can be repeated twice until the serum sodium concentration increases by 5 mmol/L or until the symptoms improve, whichever comes first. If successful, then the 3% hypertonic saline solution is stopped and the smallest feasible volume of 0.9% saline is given to keep the IV line patent until cause-specific treatment is started.

Increases in serum sodium concentration should be limited to less than 10 mmol/L within the first 24 hours of treatment (including the initial 5 mmol/L). Subsequently, increases in serum sodium concentration should be limited to 8 mmol/L every 24 hours until it reaches 130 mmol/L.

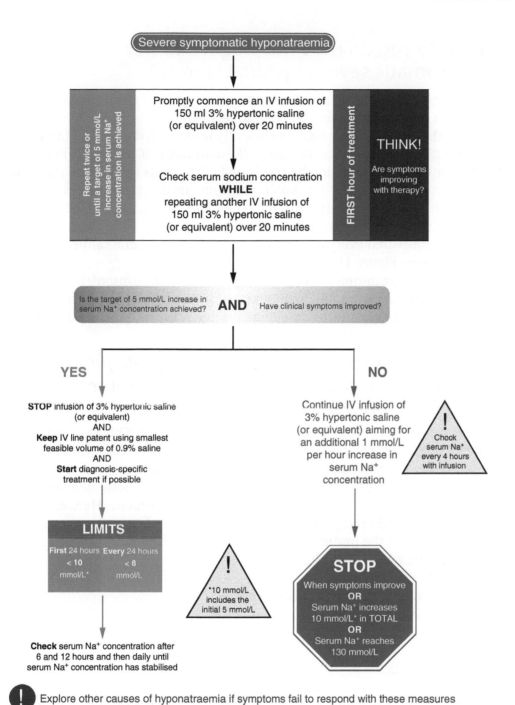

Figure 11.2: Management algorithm for severe symptomatic hyponatraemia. Ideally, pre-prepared 150 mL bags of 3% hypertonic saline should be readily available. Preparing a solution of 3% hypertonic saline solution is time-consuming and prone to errors in calculating the correct amount of NaCl required. See text for symptoms of severe hyponatraemia.

Source: Theophilus Samuels.

Gladys receives the treatment as outline above, and her serum sodium increases by 5 mmol/L within the first hour of treatment. However, her clinical symptoms do not improve. Through clinical assessment, you have not found any other obvious cause for a low GCS.

What do you do next with regard to her symptomatic severe hyponatraemia?

Bear in mind that patients with severe symptoms may not improve immediately, as it may take time for the brain to recover.

Nevertheless, as Gladys has not clinically improved, despite the increase in serum sodium concentration by 5 mmol/L, an infusion of 150 mL 3% hypertonic saline (or equivalent) should be continued. The aim is to increase the serum sodium concentration by 1 mmol/L per hour until the symptoms improve, the serum sodium concentration increases 10 mmol/L in total, or it reaches 130 mmol/L, whichever occurs first. The serum sodium concentration should ideally be measured every 4 hours while the 3% hypertonic saline infusion is continued (see Figure 11.2).

Should her symptoms still fail to improve after a 10 mmol/L increase in serum sodium concentration (including the first 5 mmol/L), then it is likely that her symptoms are not due to hyponatraemia and other causes should be sought.

What are the concerns surrounding delayed and overly rapid correction of hyponatraemia?

Delayed correction of profound hyponatraemia from a rapid decrease in sodium level can surpass the brain's ability to osmotically adapt. This can lead to irreversible brain damage and death from persistent cerebral oedema. *Overly rapid* correction without considering the need to protect the patient from the neurological sequelae of cerebral oedema can result in osmotic demyelination syndrome (OMS) approximately 3–10 days after treatment. Hence, this can occur following discharge from critical care. OMS is characterised by specific abnormalities in the brainstem seen on magnetic resonance imaging (MRI) and indicated clinically by:

- Fluctuating levels of consciousness
- Pseudobulbar palsy
- Dysarthria
- Ataxia
- Dysphagia.

OMS can be devastating for the patient and their families and is often irreversible.

List risk factors for developing osmotic demyelination syndrome

The acronym CCHASM can be used as defined below:

- **C**hronic hyponatraemia
- **C**irrhosis
- **H**ypokalaemia
- **A**lcoholism

- **S**erum sodium <105 mmol/L
- **M**alnutrition

What can be done if the serum sodium concentration rises too rapidly (i.e. rapid overcorrection)?

Evidence is lacking with regard to managing the rapid overcorrection of serum sodium concentration. The use of electrolyte-free water (e.g. 5% glucose solutions) and/or desmopressin can reduce serum sodium concentration in cases of rapid overcorrection.

However, it is *strongly recommended* that expert advice is sought before any attempt is made to re-lower serum sodium concentration in the presence of a rapid overcorrection. In addition, overcorrection may indicate the presence of a complex case. Therefore, the effect of further treatment may be even more difficult to predict, and these cases should be discussed with medical professionals experienced in managing these patients.

> Within 3 hours of ongoing treatment, Gladys's level of consciousness improves and she becomes much more alert and responsive. Over the next 24 hours, her serum sodium concentration continues to rise accordingly. Your consultant asks you to investigate the cause of her hyponatraemia.

Explain how serum and urinary concentration of electrolytes can help clinically in determining the aetiology of sodium disorders

First, it is important to understand that it is the *concentration* of the electrolytes within the urine and not its osmolality that ultimately determines the net excretion of water. So, for example, a net loss of free water may still occur in the presence of a high urine osmolality, which itself is the result of excess solutes (e.g. urea) with few electrolytes present. Therefore, if the concentration of electrolytes within the urine is *less* than that of the serum, it suggests that free water is being excreted. Conversely, when free water is not excreted in the urine, it will tend to have a concentration of electrolytes (e.g. sodium and potassium) greater than that in the serum.

Which urinary tests can aid in diagnosing the causes of hyponatraemia?

The urine osmolality and urine sodium concentration can be used for this purpose (Figure 11.3). Performing these tests must not take precedence over treating patients with symptomatic hyponatraemia and can be requested once the patient has stabilised.

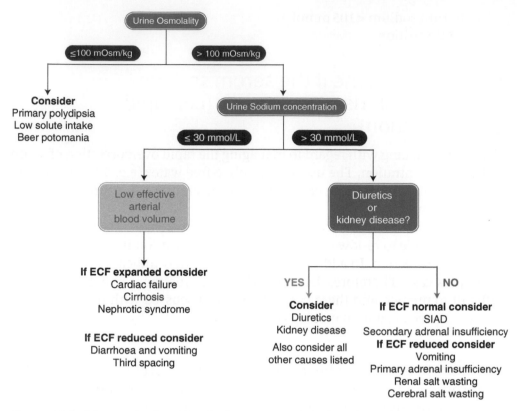

Figure 11.3: Diagnostic algorithm for hyponatraemia. ECF, extracellular fluid; SIAD, syndrome of inappropriate antidiuresis.

Source: Adapted from *Spasovski, G., et al. (2014). Clinical practice guideline on diagnosis and treatment of hyponatraemia. Eur. J. Endo. 170: G1-G47.*

Urine osmolality

- As a simple method, it can be easily and rapidly used to confirm an excess of fluid intake relative to solute intake.
- It is recommended as a first step in the diagnostic work-up of hyponatraemia.
- A urine osmolality ≤100 mOsm/kg on a spot urine sample always indicates maximally dilute urine (e.g. excess water intake or beer potomania).
- If the urine osmolality is >100 mOsm/kg then determining the urine sodium concentration on a spot urine sample is the next step in identifying the underlying cause.

Urine sodium concentration

- Both the urine and serum samples should be collected around the same time to allow correct interpretation of the value.
- A urine sodium concentration threshold of 30 mmol/L provides good sensitivity and acceptable specificity in determining volume status.
- A value less than or equal to 30 mmol/L suggests that, even in patients on diuretics, the effective arterial blood volume is low.

■ Concurrent use of diuretics may make interpreting urine sodium concentrations difficult, but diuretics should still be considered a contributing factor to the hyponatraemia.

> On day 4 of admission, Gladys's serum sodium from the morning set of bloods was reported as 136 mmol/L. You are asked to review her as she has become acutely confused and agitated, and appears to be hallucinating. You and the nursing staff consider that Gladys is now suffering with delirium. Her RASS (Richmond Agitation-Sedation Scale) is +3.

Describe the RASS

The RASS is one example of a scale that can be used to assess the level of alertness and agitated behaviour in a critically ill patient. The scale ranges between −5 and +4 (Table 11.3). Even though the RASS can be used in all hospitalised patients, it is more frequently utilised in patients who are mechanically ventilated to avoid over- or undersedation. A RASS between −2 and 0 in mechanically ventilated patients:

■ Minimises sedation
■ Reduces mortality
■ Decreases the duration of mechanical ventilation
■ Shortens the length of stay in the ICU.

The RASS has been validated for use with the Confusion Assessment Method for ICU (CAM-ICU) (discussed later).

Table 11.3: Richmond Agitation-Sedation Scale (RASS).

+4	**Combative**	Overtly combative or violent, immediate danger to staff
+3	**Very agitated**	Pulls on or removes tube(s) or catheter(s) or displays aggressive behaviour towards staff
+2	**Agitated**	Frequent non-purposeful movement or patient–ventilator dyssynchrony
+1	**Restless**	Anxious or apprehensive but movements not aggressive or vigorous
0	Alert and calm	
−1	**Drowsy**	Not fully alert, but sustained (>10 s) awakening to voice, with eye contact
−2	**Light sedation**	Briefly (<10 s) awakens with eye contact to voice
−3	**Moderate sedation**	Any movement (but no eye contact) to voice
−4	**Deep sedation**	No response to voice, but any movement to physical stimulation
−5	**Unarousable**	No response to voice or physical stimulation

What is delirium?

Delirium is defined as a disturbance in awareness, attention and cognition that develops over a short period of time, is fluctuating and is associated with perceptual changes (e.g. hallucinations).

What are the different subtypes of delirium?

Clinically, three subtypes have been established:

- *Hypoactive* delirium is probably the most common form as it is often misdiagnosed and reportedly unrecognised in 66–84% of patients. Typically, the patient appears co-operative and passive but will show signs of inattention and decreased responsiveness and be unable to organise thoughts.
- *Hyperactive* delirium is the more familiar and recognisable form of delirium but is much less common than the other types and in its pure form is even rarer. Incidentally, this subtype has a better overall prognosis. The patient can hallucinate and be agitated, combative, aggressive and uncooperative, which can potentially put the patient and staff at risk of physical harm.
- *Mixed* delirium, as the name suggests, often presents as alternating periods of aggressive behaviour and quiet confusion.

How common is delirium in critical care patients?

The incidence of delirium varies according to specific patient populations in critical care but can affect up to 80% of patients in medical intensive care units. Postoperative neurosurgical and trauma patients are also at increased risk. Patients in critical care tend to have the highest incidence of delirium compared to other clinical areas of a hospital. The incidence of delirium in ventilated patients can approach 70%, with a mixed delirium presentation predominating, followed by the hypoactive subtype.

Broadly speaking, what are the risk factors for delirium?

Modifiable risk factors

- Hypoxia
- Hypercarbia
- Acidosis
- Infection
- Dehydration or constipation
- Polypharmacy (including use of opiates, benzodiazepines and anticholinergic medications)
- Urinary catheter irritation
- Urinary retention
- Metabolic disturbances (e.g. hyponatraemia)

Non-modifiable risk factors

- Age
- Cognitive decline
- Dementia
- Depression
- Liver impairment

What role do benzodiazepines have in the development of delirium?

Benzodiazepines are considered an independent risk factor for delirium during critical illness, with little variation in risk between the different classes. With lorazepam, evidence suggests that the probability of transitioning to delirium is great even at low doses.

How can we screen for delirium in critical care?

Two methods are available in critical care for delirium screening. These have also been validated in intubated patients.

- The *CAM-ICU* is a snapshot assessment of delirium and can be easily carried out at the bedside by healthcare professionals (its specificity and sensitivity are reported as 81% and 96% respectively). In critical care, sedation must be assessed before carrying it out, and the assessment can occur if the RASS is greater than or equal to −3. Features of delirium are assessed sequentially in the following four stages:
  - **Is there an acute onset and fluctuating course?** This information can be obtained from a family member or nurse by asking if there has been any change in the patient's baseline mental status and whether the change has fluctuated throughout the day. If this has occurred then proceed with the next step; if this is absent then the patient is CAM-ICU negative.
  - **Does the patient have difficulty focusing their attention?** The patient can be asked to squeeze your hand when they hear the letter 'A' upon spelling out the phrase 'S A V E A H A A R T' or 'C A S A B L A N C A'. If three or more errors occur (i.e. fails to squeeze your hand on hearing the letter 'A' or squeezes your hand on another letter), then the assessment is continued. If two or fewer errors occur, then the patient is CAM-ICU negative.
  - **Does the patient have an altered level of consciousness?** This is essentially the RASS score taken from the first stage. If it is anything except 0 (e.g. alert and calm) then the patient is considered CAM-ICU positive, otherwise the next and last stage of assessment is undertaken.
  - **Does the patient have disorganised thinking?** This stage attempts to determine if the patient has incoherent thoughts (e.g. rambling or irrelevant conversation), disordered flow of ideas or unpredictable switching from one idea to the next. If at this stage the patient has more than one error, they are considered CAM-ICU positive.

- The *Intensive Care Delirium Screening Checklist (ICDSC)* assesses eight features:
  - Altered level of consciousness
  - Inattention
  - Disorientation
  - Hallucinations
  - Psychomotor agitation/retardation
  - Inappropriate mood/speech
  - Sleep/wake cycle disturbance
  - Symptom fluctuation

The specificity and sensitivity for the ICDSC have been reported as 99% and 66% respectively. It requires information to be gathered over a period and therefore takes longer to complete than the CAM-ICU.

> Gladys is becoming increasingly agitated and crying out for her husband. She is CAM-ICU positive. The result of the repeat urgent serum sodium concentration that you requested is 136 mmol/L. This has remained stable over the last 24 hours.

How can we manage delirium?

Primary prevention remains the most effective strategy to reduce delirium and its associated complications. However, some delirium is virtually inevitable in many critical care patients. We can categorise the management of delirium into non-pharmacological and pharmacological measures.

Non-pharmacological measures

It is important to apply basic patient management principles early and liberally.

- Early mobilisation.
- Reduce unnecessary noise and stimulation (especially at night).
- Frequent reorientation.

Reducing the exposure of critical care patients to sedatives and analgesics (e.g. propofol and fentanyl) through focused daily interruptions ('sedation holds') to achieve a RASS score of 0 (alert and calm) to −1 (drowsy) and target-based sedation have also been shown to improve patient outcomes. However, this needs to be balanced against reducing pain, especially in postoperative patients, which makes the use of regional anaesthetic techniques potentially useful although this has yet to be fully validated. Involving family members in the care of the patient while in hospital may also be of some benefit, not only for the patient but for the family members as well by teaching them to identify episodes of delirium.

Pharmacological measures

Drugs are used to treat the troublesome symptoms of delirium (usually the hyperactive type). They do not treat the delirium itself. Ideally, medications should only be employed when non-pharmacological measures have been exhausted or are considered inappropriate (e.g. the severely agitated patient who poses a risk to themselves and others). A common choice in this context is the butyrophenone haloperidol, which does not suppress respiratory drive and works by partially blocking the dopamine D_2 receptor. As with all agents used to treat delirium, there is little evidence for its safety and efficacy, and it will potentially have psychoactive effects that will increase the duration of cognitive impairment and potentially reduce the patient's level of consciousness.

What is the ICU Liberation Bundle?

This bundle has been shown to help reduce delirium, improve pain management and reduce the long-term consequences for adult critical care patients. The components of this evidence-based bundle are described using the acronym ABCDEF:

- **A**ssess, Prevent and Manage Pain
- **B**oth Spontaneous Awakening Trials (SAT) and Spontaneous Breathing Trials (SBT)
- **C**hoice of Analgesia and Sedation
- **D**elirium: Assess, Prevent and Manage
- **E**arly Mobility and Exercise
- **F**amily Engagement and Empowerment

The use of this ABCDEF bundle (www.iculiberation.org) has been shown to improve survival and increase the number of delirium-free days after adjusting for age, severity of illness and presence of mechanical ventilation. However, strong evidence is still lacking on whether delirium prevention protocols can prevent delirium in critical care patients.

Do patients who experience delirium in the ICU have a poorer outcome?

Yes. In critical care patients, delirium has been shown to be an independent predictor of mortality, increased length of stay, increased length of mechanical ventilation and long-term cognitive impairment. Critical care patients who have a prolonged period of delirium are at highest risk for long-term cognitive impairment.

> The nursing staff suspect that Gladys was becoming delirious due to disorientation and lack of family contact (as she keeps asking for her husband of 55 years). Later that same day, her husband comes to visit. With him sitting by her side, holding her hand and talking gently to her, Gladys becomes much more relaxed and co-operative. Medication was not required to treat her delirium and she is discharged to the ward the following day.

Further reading

■ Spasovski, G., Vanholder, R., Allolio, B. et al. (2014). Clinical practice guideline on diagnosis and treatment of hyponatraemia. *Eur. J. Endo.* 170: G1–G47. Excellent evidence-based guideline for the management of hyponatraemia developed in conjunction with the European Society of Intensive Care Medicine.

■ Sessler, C., Gosnell, M., Grap, M. et al. (2002). The Richmond Agitation-Sedation Scale. *Am. J. Respir. Crit. Care Med.* 166: 1338–1344. Seminal paper evaluating the RASS in adult intensive care patients.

12 The Patient in Status Epilepticus

You are called to review a young man in the resuscitation department. He was found outside a pub earlier this evening having seizures. A bystander placed him in the recovery position and an ambulance was called. He carried no identification, appeared unkempt and had no friends with him. Paramedics sited both a nasopharyngeal (NP) and an oropharyngeal (OP) airway and administered two doses of lorazepam. He arrived with a GCS of 3 without demonstrating obvious seizure activity. However, he has now started seizing again.

What could be causing his seizures?

- *Known epilepsy* – approximately 60 million people throughout the world have epilepsy, around 500 000 in the UK. It is unknown whether this man has epilepsy. He may suffer regular breakthrough seizures or he may be non-compliant with medication. He may have a lowered seizure threshold for an unknown reason such as infection or toxins.
- *Isolated seizure or new-onset epilepsy* – approximately 1 in 20 adults will have a seizure at some point in their life. This may or may not progress to epilepsy which may or may not continue throughout the individual's life. New-onset epilepsy is most likely to develop in those under 20 or over 65 years of age.
- *Pseudoseizures, factitious seizure disorder or non-epileptic seizures* – it can be extremely difficult to differentiate factitious seizures from epileptiform seizures. Often, those patients who present with factitious seizures also have co-existent epilepsy. Managing these cases is challenging since overtreatment exposes patients to the risk of iatrogenic injury (e.g. unnecessary treatment with benzodiazepines leading to airway compromise and the need for intubation). However, avoiding treatment may expose the patient to the risks of airway obstruction (i.e. where non-epileptic seizures are suspected but the patient does in fact have reduced GCS due to genuine seizure activity).

Clinical Cases in Critical Care, First Edition. Alice Myers and Theophilus Samuels.
© 2023 John Wiley & Sons Ltd. Published 2023 by John Wiley & Sons Ltd.

- *Meningitis/encephalitis* – meningitis is inflammation of the meninges. Encephalitis is inflammation of the brain itself. Infective causes include bacteria, viruses, fungi and parasites. Non-infective causes include SLE (systemic lupus erythematosus) and, rarely, drug reactions (such as with NSAIDs). Meningococcal sepsis is a diagnosis not to be missed. Presentation is most commonly with altered mental status, headache, neck stiffness, photophobia and seizures. Purpuric or petechial rash may be a sign of the intradermal haemorrhage associated with sepsis secondary to *Neisseria meningitidis*.

- *Intracranial haemorrhage* – sudden spontaneous events such as subarachnoid or intracerebral bleeding can occur secondary to aneurysm (see Case 15).

- *Space-occupying lesion* – seizure could be the manifestation of a progressive pathology such as solid tumour (primary or secondary), lymphoma or abscess. Small lesions may be tolerated with few or no symptoms. With increasing size, the lesion itself, the surrounding oedema or resultant mass effect can lead to symptoms. Examine the patient for focal neurological signs and perform imaging of the brain to look for tumour and ring enhancing lesions.

  The WHO reclassified CNS tumours in 2016, integrating molecular data with histopathology. The 2007 grading system, based on characteristics such as growth rate and likelihood of metastasis, is still commonly used. In the UK >4000 people are diagnosed annually with lower grade tumours (I and II) and approximately 5000 with the more malignant grades III and IV. Glioblastoma multiforme, a grade IV tumour, is the most common primary brain tumour accounting for approximately 15% of all intracranial tumours with an incidence of about 2 per 100 000. It has a median survival of 15 months and a 5-year survival rate of 4%.

- *Traumatic brain injury* – the patient may have been involved in an altercation or be the subject of assault. Inspect for signs of trauma and examine the scalp as carefully as possible. Haematomas can be hidden beneath hair. If there is reason to suspect trauma, state this clearly to the attending team and re-call this incident as a trauma call, proceeding according to ATLS® guidance.

- *Drugs/toxins/overdose/withdrawal* – the patient was found outside a pub. He has not necessarily been drinking alcohol, but this possibility should be borne in mind. Severe alcohol withdrawal can be associated with seizures, delirium tremens and hallucinations. Without careful management, this can be fatal. Nearly 10% of cases of status epilepticus are due to drugs and poisons including antidepressants, opioids, recreational drugs, stimulants and insecticides. Neurotransmitters implicated in the process can include GABA and glutamate. Drugs such as amphetamine derivatives and cocaine can cause hyperpyrexia which itself can also lead to seizures.

- *Metabolic causes* – other occult causes of seizure should be considered, including hyper- and hypoglycaemia, electrolyte imbalance and uraemia secondary to renal failure. Many inborn errors of metabolism require careful management to avoid accumulation of neurotoxins. For instance, phenylketonuria requires meticulous diet control due to deficiency of phenylalanine hydroxylase. In the absence of diet control, accumulation of phenylalanine can result in intellectual impairment or even seizures. Fortunately, this disease is rare (approximately 1 in 10 000) and usually detected in infancy, with careful management preventing symptom development.

> On examination, the man has tonic-clonic movements of his upper and lower limbs. There is vomitus around his mouth and a large boggy haematoma on the back of his head with some grazes around his elbows. His BP before the current seizure was 135/89 mmHg, HR 110 bpm sinus rhythm, RR 24 breaths per minute, temperature 35.8 °C, blood glucose 6.4 mmol/L, lactate 6.5 mmol/L, pH 7.14, PaO_2 9.3 kPa on 15 L/min via non-rebreathe mask, $PaCO_2$ 7.6 kPa, base excess −7 mmol/L.

What are your main concerns?

Life-threatening issues

- Ongoing seizures with an unprotected airway.
- Hypoxia and signs suggestive of aspiration.
- Evidence of trauma to the head which could be the cause of his seizure or sustained secondary to falling during a seizure.
- Potential for occult injuries such as broken limbs or spinal injury.

Establishing the underlying cause(s) of seizures

- No available collateral history.
- Lactataemia with a mixed metabolic and respiratory acidosis.

Serum lactate can be raised subsequent to the sustained and excessive muscular activity in tonic-clonic seizures. If the lactate is raised due to seizures, this would decrease rapidly following seizure control. If it does not, consider other causes.

What are your management priorities?

Take an ABCDE approach, give oxygen and call for help. This patient is likely to need intubation and his airway may be difficult. Call for assistance early. Management priorities are:

- Airway management with cervical spine control
- Terminate seizures
- Investigate and treat the cause of his seizures (including traumatic head injury)
- Investigate and treat any problems resulting from his seizures.

What is the definition and pathophysiology of status epilepticus?

Status epilepticus can be convulsive or non-convulsive. The International League Against Epilepsy (ILAE) redefined status epilepticus in 2017. Status epilepticus is continuous seizure activity or repeated seizures without intervening recovery of consciousness lasting 5 minutes or more.

Dysregulation of neurotransmission occurs, involving excitatory neurotransmitters like aspartate, glutamate and acetylcholine, and inhibitory transmitters such as GABA. Status epilepticus (convulsive and non-convulsive) is associated with cognitive problems and even neuronal necrosis, possibly due to depletion of ATP and lactate accumulation.

What is the pharmacological management of refractory convulsive status epilepticus?

NICE guidance CG137 (updated 2021) specifies the use of oxygen, glucose and IV thiamine, and refers users to the BNF regarding antiepileptic drugs. Appropriate antiseizure medications include IV lorazepam, IV diazepam, IV phenobarbital and rectal diazepam. At the time of writing, there is no evidence-based preferred second therapy of choice, but options include IV levetiracetam, IV valproic acid and IV phenytoin.

Classify epilepsy

The ILAE revised the classification of epilepsy in 2017 (terms such as 'complex partial' and 'secondarily generalised' are no longer used).

Seizure types

- Focal onset – aware vs impaired awareness, motor onset vs non-motor onset
- Generalised onset – motor (tonic-clonic) vs non-motor onset (absence)
- Unknown onset – motor vs non-motor, unclassified

Epilepsy types

- Focal
- Generalised
- Combined generalised and focal
- Unknown

Aetiology

- Structural, e.g. traumatic brain injury, post craniotomy, stroke
- Genetic, e.g. point mutations, mosaicism, polymorphisms or syndromes such as neurofibromatosis
- Infectious, e.g. HIV, malaria, TB

- Metabolic, e.g. mitochondrial disorders, creatine disorders, pyridoxine disorders
- Immune, e.g. Rasmussen syndrome
- Unknown

> You alert the team that this should be managed as a trauma scenario. You intubate the patient with manual in-line stabilisation. You elect to use thiopentone as the induction agent for its antiseizure properties. On primary survey, there do not appear to be any further life-threatening injuries. You commence loading the patient with phenytoin and transfer him to the CT scanner for CT head and neck. There are no radiological abnormalities of the neck. The only abnormalities noted on the CT head are an extracranial soft tissue swelling over the occiput. Right basal consolidation is seen on plain chest radiograph. You transfer the patient to intensive care for further management.
>
> Some initial blood results are available: Hb 124 g/L, WBC 24×10⁹/L, CRP 106, platelets 134×10⁹/L, INR 1.4.

Would you give this patient antimicrobials?

Meningitis is a possible diagnosis so treat with antimicrobials until this has been ruled out. There is also radiological evidence of lower respiratory tract infection (LRTI). Pre-existing infection could have lowered his seizure threshold. In this context, antimicrobial cover for bacterial and viral meningitis according to local protocol would be reasonable, e.g. ceftriaxone 2 g IV bd with aciclovir 10 mg/kg IV tds.

Which organisms commonly cause meningitis?

Although meningitis can occur in anyone, certain pathogens are more common in particular groups.

- *Neonates* – the most common bacterial causes are Group B strep, *E. coli*, *S. pneumoniae*, *Listeria* and *Salmonella*.
- *Children and younger adults (such as our patient)* – the most common bacterial causes are *N. meningitidis* (Men B is the most common strain in the UK), *S. pneumoniae* and *H. influenzae* type b. Common viral causes include herpes viruses, enteroviruses, flaviviruses and measles.
- *Immunocompromised* – other causes such as TB and fungal infection should always be considered, particularly in a patient like ours for whom we have limited background history and who may be immunosuppressed.
- Older adults (aged >60 years) – similar causes to those in younger adults with the addition of *Listeria*. Susceptibility is increased due to a waning immune system.

What are the causes of encephalopathy?

- *Infection* – bacteria, viruses, fungi, parasites, prions
- *Hypoxia/anoxia* – hypoxic ischaemic encephalopathy

- *Metabolic* – e.g. derangement of calcium, glucose, sodium, etc.
- *Alcohol, drugs, poisons* – e.g. cyanide, carbon monoxide and heavy metals such as mercury and lead. Chemotherapy agents can induce encephalopathy which may present much like hypoxic ischaemic encephalopathy.
- *Hepatic* – ammonia
- *Renal* – urea
- *Tumour*
- *Autoimmune* – e.g. Hashimoto' disease
- *Nutritional deficiencies* – e.g. lack of vitamin B1/Wernicke
- *Hypertension*
- *Traumatic* – chronic traumatic encephalopathy

Would you give steroids?

A Cochrane review in 2015 (Brouwer et al.) reviewed evidence on the effect of corticosteroids in acute bacterial meningitis. After analysing 25 studies, there is moderate-quality evidence to support corticosteroids reducing hearing loss and neurological sequelae in bacterial meningitis but there was no impact on mortality.

This is not a classic presentation of bacterial meningitis. However, there is sufficient concern that it would be reasonable to start dexamethasone 10 mg IV qds. If *S. pneumoniae* meningitis is confirmed, steroids should continue for 4 days. However, if an alternative cause is found or pneumococcal meningitis is unlikely, dexamethasone can be stopped.

What is your plan in intensive care?

Provide appropriate organ support, investigate the cause, then try to wake the patient up and assess neurology as soon as it is safe to do so.

Organ support

- Invasive monitoring as required – intra-arterial monitoring as a minimum.
- Lung-protective ventilation.

Manage pathology

- Seizure control and neuro observations with regular frequent pupil assessment.
- Treat for meningitis until ruled out.
- Consider treating for LRTI. Do not treat suspected aspiration pneumonitis with antibiotics.
- As soon as it is safe to do so, stop the sedative agents and assess the patient's neurology.
- Although his cervical spine is radiologically clear, the patient needs to be awake and co-operative to be fully assessed and cleared neurologically. While he is sedated, he can be managed with inline C-spine stabilisation.
- Clean the wound and request surgical review.

Investigate underlying cause

- Full septic screen including urinary antigen screen for *S. pneumoniae* and *Legionella*, viral influenza swab, wound swabs, sputum sample, lumbar puncture with viral PCR.
- Metabolic screen with LFTs, ammonia.
- Drug levels – paracetamol, salicylate, alcohol, toxicology screen.
- Collateral history focusing particularly upon drug history, history of seizures and presence of other risk factors for seizures (e.g. exposure to meningitis, etc.).
- Complete secondary trauma survey.

Basic intensive care management

- Venous thromboembolism prophylaxis following lumbar puncture.
- Stress ulcer prophylaxis.
- Replace vitamins B and C to prevent refeeding syndrome given this patient looks unkempt and malnourished.
- Insert an NG tube and start feed.
- Temperature management.
- Attempt to locate next of kin if possible.

After 24 hours following sedation hold, the patient remains intubated and has displayed no seizure activity but does not appear to be waking. His GCS is 3, his pupils are equal and reactive at 3 mm each. The initial lumbar puncture results were as follows: WBC 4 cells/microlitre, RBC 1 cells/microlitre, no organisms seen, no xanthochromia. He is breathing spontaneously on the ventilator with a pressure support 10 cm H_2O, PEEP 6 cm H_2O, FiO_2 0.30 to achieve a PaO_2 8.4 kPa, $PaCO_2$ 6.3 kPa. He has not required any cardiovascular or renal support. His plasma WBC is 18×10^9/L and his CRP is 64. Temperature 37.1 °C.

The police tell you his name is Bruce. He is a 19-year-old homeless man with no next of kin. He is known to have problems with substance misuse and epilepsy for which he takes phenytoin.

What are your concerns regarding his slow neurological progress?

- This could be non-convulsive status epilepticus.
- He might have sustained significant brain injury which was not visible on the initial CT head scan.
- There could be unknown circulating toxins or an as yet unidentified metabolic cause.
- Bruce is homeless and has a history of drug misuse, making him vulnerable to HIV and TB meningitis.
- He may be non-compliant with medications or have taken an overdose of his medication.

What do you do about the antimicrobials?

The viral PCR results remain outstanding. Bruce's white blood count is elevated. He has not made significant neurological recovery.

A viral cause of meningitis remains a possibility so continue aciclovir. Although no organisms were seen on gram stain of the CSF, it would be reasonable to continue antibiotics while the sample is processed and re-discuss the case with microbiology in 24 hours.

What are the next steps in management?

Neurological management

- Neurology consultant review.
- Remain without sedation with frequent neuro observations.
- Add an additional anticonvulsant.

Investigations

- Send blood sample to measure phenytoin level.
- Request electroencephalogram (EEG).
- Send blood for HIV.
- Consider sending samples for acid-fast bacilli.

Safeguarding

- Bruce has no next of kin so an IMCA (independent mental capacity advocate) is required.

What is the role of EEG in intensive care and how does it work?

Electroencephalographic data is essential for identifying non-convulsive status epilepticus. Beyond this, EEG can help differentiate types of epileptiform activity and also assist in the diagnosis and investigation of encephalopathy. Certain patterns within the EEG trace can suggest different causes of metabolic encephalopathy.

Continuous EEG is not available in every centre but is often used in specialist neuro-intensive care units. EEG produces large volumes of data which require expert interpretation. Many centres utilise modified EEG systems such as BIS (Bispectral index) and E-entropy which are used for depth of anaesthesia monitoring. These monitors use algorithms to integrate and interpret EEG data to generate fewer, simplified variables.

EEG waves can be broadly described as follows:

- *Alpha*, 8–15 Hz – these predominate in the normal resting state but are also detected in comatose patients.
- *Beta*, 16–31 Hz – these predominate where the patient is alert. They may also be seen following administration of benzodiazepines.

- *Theta*, 4–7 Hz – these waves are often detected in those who are idle or drowsy. Changes in theta waves can suggest specific forms of encephalopathy or lesions in particular territories of the brain.
- *Delta*, <4 Hz – these predominate in slow-wave sleep. Specific changes can suggest encephalopathies or lesions in particular territories of the brain.
- *Gamma*, >32 Hz – originating in the somatosensory cortex, changes in gamma wave patterns can be associated with cognitive decline.
- *Mu*, 8–12 Hz – these originate in the sensorimotor cortex and are usually most evident in a state of drowsiness.

In some countries such as the United States, EEG is one of the investigations used in the diagnosis of brain death. In the UK, EEG may be used as part of prognostication when dealing with patients with hypoxic ischaemic encephalopathy. For further discussion on brain death, see Case 16.

What is an IMCA and why might you want one in this case?

Independent mental capacity advocates were introduced in the Mental Capacity Act 2005 to provide legal safeguarding for those people who are unable to make specific important decisions for themselves. Bruce is unable to make decisions for himself because he is unconscious. He does not have any relatives who would be able to represent him, so an IMCA is required to fulfil this role.

> Phenytoin levels are within the normal range. The EEG findings are consistent with non-convulsive status epilepticus. You add another anticonvulsant, levetiracetam. Microbiological investigations are, thus far, negative and the HIV test is negative.
>
> After a further 24 hours with drug levels within the therapeutic range and off all sedation, Bruce is still not waking. You discuss with the neurology consultant and decide to attempt burst suppression.

What is burst suppression and how do you do it?

This technique has been used in a variety of situations, including trying to achieve neuroprotection during neurosurgery. It is most utilised to treat refractory status epilepticus. There is limited strong supporting evidence and no widely agreed protocol for carrying it out. Theoretically, burst suppression allows resetting of the disordered neurotransmission within the brain.

Generally, patients are sedated using an intravenous or inhalational agent, e.g. thiopentone, propofol or a volatile anaesthetic. Continuous EEG is mandatory, and depth of anaesthesia is titrated, aiming for a 1:10 burst suppression ratio in EEG activity. Intra-arterial monitoring is required with careful blood pressure control since deep anaesthesia may induce hypotension.

Burst suppression is usually maintained for 24 hours (depending on local practices). Following this, sedation is lightened and neurology can be reassessed.

> Your team successfully burst suppresses Bruce for 24 hours. On sedation hold, he wakes up and gross neurological examination is normal, and you are able to clinically clear his cervical spine. You extubate him on day 6 of his admission and send him to the ward having had no further seizures.

What outstanding issues do you need to highlight for follow-up on discharge to the ward?

- This is a vulnerable young man who would benefit from safeguarding or social services input.
- Compliance may remain an issue, particularly if he remains homeless and without a resilient support network.
- Neurology follow-up and medication review are warranted.
- Viral PCR on lumbar puncture still not back, continue aciclovir until the results are available and can be reviewed by the medical team.

Further reading

- NICE Epilepsy: Diagnosis and Management. CG137 (2012) London: NICE.
- Robinson, C. and Busl, K. (2019). Meningitis and encephalitis management in the ICU. *Curr. Opin. Crit. Care* 25 (5): 423–429. Informative review article on ICU management of meningitis.
- Lapointe, S., Perry, A., and Butowski, N. (2018). Primary brain tumours in adults. *Lancet* 392 (10145): 432–446. Excellent summary of primary brain tumour pathology and management.

13 The Patient Who is Hypotensive

You attend a peri-arrest call on the ward. Joan is 86 years old and has been an inpatient since yesterday morning. She was admitted following a collapse at home and is being treated for a urinary tract infection (UTI). This afternoon, she became unresponsive and was found to have a BP of 62/35 mmHg, HR 145 bpm and RR 35 breaths per minute.

What could be some of the potential causes for Joan's sudden deterioration?

- *Sepsis* – since she was being treated for a UTI, the source would most likely be urosepsis.
- *Cardiovascular event* – acute myocardial infarction (AMI), arrhythmia (e.g. atrial fibrillation).
- *Pulmonary embolus (PE)* – massive PE can present with haemodynamic collapse.
- *Intracranial event* – acute stroke or intracerebral haemorrhage, seizures.
- *Metabolic or hypoglycaemic event* – severe hyponatraemia may result in a cardiac arrhythmia. Hypoglycaemia could precipitate a seizure.
- *Drug reaction* – severe anaphylaxis occurring in response to her medication.
- *Occult bleed* – ensure the patient is adequately exposed to assess for melaena/haematochezia (fresh PR bleed) in the initial evaluation.

How do we define shock?

Shock is a generalised form of acute circulatory failure associated with inadequate cellular utilisation of oxygen that is life-threatening. Cellular dysfunction occurs when the circulation is unable to deliver enough oxygen to meet the metabolic demands of the tissues.

Clinical Cases in Critical Care, First Edition. Alice Myers and Theophilus Samuels.
© 2023 John Wiley & Sons Ltd. Published 2023 by John Wiley & Sons Ltd.

How can we classify the different types of shock?

- *Hypovolaemic* – circulating volume loss that effectively leads to a decrease in venous return to the heart (e.g. haemorrhage, persistent diarrhoea and vomiting with inadequate fluid intake).
- *Distributive* – considered a relative hypovolaemia that has resulted from maldistribution of the absolute intravascular volume (e.g. sepsis, anaphylaxis or spinal injury).
- *Obstructive* – occurs when elevated resistance to blood flow leads to tissue hypoperfusion (e.g. pulmonary embolism, cardiac tamponade or tension pneumothorax).
- *Cardiogenic* – inadequate contractility of the myocardium (e.g. ischaemia, infarction or major arrhythmia).

While the classification of shock can be invaluable for the clinician, a patient may develop one or more of these types of shock at the same time or at different times during their presentation (e.g. the septic shock patient who develops cardiogenic shock due to a septic cardiomyopathy).

> The medical team have given Joan 500 mL of fluid that resulted in her becoming slightly more responsive but with confused speech. With the bed positioned so her legs are raised, Joan's BP is now 83/40 mmHg. Her HR is 135 bpm, temperature 38.3 °C and blood sugar 6.7 mmol/L. Her respiratory rate remains elevated at 30 breaths per minute with SpO$_2$ 96% on 10 L/min oxygen.

What do you now think is the most likely cause?

The most likely cause of her deterioration is sepsis and potentially septic shock.

Define sepsis

The Third International Consensus Definitions for Sepsis and Septic Shock (Sepsis-3) defined sepsis as life-threatening organ dysfunction caused by a dysregulated host response to infection.

Define septic shock

Sepsis-3 defines septic shock as a subset of sepsis, where profound circulatory, cellular and metabolic abnormalities are associated with an increased risk of mortality compared with sepsis alone (hospital mortality rates greater than 40%). Clinically, these patients can be identified by a vasopressor requirement to maintain a mean arterial pressure of greater than 65 mmHg and the presence of a serum lactate level greater than 7 mmol/L in the absence of hypovolaemia.

Describe the qSOFA Score

The quick Sequential Organ Failure Assessment (qSOFA) score consists of the following three easily measured and repeatable criteria (with a score of 2 or 3 being associated with a poor outcome due to sepsis, and the patient is considered qSOFA positive):

- Low systolic blood pressure <100 mmHg
- Respiratory rate >22 bpm
- Altered mentation (GCS <15)

A patient outside of ICU with a positive qSOFA should alert the clinician to the possibility of sepsis. While the score appears attractive and very simple to use (e.g. does not rely on laboratory tests, but uses bedside measurements), it should be considered a predictive rather than a diagnostic tool. It should also not be used in patients once they are admitted to critical care, as it has been shown to be inferior to other scoring systems for predicting outcome. qSOFA had a key role in screening for sepsis in Sepsis-3 (2016). However, updated guidance (2021) *no longer recommends* it to be used as a single screening tool for sepsis or septic shock.

Describe NEWS2

NEWS2 is an aggregate scoring system based upon the following six simple physiological parameters (Table 13.1).

- Respiration rate
- Oxygen saturation

Table 13.1: NEWS2 (Royal College of Physicians).

Physiological parameter	3	2	1	0	1	2	3
				Score			
Respiration rate (per minute)	≤8		9–11	12–20		21–24	≥25
SpO$_2$ Scale 1 (%)	≤91	92–93	94–95	≥96			
SpO$_2$ Scale 2 (%)	≤83	84–85	86–87	88–92 ≥93 on air	93–94 on oxygen	95–96 on oxygen	≥97 on oxygen
Air or oxygen?			Oxygen	Air			
Systolic blood pressure (mmHg)	≤90	91–100	101–110	111–219			≥220
Pulse (per minute)	≤40		41–50	51–90	91–110	111–130	≥131
Consciousness				Alert			CVPU
Temperature (°C)	≤35.0		35.1–36.0	36.1–38.0	38.1–39.0	≥39.1	

CVPU, confusion, voice, pain, unresponsive.
SpO$_2$ Scale 2 is used when the target range is between 88% and 92% (e.g. in hypercapnic respiratory failure).

- Systolic blood pressure
- Pulse rate
- Level of consciousness or new confusion
- Temperature

The further away the parameter is from the normal value then the higher the score allocated. In addition, if supplementary oxygen is being given then a further two points are added to the aggregated score. Since 2017, NHS England (NHSE) has recommended using NEWS2 as the early warning score to detect clinical deterioration in patients with suspected sepsis. Evidence suggests that it is superior to qSOFA in predicting adverse outcomes in both the emergency department and general ward setting. A raised NEWS2 score of 5 or more in a patient with signs and symptoms of infection, or in a patient at high risk of infection who clinically deteriorates, should trigger urgent review. Currently, Joan scores a total of 15 using this scoring system.

How can organ dysfunction be identified in sepsis?

This can be identified by an increase in the Sequential (Sepsis-related) Organ Failure Assessment (SOFA) score of two points or more.

Describe the SOFA Score

The SOFA score is well recognised within the critical care community, with increased risk of mortality being associated with higher scores. This score is not diagnostic for sepsis but enables the clinician to identify patients with a high risk of dying from infection. Calculating the total score requires time and therefore potentially delays recognition of acute organ dysfunction (Table 13.2).

Table 13.2: SOFA score.

	Points				
	0	**1**	**2**	**3**	**4**
PaO_2/FiO_2 (mmHg)	≥400	300–399	200–299	100–199 and mechanically ventilated	<100 and mechanically ventilated
Platelets (× 10³/μL)	≥150	100–150	50–99	20–49	<20
Glasgow Coma Scale	15	13–14	10–12	6–9	<6
Bilirubin (μmol/L)	<20	20–32	33–101	102–204	>204
Mean arterial pressure (MAP) or use of vasoactive agents (mcg/kg/min)	No hypotension	MAP <70 mmHg	Dopamine ≤5 or dobutamine (any dose)	Dopamine >5, adrenaline <0.1 or noradrenaline ≤0.1	Dopamine >15, adrenaline >0.1 or noradrenaline >0.1
Creatinine (μmol/L) or urine output (UOP)	<110	110–170	171–299	300–440 or UOP <500 mL/d	>440 or UOP <200 mL/d

How does sepsis lead to hypotension?

There are several factors that can lead to hypotension in sepsis, and it remains one of the most challenging tasks for clinicians to manage.

- *Hypovolaemia and decreased cardiac filling* – endothelial cell surface integrity becomes compromised by the release of proinflammatory mediators. This results in severe capillary leak and extravasation of fluid into the tissues along with reduced venous return due to venodilation. This redistribution of blood volume leads to the inability to maintain vascular wall tension, mean systemic filling pressure, venous return, cardiac filling, cardiac output and arterial blood pressure. Hypovolaemia may continue to be difficult to manage despite adequate fluid resuscitation due to the ongoing capillary leak that occurs.
- *Vasodilation* – peripheral maldistribution of blood can persist despite a normal or high cardiac output and is referred to as 'distributive shock'. Both the micro- and macrocirculation are affected. For example, blood is shunted away from the splanchnic circulation to preserve blood flow to the myocardium, brain and skeletal muscles.
- *Myocardial dysfunction* – biventricular function can be depressed with a decrease in ejection fraction. Potential causes include disruption to myocardial bioenergetics, circulating inflammatory cytokines and altered cardiac adrenergic signalling. Despite this, if adequate volume resuscitation is achieved, the resulting tachycardia, arteriolar dilation and biventricular dilation (which increases stroke volume through the Frank–Starling Law) can still produce a high cardiac output.

> Joan's urine dip on admission was positive for leucocytes and nitrites (a specimen was sent to the laboratory, results are outstanding) and she has received four doses of intravenous co-amoxiclav. There are no previous urine samples in the lab. Over the past 24 hours, her WBC and CRP have increased from 16 to 32×10^9/L and 35 to 186 respectively. Her NEWS2 remains elevated at 15.

What is the 'hour-1 bundle'?

In 2018 the Surviving Sepsis Campaign (SSC) published the initial resuscitation for sepsis and septic shock bundle that should be completed within the first hour (the 'hour-1 bundle'). In addition to ongoing resuscitation:

- Measure lactate level
- Obtain blood cultures before administering antibiotics
- Administer broad-spectrum antibiotics (according to your local guidelines)
- Begin rapid administration of 30 mL/kg crystalloid for hypotension or lactate ≥ 4 mmol/L
- Commence vasopressors if hypotensive during or after fluid resuscitation to maintain a MAP ≥ 65 mmHg.

Even though these goals are highly desirable, in real-world practice this timeframe is not always met, especially if the diagnosis of sepsis is not considered at the time of initial presentation.

What is the significance behind developing the 'hour-1 bundle'?

Sepsis and septic shock, just like an AMI or acute stroke, should be considered a medical emergency. It has been shown extensively that rapid assessment and treatment lead to improved patient outcomes. Even though more than 1 hour may be needed to complete resuscitation efforts, it is of paramount importance that the resuscitation and treatment measures, as outlined in the 'hour-1 bundle', begin immediately.

Which antibiotics would you start?

Joan has developed septic shock despite already receiving four doses of co-amoxiclav (amoxicillin and clavulanic acid). Therefore, depending on your local guidelines and advice from your microbiologist, following blood cultures, one option would be to change this to another beta-lactam beta-lactamase inhibitor combination (e.g. piperacillin-tazobactam [Tazocin®]) with an aminoglycoside (e.g. gentamicin) for synergistic activity.

> You arrange for Joan to be transferred to your ICU. As you are informed that this will take at least an hour due to lack of an immediate bed space, you decide to perform point-of-care echocardiography whilst resuscitative measures and preparations for her transfer are ongoing.

How can focused echocardiography help in differentiating the causes of shock?

- *Hypovolaemic or distributive shock* – when imaging the inferior vena cava (IVC) using a subcostal approach, a small (<1 cm) and collapsing IVC may suggest that fluid administration might be beneficial (for further details see Case 1). In addition, a hyperdynamic left ventricle (LV) with near total or complete effacement of the papillary muscles seen on a parasternal short-axis view also may suggest fluid responsiveness.
- *Cardiogenic shock* – assessment of LV systolic function can be rapidly achieved via parasternal and apical windows. Attention should be directed to how well the ventricular walls contract and move inwards towards the centre of the chamber. Recognising a significantly impaired LV strongly suggests cardiogenic shock, especially if it is a new finding. RV function can also be assessed well using the apical view, with its chamber size visually compared to the LV chamber (RV is considered dilated if > two-thirds the width of the LV).

- *Obstructive shock* – pericardial effusion with compression of the RA and RV during diastole would suggest cardiac tamponade. Conversely, a dilated RV with or without poor contraction of the free wall and absence of hypertrophy might indicate a massive pulmonary embolism.

For the different types of shock, focused echocardiography can provide valuable information that should be used in conjunction with other clinical findings to aid in diagnosis and ongoing management. But remember that ultrasonography is no substitute for a thorough history and physical examination. This amalgamation of all the available evidence is much more useful than making an inference from a single finding. For example, a patient with known malignancy developing significant hypotension with a normally functioning RV on echocardiography makes the probability of a massive pulmonary embolism extremely low.

> You have given Joan a litre of fluid intravenously in 250 mL boluses while still on the medical ward. With the last bolus of fluid, her blood pressure did not improve. Her BP is now 89/45, MAP 60 mmHg, HR 134 bpm sinus rhythm, RR 28 breaths per minute. Her lactate on the arterial blood gas is 4.6 mmol/L.

How do you proceed at this point?

- Increase the flow of oxygen from 10 to 15 L/min.
- Site an arterial catheter for invasive blood pressure monitoring and repeat lactate measurement.
- Ideally, site a central venous catheter (CVC) and commence an infusion of noradrenaline aiming for a MAP of at least 65 mmHg or higher if the patient is a known hypertensive. However, if it is impractical to site a CVC, then starting vasopressors peripherally to restore MAP is increasingly accepted practice. But only for a short period of time (consult your local guidelines).
- Insert a urinary catheter and monitor hourly urine output.
- Perform a complete septic screen.
- Liaise with your microbiologist to discuss your antibiotic choice, taking into consideration the most likely pathogens and local resistance patterns.
- Continue to bolus IV fluid up to the recommended limit of 30 mL/kg.
- Liaise with your consultant regarding admission to ICU.

Which vasopressors are recommended in sepsis?

Noradrenaline (NA) is the preferred first-line vasopressor in sepsis. It should be borne in mind that at high doses, NA can cause intense vasoconstriction, which may result in reduced tissue perfusion despite maintaining blood pressure. For second-line agents to maintain a MAP > 65 mmHg, instead of escalating the dose of NA, vasopressin should be commenced (usually when NA dose is in the range of 0.25–0.5 mcg/kg/min). If both NA and vasopressin fail to reach the target MAP, then adrenaline can be added.

Describe how these vasopressors work

- *Noradrenaline* is an endogenous catecholamine that exerts its effects via alpha-1 and beta-1 adrenergic receptors (it has little effect on beta-2 receptors) and is the initial agent of choice for sepsis. Alpha-1 receptor activation is cyclic adenosine 3,5-monophosphate (cAMP) independent and beta-1 adrenergic receptor activation is cAMP dependent. Like other natural and synthetic catecholamines, NA increases the amount of intracellular calcium, which leads to shortening of the contractile apparatus. NA has a short half-life between 1 and 2 minutes and achieves a steady-state plasma concentration within 5–10 minutes following a constant infusion. NA results in increased stroke volume (beta-1 adrenergic effect), mean arterial pressure and left ventricular afterload. More importantly, by constricting the venous circulation which contains most of the intravascular volume, this also increases preload and cardiac filling pressures with minimal effect on heart rate. NA enhances coronary blood flow due to coronary vasodilation secondary to improved cardiac metabolism and increases in diastolic blood pressure.
- *Vasopressin* is an endogenous hormone secreted from the neurohypophysis in response to arterial hypotension and hypovolaemia. Vasopressin acts on specific vasopressinergic receptors (V_1, V_2) located within the sympathetic nervous system. Interestingly, vasopressin levels are low in patients with septic shock, and exogenous administration of vasopressin, or its analogues, quickly restores MAP and vascular tone, and reduces noradrenaline requirements. However, the Vasopressin And Septic Shock (VASST) study demonstrated no significant difference in mortality when low-dose vasopressin was compared to noradrenaline.
- *Adrenaline* is a potent beta-1 adrenergic agonist with moderate beta-2 and alpha-1 adrenergic receptor activity. It increases both the cardiac index and MAP by vasoconstriction. Adrenaline is very effective at raising arterial pressure, but potentially at the cost of significantly impairing splanchnic circulation.

What role do corticosteroids have in the management of sepsis?

When at least 4 hours of noradrenaline or adrenaline at a dose ≥0.25 mcg/kg/min have been required to maintain the target MAP, intravenous hydrocortisone should be given in a divided dose of 200 mg per day.

Increased vigilance may be required to prevent associated hypernatraemia and hyperglycaemia. Interestingly, even though the evidence consistently demonstrates that steroid therapy leads to a faster resolution of shock, there appears to be minimal or no effect on mortality.

When you and Joan arrive in intensive care, you administer two further boluses of 250 mL intravenous fluid and site the CVC into the right internal jugular vein. Around 20 minutes after you have completed the procedure, Joan complains that her breathing is becoming more difficult. On auscultation of her chest, you find bilateral widespread crepitations. She denies chest pain. Her BP is unchanged, her HR is 135 bpm sinus rhythm, her RR is now 35 breaths per minute and her saturations are 88% on 8 L/min oxygen via a Hudson mask.

What do you think has happened based on her clinical findings?

- *Cardiogenic pulmonary oedema (CPO)* – this is the most likely cause of her current breathing problems. Either the volume, infusion rate or both can lead to CPO in these situations, especially if there is underlying cardiac disease.
- *Iatrogenic pneumothorax* – pneumothorax is a known complication of central line insertion into the internal jugular veins and should be ruled out. However, given her clinical findings, the probability of this having occurred remains relatively low.

How can lung ultrasonography help you differentiate between these two potential causes?

As already stated, history and clinical examination are essential to fully interpret ultrasonographic findings. Nevertheless, lung ultrasonography can help distinguish between these two clinical entities as follows:

- *A- or B-line patterns* – when the predominant findings change from an A-line to a B-line pattern, this suggests that the patient has developed new-onset interstitial oedema alongside fluid resuscitation. If ultrasonography is only performed following aggressive fluid administration and bilateral B-lines are found, then it is possible this could represent pre-existing CPO. However, other causes should also be considered such as chronic lung disease and infection.
- *Lung point/lung sliding* – see Case 5.

You request a chest radiograph and perform lung ultrasound (US). Both confirm that this is CPO. After successfully treating the CPO, Joan begins feeling better. Her blood pressure has increased to 124/53 (MAP 77) mmHg with noradrenaline. The ECG remains unchanged, and bedside focused echocardiography shows a hyperdynamic LV. Her HR is now 112 bpm and RR 19 breaths per minute. Microbiology informs you the following morning that blood cultures taken on admission have grown gram-negative bacilli. She currently requires 0.25 mcg/kg/min noradrenaline.

What is the significance of gram-negative bacilli in a blood culture?

The presence of gram-negative bacilli is always a significant finding that needs to be acted upon. Discussing the likely pathogen, possible sources and any previous/current antimicrobial therapy with a microbiologist is of paramount importance. Your microbiology laboratory will hopefully be able to identify the pathogen within 24 hours of receiving the sample, which will enable you to target your antimicrobial therapy.

Which organisms are most likely to be responsible for gram-negative sepsis in this case?

There are many gram-negative bacilli that can cause bacteraemia. However, in this case the most common organisms include *Escherichia coli*, *Proteus* spp., *Enterococcus* spp. and *Klebsiella* spp.

Briefly describe the differences between gram-positive and gram-negative bacteria

In gram-positive bacteria, the cell membrane is covered by a thick (20–80 nm) protective cell wall made from peptidoglycan. This wall forms the external surface of the cell and disrupting its integrity constitutes one of the targets for antimicrobial therapies (e.g. beta-lactam antibiotics). However, in gram-negative bacteria the peptidoglycan layer is thin (5–10 nm) and there is an additional outer layer rich in lipopolysaccharides (LPS) and lipoproteins. This extra layer offers protection against antibiotics and the host's immune system. LPS in the membrane has both antigenic properties (e.g. carbohydrate chain *O antigens*) and toxic properties (e.g. lipid A component *endotoxin*).

The microbiologist calls back to say that they have isolated *E. coli* from the urine culture and that it is sensitive to meropenem only.

To which class of antibiotics does meropenem belong and what is its general spectrum of activity?

Meropenem (along with ertapenem and imipenem) is classed as a carbapenem. These carbapenem drugs belong to the much larger family of beta-lactam bactericidal compounds (i.e. they all contain the beta-lactam ring). Carbapenems are active against both gram-positive and gram-negative bacteria.

Briefly describe the other beta-lactam antibiotics and how they work

Beta-lactam antibiotics are differentiated according to the structure of the chemical ring that is attached to the beta-lactam ring. They bind to and inhibit the enzymes responsible for the final stages of cross-linking of the bacterial peptidoglycan cell wall subunits once they have been transported across the cell membrane. Apart from the carbapenems, the other beta-lactam drugs are as follows:

- *Penicillins* – these include naturally occurring compounds such as penicillin V or G, and semisynthetic compounds such as amoxicillin, ampicillin and piperacillin. Effective mainly against gram-positive bacteria, some of the semisynthetic penicillins have been developed for their activity against gram-negative rods (e.g. piperacillin).
- *Cephalosporins* – currently, there are five generations of cephalosporins that can be used. The first three generations (that contain cephalexin, cefuroxime and ceftriaxone) are effective against gram-positive bacteria. However, fourth- and fifth-generation cephalosporins (such as cefepime and ceftrolozane) have improved activity against gram-negative bacteria, with the fifth generation also being effective against methicillin-resistant *Staphylococcus aureus* (MRSA).
- *Monobactams* – aztreonam is generally effective against gram-negative bacteria including *Haemophilus influenzae* and *Pseudomonas aeruginosa*.
- *Cephamycins* – these drugs are often classified as second-generation cephalosporins. However, both cefotetan and cefotixin are effective against gram-positive bacteria as well as *Bacillus fragilis*.

What does the term extended-spectrum beta-lactamase (ESBL) mean?

Ongoing mutations in the beta-lactamase genes confer resistance against the beta-lactams in gram-negative bacteria. Enterobacteriaceae (e.g. *E. coli* and *Klebsiella* spp.) are the most often identified bacteria that produce ESBLs. The ESBLs that *E. coli* produces most often are called CTX-M enzymes, which inevitably make these infections much harder to treat. With ever increasing resistance to beta-lactam beta-lactamase inhibitor combinations, there remain few options in our arsenal to tackle these challenges. Carbapenem-resistant ESBL-producing Enterobacteriaceae are a major and constant health problem worldwide.

By day 6 on critical care, Joan has been over 48 hours without the need for noradrenaline and she is only requiring nasal oxygen therapy. As she no longer requires any organ support, she is transferred back to the ward, and you're informed when she is successfully discharged home the following day.

Further reading

■ Singer, M., Deutschman, C., Seymour, C. et al. (2016). The third international consensus definitions for sepsis and septic shock (sepsis-3). *JAMA* 315: 801–810. World leading experts define sepsis.

■ Evans, L., Rhodes, A., Alhazzani, W. et al. (2021). Surviving sepsis campaign: international guidelines for management of sepsis and septic shock 2021. *Intensive Care Med* 47: 1181–1247. Important updates to sepsis and its management by the ESICM and SCCM.

■ Goering, R., Dockrell, H., Zuckerman, M. et al. (2019). *MIMS' Medical Microbiology and Immunology*. St Louis: Elsevier. Invaluable textbook when dealing with infectious diseases.

14 The Patient Who Deteriorates Post Intubation

You are asked to review Michael, a 75-year-old man who has just been admitted to your ICU with shortness of breath, a productive cough, oliguria and pyrexia. The presenting ECG demonstrates left ventricular hypertrophy and a chest radiograph demonstrates bilateral consolidation. On examination, a late peaking systolic ejection murmur is detected, but accurate assessment of heart sounds is not possible. Following initial fluid resuscitation, lactate is 2.4 mmol/L and urine output improved to >0.5 mL/kg/h. He requires noradrenaline at a dose of 0.05 mcg/kg/min. However, due to his deteriorating respiratory function, Michael is intubated and mechanically ventilated with propofol/fentanyl sedation. Within 20 minutes, the noradrenaline requirement has increased to 0.6 mcg/kg/min to maintain a MAP >65 mmHg, and despite this increase he remains haemodynamically unstable: BP 78/58 mmHg, HR 130 bpm sinus rhythm.

What could be the causes of his persistent hypotension despite increases in noradrenaline and adequate fluid resuscitation?

- Acute coronary syndrome
- Acute heart failure (AHF)
- Pulmonary embolism
- Tension pneumothorax
- Severe aortic stenosis
- Septic shock
- Artefact (e.g. equipment failure or user error)
- Effects of anaesthetic agents used for intubation

Clinical Cases in Critical Care, First Edition. Alice Myers and Theophilus Samuels.
© 2023 John Wiley & Sons Ltd. Published 2023 by John Wiley & Sons Ltd.

The focused echocardiogram demonstrates LV impairment. A subsequent formal echocardiogram is performed that demonstrates moderate left ventricular hypertrophy with a small cavity, a peak velocity through the AV of 3.5 m/s, mean pressure gradient of 33 mmHg but with an estimated AV area of 0.8 cm². The report also states that the valve appears severely calcified with severely reduced leaflet motion. Ejection fraction is estimated to be 40%, indicating impaired LV systolic function.

What is the normal range for aortic valve area and peak transvalvular flow?

The normal area is considered to be between 3 and 4 cm² and under normal circumstances, the flow velocity through the aortic valve (transvalvular flow) should be less than 2 m/s.

What are the echocardiographic criteria for diagnosing severe aortic stenosis?

The British Society of Echocardiography defines severe aortic stenosis (Table 14.1) as follows:

- Aortic valve area (AVA) <1.0 cm²
- Aortic valve area indexed (AVAi) <0.6 cm²/m²
- Peak velocity (Vmax) between 4.0 and 4.9 m/s
- Mean pressure gradient 40–59 mmHg
- Dimensionless Index (DI) is obtained from the ratio of left ventricle outflow tract (LVOT)/AV velocities, and a ratio <0.25 is consistent with severe AS

How would you interpret the reported echocardiogram?

The estimated aortic valve area suggests severe aortic stenosis (AS). However, the mean pressure gradient and peak velocity through the valve do not meet the definition of severe AS. Considering that the report states:

- 'severely calcified'
- 'severely reduced leaflet motion'
- 'left ventricle appears hypertrophied'

Table 14.1: Grading aortic stenosis severity.

	Aortic sclerosis	Mild	Moderate	Severe	Very severe
AV V$_{max}$ (m/s)	<2.5	2.5–2.9	3.0–3.9	4.0–4.9	≥5.0
Mean gradient (mmHg)	–	<20	20–39	40–59	≥60
AVA (cm²)	–	>1.5	1–1.5	<1	≤0.6

you would conclude that even though most of the reported parameters fit with moderate AS, you cannot exclude severe AS at this point.

How might you explain the inconsistencies in the reported echocardiogram regarding the estimated AV area and pressure measurements?

The impaired LV systolic function decreases the gradient across the valve. This is classified as a low-gradient AS with impaired LV ejection fraction (LVEF). This can lead to the clinical picture of non-severe AS and potentially underestimates severity. Also, measurement error must be excluded, and this requires the operator to recheck all measurements (e.g. LVOT diameter) and indices to ensure the information is accurate.

What is low-gradient aortic stenosis?

Attempting to diagnose severe AS in critical care patients with low cardiac output and a non-severe gradient across the valve can be challenging. Low-gradient AS is divided into the following two possibilities:

Low-gradient AS with impaired LVEF
This is defined as follows:

- AVA $<1.0\,cm^2$
- AVAi $<0.6\,cm^2/m^2$
- Mean gradient $<35\,mmHg$
- LVEF $\leq40\%$

Measurement error must be excluded first in these cases. As these patients have reduced cardiac output, they can be distinguished from the other type of low-gradient AS by examining the response of the left ventricle to low-dose dobutamine. If LV systolic impairment can be improved using inotropes, then the mean pressure gradient will exceed 40 mmHg in the presence of true severe AS. Formal dobutamine stress echocardiography is not routinely performed in critical care.

Low-gradient AS with LVEF $\geq50\%$
This is defined as follows:

- AVA $<1.0\,cm^2$
- AVAi $<0.6\,cm^2/m^2$
- Mean gradient $<40\,mmHg$
- AV V_{max} $<4\,m/s$
- LVEF $\geq50\%$

Ensuring that accurate measurements have been taken is again an important first step in preventing misdiagnosis. Additionally, examining the echocardiography report is essential. If the AV is *not* described as being both heavily calcified and restricted, then significant AS is unlikely. Calculating an indexed stroke volume (SVi) is the next step. Patients with a 'normal' SVi ($\geq 35\,mL/m^2$) have a prognosis similar to conventional 'moderate AS' and usually only require observation. Patients with a 'low' SVi ($< 35\,mL/m^2$) are very challenging to differentiate between truly severe AS and non-severe AS and this is beyond the scope of this book.

> The measurements and indices from the formal echocardiogram are rechecked and confirmed to be accurate. You discuss this with your critical care lead for echocardiography. Given that the valve appears severely calcified with severely reduced leaflet motion and an estimated AVA of $0.8\,cm^2$, it is likely that this is a low-gradient AS with impaired LVEF.

What is the prevalence of AS in the general population?

As the population continues to age, the prevalence of valvular heart disease increases, with AS being the most common in developed countries. AS is present in about 3% of patients over the age of 75 years. The increasing use of echocardiography in critical care will continue to increase the detection of AS.

What are the main causes of aortic stenosis?

Acquired causes

- *Calcific AS* – this is the most common cause of AS and should be considered an active and progressive disease process characterised by inflammation, fibrosis, lipid infiltration and calcification. Predisposing factors include male sex, age and hypercholesterolaemia.
- *Rheumatic heart disease* – this remains the most common cause of valvular heart disease worldwide but is rarely the cause in Europe and North America. Rheumatic AS most commonly coincides with mitral valve disease.

Congenital causes

Bicuspid AV – as a congenital abnormality, there is a great deal more mechanical stress placed on these structures and therefore the average age at presentation of patients with bicuspid AV stenosis is significantly lower than that seen in the elderly population with normal AV morphology.

What is aortic sclerosis?

In aortic sclerosis, there is calcification and thickening of the aortic leaflets but without significant outflow obstruction (maximum velocity across the aortic valve $< 2.5\,m/s$). In patients over age 65, aortic sclerosis is present in nearly 30%, which increases to 50% by the age of 85. Aortic sclerosis suggests the presence of vascular disease and, more importantly, coronary artery disease. Therefore, the critical care clinician should be wary of vascular disease in any patient who is reported to have aortic sclerosis.

Describe the morphological changes to the LV that can occur with severe aortic stenosis

In the presence of a fixed outflow obstruction causing pressure overload, the left ventricle undergoes remodelling. This results in compensatory hypertrophy in most cases. However, if the hypertrophic response is inadequate, the LV is placed under extreme wall stress that can result in dilation and dysfunction of the cavity.

What is the physiological role of LV hypertrophy?

According to the principle of LaPlace regarding wall tension, the left ventricle wall stress (σ) is proportional to the pressure (P) multiplied by the radius (r) of the cavity divided by the wall thickness (T)

$$\sigma \propto \frac{P \times r}{T}$$

Hence, as pressure increases, the heart attempts to keep wall stress constant by increasing the wall thickness of the LV.

What are the problems that can arise with LV hypertrophy?

While the physiological response to increased pressure overload is hypertrophy, this is associated with the following deleterious effects:

- *Increased myocardial oxygen demand* – the increased muscle mass and wall stress can potentially lead to a relative reduction in delivery of oxygen and nutrients to cardiac myocytes.
- *Increased LV filling pressures* – decrease in LV compliance, diastolic dysfunction and increased diastolic filling pressures can impair subendocardial blood flow and give rise to ischaemia.

What do we mean by the term 'preload'?

The force or load acting to stretch the cardiac myofibril defines preload. It is commonly estimated using the LV end-diastolic pressure, diameter or volume (e.g. normal LV diastolic volume indexed to body surface area is between 35 and 75 mL/m^2). The inherent stiffness of cardiac muscle attempts to counteract the stretching caused by preload, and therefore the actual degree to which the myofibril is stretched depends on this interaction. And note, since LV systolic performance is related to this initial length (as demonstrated by the Frank–Starling mechanism), it is also affected by preload.

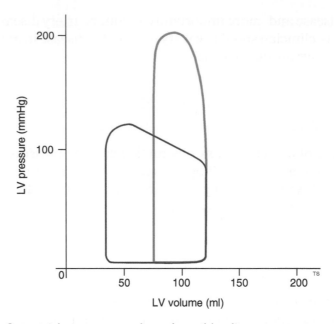

Figure 14.1: Left ventricle pressure–volume loop (blue line represents normal LV).
Source: Theophilus Samuels.

How is preload affected in AS?

As shown in Figure 14.1, the pressure–volume loop in AS (red curve) demonstrates an increased peak systolic pressure within the ventricle due to the high outflow resistance and large pressure gradient that occurs across the AV. This increased afterload, when cardiac myofibrils are exposed to greater stress during systole, decreases SVi and increases end-systolic volume. As venous return occurs, this increase in end-systolic volume leads to an increase in end-diastolic volume with a resultant increase in preload. And as described, as preload increases so does the stretch on the myofibrils, which then through the Frank–Starling mechanism increases the force of contraction to overcome the outflow resistance of AS.

What is meant by the term 'afterload'?

Afterload is the force or stress developed by the myocardium after the onset of contraction and consequently varies with time. It can be measured at any point during systole. It is important to note that while systemic vascular resistance and LV systolic pressures can *affect* afterload, they should not be considered *equal to* afterload, which is often a misconception.

How is afterload affected in the presence of severe AS?

As the LV becomes hypertrophied in clinically significant AS, this reduces wall stress and therefore decreases the force exerted on each cardiac muscle unit so that afterload remains near normal. As afterload is a key determinant of ejection performance, this attempt at its normalisation is important in maintaining normal ejection fraction and SVi.

What treatment options are available for severe AS?

Percutaneous interventions

- *Balloon valvuloplasty (BV)* – as a temporising measure for those patients who are haemodynamically unstable, BV can be considered. It should be noted that this technique mainly exerts its effects by creating multiple microscopic fracture lines in the calcified leaflets and thereby temporarily improves leaflet compliance. Hence, any haemodynamic benefit only lasts a few hours and within a few weeks to months, the AV returns to its original calcified pre-valvuloplasty state. The use of BV alone has not been shown to improve long-term outcomes. However, in a few cases with severe haemodynamic compromise, it has been successfully performed with haemodynamic support devices such as an intra-aortic balloon pump.
- *Transcatheter aortic valve replacement (TAVR)* – being able to site a tissue valve without the need for major surgery has dramatically altered the management of AS in high-risk patients. The Placement of Aortic Transcatheter valves study (PARTNER) demonstrated that the use of TAVR in these types of patients produced results that were like surgical aortic valve replacement (SAVR) at 2 years follow-up. TAVR is associated with more vascular complications and stroke, whilst SAVR is associated with more bleeding complications and atrial fibrillation. In addition, in a small number of cases with pre-existing conduction disturbances (especially right bundle branch block), the use of TAVR is associated with permanent pacemaker placement. Patients are usually given 3 months of anticoagulation due to supporting evidence of thrombus formation following TAVR.

Surgical intervention

- *SAVR* – this option remains the treatment of choice for the following patients:
  - Symptomatic severe AS (valve area <1 cm^2) and low operative risk.
  - In addition, irrespective of symptoms, the following patients should be considered for SAVR (class I recommendation):
    - Severe AS undergoing coronary artery bypass
    - Severe AS with LV dysfunction
    - Severe AS undergoing surgery for other heart valves or the aorta

What are the risk factors for increased surgical mortality?

- Renal failure
- Age over 75 years
- Reduced LV function
- Congestive cardiac failure
- Pulmonary hypertension

And like TAVR, these patients will require anticoagulation post surgery.

What is the prognosis for patients with symptomatic severe AS?

Once patients with AS begin to develop symptoms (classically angina, dyspnoea and syncopal episodes), prognosis is poor without valve replacement: 50% mortality within the next 12–18 months.

Michael's clinical condition improves, and his noradrenaline requirements reduce with additional inotropic support and further IV fluid boluses. His blood pressure increases to 100/40 mmHg and his tachycardia reduces to 110 bpm. With ongoing treatment, Michael begins to improve over the next 72 hours. After a total of 10 days in your ICU, he is successfully extubated with no further cardiac or respiratory support required. A repeat echocardiogram confirms that he does have severe AS now that his LV systolic function has returned to normal.

On day 11, during your night shift, the nurse looking after Michael is concerned that his breathing has become more laboured, his chest has widespread crackles throughout, and his BP is approximately 170/110 mmHg. You suspect that Michael has gone into acute heart failure (AHF). Focused ultrasonography demonstrates impaired LV systolic function and multiple B-lines throughout.

Define acute heart failure (AHF)

AHF 'presents suddenly' and results from any functional or structural impairment of ventricular filling or ejection of blood, producing a complex clinical syndrome. Heart failure may be classified as:

- *heart failure with **reduced** ejection fraction (HRrEF)* – characterised by reduced cardiac contractility, or
- *heart failure with **preserved** ejection fraction (HRpEF)* – commonly the result of diastolic dysfunction represented by impaired LV relaxation and/or increased LV filling pressures.

What are the treatment principles for managing AHF?

Urgent treatment is designed to relieve symptoms, reverse acute haemodynamic instability and preserve myocardial function as well as possible. The main interventions include the following:

- *Intravenous diuretics* – the loop diuretic furosemide is most used in the acute setting and increases renal excretion of salt and water (other loop diuretics include bumetanide and torsemide). The onset of action is approximately 30 minutes, with a peak effect occurring at between 1 and 2 hours, and a half-life of 6 hours. Loop diuretics also enhance prostaglandin synthesis, which can lead to renal and venous dilation, which may in turn reduce preload and relieve pulmonary congestion.

- *Vasodilators* – drugs such as glyceryl trinitrate (GTN) are often given in combination with diuretic therapy. This effective systemic and coronary vasodilator can be particularly useful in cases of coronary ischaemia. At low doses, it is a venodilator and can also relieve symptoms of pulmonary oedema. After 24 hours of continued use, GTN is subject to tachyphylaxis, which is the rapid development of tolerance to its actions. Sodium nitroprusside is also used and is a potent vasodilator of both arterial and venous circulations. It is the drug of choice in patients with severe heart failure due to mitral regurgitation with associated hypertension and pulmonary oedema. Caution should be exercised in patients with renal or hepatic impairment as its toxic metabolites thiocyanate and cyanide may accumulate.
- *Inotropic drugs* – dobutamine can be used in these patients to increase contractility and cardiac output but may also cause tachyarrhythmias, limiting its use. Of note, by exerting these inotropic effects, it should be appreciated that myocardial oxygen demand increases and therefore it can be detrimental in patients where the cause of the heart failure is ischaemic in origin (e.g. following myocardial infarction). It should also be noted that beta-receptors are downregulated in patients with chronic heart failure and therefore its effects may be attenuated. Another drug that may be used is milrinone, which is a phosphodiesterase-3 inhibitor that increases intracellular calcium levels and may be more efficacious in patients on beta-blockers. It increases cardiac output and SVi but does also result in a decrease in systemic vascular resistance due to its vasodilatory properties. While it acts as a coronary vasodilator, it does not increase myocardial oxygen demand.
- *Vasopressors* – noradrenaline is commonly used, and its main aim is to restore systemic arterial pressure through peripheral vasoconstriction with little effect on cardiac output. It is generally only used in those patients who have severe hypotension and/or complicating conditions such as sepsis.
- *Non-invasive ventilation* – mortality and the need for endotracheal intubation are reduced by the early use of non-invasive positive pressure ventilation in those patients presenting with acute cardiogenic pulmonary oedema.

How might you adjust your treatment for AHF in Michael given that he has severe AS?

Your treatment would still follow the principles described for managing acute cardiac failure, but you would need to be cautious in severe AS.

- *Diuretics and vasodilators* – these drugs may cause refractory shock due to their effect on reducing preload (especially if the LV cavity appears small and hypertrophied as cardiac output in this setting is very much preload dependent). However, nitroprusside can increase cardiac output significantly in patients with both severe LV dysfunction and severe AS but who are not dependent on inotropes.
- *Inotropes* – these may be required but patients may show little improvement if their contractile reserve is limited.

Michael stabilises with your acute cardiac failure management. He is seen the next day by the cardiothoracic team to assess for aortic valve replacement.

Further reading

■ Ring, L., Shah, B., Bhattacharyya, S. et al. (2021). Echocardiographic assessment of aortic stenosis: a practical guideline from the British Society of Echocardiography. *Echo. Res. Pract.* 8: G19. Detailed guideline regarding the echocardiographic assessment of aortic stenosis, and includes haemodynamic considerations and other useful information.

■ Anderson B. (2017). The Normal Examination and Echocardiographic Measurements. Echotext Pty Ltd. Essential reading for anyone learning advanced echocardiography.

15 The Patient with Reduced Consciousness

Debbie has been brought in by ambulance to the resuscitation area of the ED. She is 45 years old. Her husband called emergency services after she collapsed at home. She is normally very fit, but this morning did not want to get out of bed due to a headache. She vomited once then became unrousable. She does not appear to have lost cardiac output at any point. She is tolerating the oropharyngeal airway inserted by paramedics. BP 162/94 mmHg, HR 86 bpm, RR 10 per minute, pulse oximetry 98% on 15 L/min oxygen via non-rebreathe mask. Glasgow Coma Scale (GCS) 8 (E1V2M5). Pupils equal and reactive to light. Temperature 36.7 °C.

What could be the cause of Debbie's low GCS?

- *Cerebrovascular event* – haemorrhagic or thrombotic. This type of rapid deterioration, associated with symptoms consistent with cerebral irritation (i.e. headache and vomiting), could be compatible with a sudden vascular event. There are more than 100 000 strokes in the UK each year and stroke is a leading cause of death (NICE CKS 2022 Stroke and TIA). Approximately 85% of strokes are ischaemic and 15% are haemorrhagic.
- *Space-occupying lesion* – tumour, lymphoma, abscess. It is possible that Debbie may have had a space-occupying lesion for some time which, due to location and size, had not caused symptoms until now.
  - Tumours can be primary or secondary. Tumours commonly leading to cerebral metastases include lung, breast, genitourinary, skin, colon and osteosarcoma.
  - Tumours can be benign or malignant depending on growth rate and likelihood of invasion into surrounding tissue. Malignant brain tumours rarely spread beyond the central nervous system:
  - Common brain tumour types include the following:
    - Gliomas (>50%), which include astrocytomas (a type of glioma originating in the cerebrum from astrocyte cells, can be any grade), oligodendrogliomas and ependymomas.

Clinical Cases in Critical Care, First Edition. Alice Myers and Theophilus Samuels.
© 2023 John Wiley & Sons Ltd. Published 2023 by John Wiley & Sons Ltd.

- Meningiomas (approximately 25%) – arise from the meninges, usually benign and slow growing. Usually occur in those older than 70 years. Can be grades 1–3.
- Intracranial abscesses are uncommon in developed countries and in non-immune suppressed populations (approximately 0.5–1 in 100 000). Causes include bacteria, fungi, protozoa and helminths. Look for systemic signs of sepsis, local sources of infection (e.g. dental infection, mastoiditis, otitis media), and ascertain whether there is a history of congenital cardiac disease, intravenous drug use or immune suppression, such as HIV.

- *Meningitis or encephalitis* – cerebral infection should be considered in a previously well person presenting with low GCS and signs of meningism.
- *Drugs* – decreased GCS with a history of vomiting could be consistent with paracetamol overdose, alcohol intoxication, opioid use, or misuse, etc. So even though Debbie is apparently normally well, explore the possibility of drug side-effects and overdose from prescription medication, over-the-counter drugs or recreational drug use. Obtain collateral history from the GP, relatives and paramedics.
- *Sepsis* – the clinical signs described here are non-specific. Sepsis can present in a variety of ways but normally, a young fit patient such as Debbie would mount more of a physiological response with raised or lowered temperature, hypotension, tachycardia and tachypnoea, etc. Consider this as a possibility, but it is less likely than some other differential diagnoses on this list.
- *Metabolic* – consider the possibility of hepatic or uraemic encephalopathy due to occult liver or renal disease. Acute liver failure and raised ammonia can lead to cerebral oedema and a rapid, dangerous increase in intracranial pressure (ICP).
  - Uraemic encephalopathy may develop when glomerular filtration rate (GFR) falls to below 10–15 mL/min. This would be a very unusual primary presentation of renal failure. However, at this early stage, consider the full range of possibilities.
  - Check electrolytes and never forget to test glucose (and sodium) in patients with a low GCS.
- *Autoimmune* – autoimmune encephalitis has an incidence of approximately 0.5–2 per 100 000. Causes include acute disseminated encephalomyelitis (ADEM), N-methyl D-aspartate (NMDA) receptor encephalomyelitis, limbic and Hashimoto' encephalitis (also, rarely, Rasmussen's in children and young adults). Some cases occur following infection but in many there is no identifiable prodrome.
- *Haematological* – thrombotic thrombocytopenic purpura classically presents with the pentad of fever, microangiopathic haemolytic anaemia, thrombocytopenia, renal impairment and neurological symptoms (including headache, confusion, seizures or focal neurological deficit). Autoantibodies against ADAMTS13 protease result in platelet aggregation and clumping, accumulation of ultra-large von Willebrand factor, and formation of microthrombi and microangiopathic haemolytic anaemia (MAHA). This life-threatening condition can be triggered by

infection, pregnancy, systemic lupus erythematosus (SLE) or drugs, and can be treated effectively with prompt plasmapheresis. Haemolytic uraemic syndrome is clinically similar but the platelet microthrombi tend to be confined to the kidneys and it is less likely to cause neurological symptoms. If the platelet count is low, this should be investigated as a potential cause of Debbie's presentation (see Case 23).

■ *Thrombus/obstruction to venous drainage of the brain* – cerebral venous sinus thrombosis accounts for less than 1% of all strokes. Thrombus can form in the deep or superficial venous systems of the brain and, depending upon location, can result in varying patterns of focal or generalised neurological deficit. Raised ICP results from several mechanisms including oedema formation due to mechanical obstruction of venous drainage, vasogenic oedema from disruption of the blood–brain barrier, and cytotoxic oedema generated as ischaemia develops with falling cerebral perfusion.

■ *Non-convulsive status epilepticus (NCSE) or a postictal state* – it is relatively common following subarachnoid haemorrhage (SAH) to see the GCS 'artificially' worsened by NCSE or a postictal period. This often worsens the WFNS (World Federation of Neurosurgical Societies) score and may lead to surprise when these patients 'do well' despite having a WFNS score of 5.

What are your main concerns at this point?

■ *Airway protection* – Debbie's GCS is 8 and she is tolerating an oropharyngeal airway. She is at high risk of aspiration and airway obstruction.

■ *Possible aspiration* – there is a history of vomiting and, given Debbie has a low GCS, she may already have aspirated. She is currently receiving 15 L/min oxygen via non-rebreathe mask with saturations of 98% but the PaO_2 is unknown at this point. Aspiration pneumonitis or superadded infection may develop over the next few hours or days.

■ *Neuroprotection* – Debbie's presentation could be consistent with meningism (look for the triad of nuchal rigidity, photophobia and headache, often accompanied by nausea and vomiting). Intracranial pathology is possible in this case. If ICP is rising, it is imperative to take control of the situation to minimise further damage.

■ *Diagnosis* – the main differential diagnoses include several problems which could require urgent neurosurgical intervention. Identify or rule these out rapidly to maximise Debbie's chances of making a good recovery.

You decide to intubate Debbie and transfer her to the CT scanner. The CTA head is shown in Figure 15.1.

Review this CT image (Figure 15.1). What is the diagnosis?

This CT head demonstrates acute subarachnoid haemorrhage (SAH).

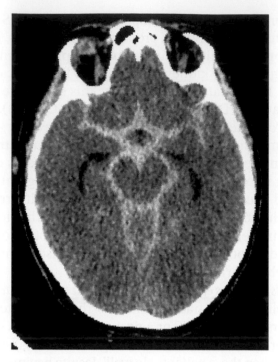

Figure 15.1: CT head demonstrating SAH.

What is the Monro–Kellie Doctrine?

The doctrine assumes that the sum of the volumes of non-compressible contents within the cranium (brain, cerebrospinal fluid (CSF) and intracranial blood) is constant. Therefore, an increase in one should result in a decrease in one or both of the other two. This pressure–volume relationship is particularly significant because the cranium can be thought of as a rigid box with one major opening (the foramen magnum) and limited capacity for accommodating changes in volume. Small increases in blood volume can be compensated for without a resultant change in pressure through a decrease in CSF volume. However, a sudden large increase in blood volume beyond this capacity for compensation will lead to a rise in ICP. The increase in pressure leads to the non-compressible contents expanding towards and possibly through the foramen magnum. Initially, this causes false localising signs due to stretching of the cranial nerves over the base of skull (i.e. sixth nerve palsy) and ultimately tonsillar herniation and coning. This process can be exacerbated by cerebral oedema development as perfusion of the brain is impaired.

The effects can be illustrated in the compliance curve (Figure 15.2).

What is cerebral perfusion pressure (CPP)?

This equation reflects the pressure gradient driving cerebral blood flow.

$$CPP = MAP - ICP$$

MAP, mean arterial pressure, *ICP*, intracranial pressure

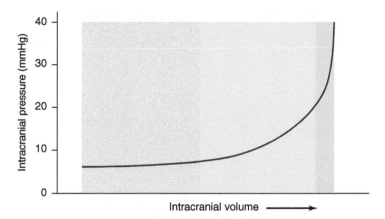

Figure 15.2: Intracranial compliance (pressure–volume) curve. Compensatory mechanisms maintain intracranial pressure (ICP) within normal range (green shaded area). As increases in volume continue to occur, there is a steady decline in compliance, causing a rise in ICP (yellow shaded area). Small increases in volume result in marked increases in ICP, causing a fall in the perfusion pressure leading to cerebral ischaemia (red shaded area).

Source: Theophilus Samuels.

This is normally under autoregulatory control but can be disrupted when either the mean arterial pressure (MAP) falls or ICP rises significantly.

Note that normal ranges vary with age. In adults, 'normal' should be between 7–15 mmHg. Between 20 and 30 mmHg would constitute mild intracranial hypertension. A pressure sustained above 40 mmHg would represent severe, life-threatening intracranial hypertension.

What is secondary brain injury and how can you minimise it?

This concept is used in trauma to describe the cellular processes which occur following initial primary injury to the brain (e.g. diffuse axonal injury or local trauma) and includes problems such as the oedema and hypoxia which result from raised ICP. These principles can also be applied in Debbie's case as sudden bleeding within the cranium exerts similar effects. The focus of clinicians is to ameliorate the damage which occurs after the initial insult. Management strategies include the following:

Conservative

- Avoid impairing cerebral venous drainage – head in neutral position, avoid tight endotracheal tube ties around the neck, 30–45° head up tilt.
- Maintain sodium >142 mmol/L, glucose 4.6–10 mmol/L.
- Aim for normothermia.

Medical

- Drugs such as mannitol and hypertonic saline can be used with caution where the blood–brain barrier remains intact.

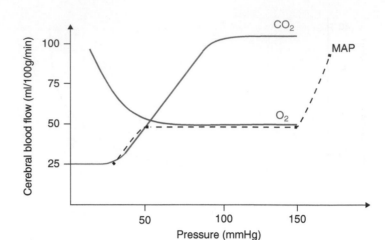

Figure 15.3: Cerebral blood flow (mL/100 g/min) relationship with partial pressure of oxygen and carbon dioxide, along with mean arterial blood pressure (MAP).

Source: Theophilus Samuels.

- Where seizures are noted, rapid pharmacological control is indicated to reduce cerebral metabolic rate and oxygen demand.

Anaesthetic

- Optimise cerebral blood flow through careful ventilator management – $PaCO_2$ 4.5–6 kPa, systolic BP >90 mmHg but less than 160 mmHg to avoid exacerbating bleeding from an unsecured aneurysm. Some centres advocate PaO_2 >10 kPa to avoid hypoxia though others would tolerate >8 kPa. Extreme hyperoxia (>40 kPa) is associated with poorer outcome (Figure 15.3).
- Deep sedation can be used to reduce straining or agitation in intubated patients, and to reduce cerebral metabolic rate and oxygen demand.

Surgical

- Decompression – craniectomy.
- Drainage of CSF.

You promptly refer Debbie to the regional neurosurgical centre while providing neuroprotection. She is accepted for transfer and neurosurgeons request that you take her straight to the operating theatres on arrival.

What is the incidence and what are the causes of subarachnoid haemorrhage (SAH)?

Incidence

SAH occurs in around 6–9 per 100 000 per year in the UK. Around 10% die before reaching hospital and approximately only a third of patients have a good outcome after treatment.

Causes

- *Spontaneous SAH* – usually caused by aneurysm rupture (85%). Approximately 5% are due to other vascular anomalies such as arteriovenous malformations. The remaining 10% are from non-aneurysmal perimesencephalic bleeding. Mean age at presentation is 50 years and there is a slight female preponderance (1.6:1). Risk factors include:
  - Hypertension
  - Smoking
  - Cocaine
  - Alcohol excess
  - Connective tissue disorders
  - Congenital syndromes including polycystic kidney disease and neurofibromatosis type 1.

  Saccular or 'berry' aneurysms occur in around 4% of the population but only those greater than 7 mm will rupture. Approximately 80% occur in the anterior circulation of the circle of Willis. Estimates of incidence vary but the most common sites are at bifurcations of the anterior and posterior communicating arteries (30–35% and 30–40% respectively). Around 20% involve the middle cerebral artery and a small percentage occur in the vertebrobasilar arteries.

  A less common form of aneurysm is the fusiform aneurysm which lacks the neck of the berry aneurysm.

- *Traumatic SAH* – occurs in around 25–50% of patients with traumatic brain injury.

Draw a diagram to represent the circle of Willis

See Figure 15.4.

What scoring systems can be used to grade the severity of SAH?

Clinical

- *GCS* – this was not developed specifically in relation to SAH. However, studies have shown that a GCS of 14 or 15 at presentation correlates with good outcomes. Progressively lower GCS is associated with worse outcomes, an impaired motor score being the most significant component.
- *World Federation of Neurosurgical Societies (WFNS)* – combines GCS on presentation with focal neurological deficit to predict outcome. Grades 1 and 2 have no motor deficit and favourable outcomes. Grades 3–5 involve either motor deficit or significantly reduced GCS and result in poorer outcomes.
- *Hunt and Hess* – the oldest of the grading systems. Predicts percentage survival based on signs and symptoms. From grade 1 (70% survival) asymptomatic or minimal headache or neck stiffness, to grade 5 (10% survival) deep coma, decerebrate rigidity.

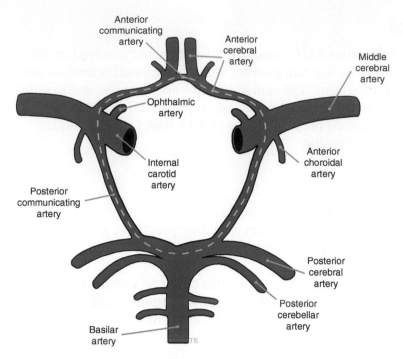

Figure 15.4: Circle of Willis (green dashed line).

Source: Theophilus Samuels.

Radiological

- *Fischer* – based on appearance of haemorrhage on CT head. Grades:
  - 1 – none evident
  - 2 – less than 1 mm thick
  - 3 – more than 1 mm thick
  - 4 – diffuse or intraventricular haemorrhage, or parenchymal extension.
- *Claassen* – Claassen modified the Fisher scale to incorporate the impact of intraventricular haemorrhage. This gives patients a score from 0 to 4.
- *Ogilvy and Carter* – this is a combined score based on the presence or absence of each of the following factors:
  - Age over 50 years
  - Hunt and Hess grade 4 or 5
  - Fisher scale 3 or 4
  - Aneurysm size more than 10 mm
  - Posterior circulation aneurysm more than 25 mm

What are the treatment options for aneurysmal SAH?

Options for management depend upon the cause of the haemorrhage, the condition of the patient on presentation as a reflection of the severity of their condition, and the previous performance status of the patient.

- *Conservative management* – where the cause is an aneurysm which is not amenable to intervention (usually through its anatomical position), or where attempting to perform the intervention is deemed too high risk, conservative management is undertaken by optimising medical therapy.

- *Medical treatment*
  - Nimodipine – a dihydropyridine which prevents calcium influx through L-type calcium channels. It is used to treat cerebral vasospasm and is given in a dose of 60 mg 4 hourly for 14–21 days post SAH (divided doses of 30 mg 2 hourly can reduce large fluctuations in blood pressure).
  - Analgesia – the headache of SAH can be severe. This is usually managed with paracetamol and codeine or morphine.
  - Antiemetics.
  - Antiseizure medication.
- *Surgical intervention*
  - Clipping – craniotomy allows direct visualisation and placement of a metal clip across the neck of the aneurysm.
  - Craniectomy – used less commonly in SAH but is employed where ICP is high and cannot be managed. The patient can be left with no bone flap to allow expansion of the brain without further damage to parenchyma from compression against the wall of the cranium.
- *Interventional radiological approach*
  - Coiling – usual approach via radial or femoral arteries. Under anaesthetic, platinum wires are coiled into the aneurysmal sac.

ISAT (International Subarachnoid Aneurysm Trial 2002) compared the outcomes of patients undergoing endovascular coiling compared with neurosurgical clipping following SAH. They found that coiling resulted in better 1-year disability-free survival. A Cochrane review published in 2018 (Lindgren et al., Cochrane Database Syst Rev) found that where patients were in good condition and the aneurysm was amenable to both management options, those patients undergoing coiling were more likely than those undergoing clipping to survive and return to independent living.

On arrival at the neurosurgical centre, Debbie is rushed to the interventional radiology suite where she undergoes coiling of an anterior communicating artery aneurysm. Following the procedure, she is moved to the neurointensive care where sedation is stopped so she can be assessed neurologically.

Apart from the issues already explored, how else will you manage Debbie in critical care?

Physiological optimisation

- *Fluids* – intravenous fluid of choice is usually 0.9% saline. Fluid management strategy is contentious. Although dehydration is to be avoided, studies have shown an association between excessive positive fluid balance and poorer functional outcomes.
- *Electrolyte and glucose management.*

- *Temperature control* – fever is common after SAH and is associated with worse outcomes.
- *Careful ventilation and oxygenation* – Debbie may have aspirated so her lungs should be protected as much as possible.

Follow-up investigations

- *12-lead ECG* – brain injury leads to massive catecholamine release. Cardiac complications occur in over 50% of patients. Myocardial ischaemia and cardiac failure can develop. Common ECG changes include large U waves, T-wave changes, prolonged QTc, high R waves and ST depression.
- *Echocardiography* – to assess for development of cardiac complications including Takotsubo cardiomyopathy.
- *Lumbar puncture* – Debbie's SAH has been demonstrated on CT and cerebral infection appears unlikely, so lumbar puncture (LP) is not necessary for diagnosis. LP could be considered after discussion with neurosurgeons if required.

Prophylactic medication

- *Ulcer prophylaxis* – neurocritical care patients are at high risk of stress ulcer development and upper gastrointestinal bleeding. Histamine-2 antagonist or a proton pump inhibitor (selective inhibitor of H^+/K^+ ATPase in gastric parietal cells) are commonly used agents.
- *Thromboprophylaxis* – this should be reviewed daily, ideally with the input of a neurosurgeon, and the daily decision documented in the patient's notes. The risk of devastating intracranial bleeding must be weighed up against the risk of deep vein thrombosis and life-threatening pulmonary embolus. These patients are at high risk of both bleeding and thrombus.

Initially, Debbie appeared to make a good recovery. On day 2 following her procedure, she had a GCS 13 (E3V4M6) and she appeared to be progressing well. However, on day 5 her motor score suddenly dropped from 6 to 4, with no sign of a seizure. You call the neurosurgeon and neurointensive care consultant to discuss the case.

What do you think might have occurred?

- *Rebleeding* – occurs in up to 25% of patients with SAH within the first 72 hours. Mortality associated with rebleeding is up to 60%.
- *Vasospasm* – most commonly 5–10 days post SAH. The mechanism is not clearly understood but the breakdown of erythrocytes appears to increase oxidative stress via activation of calcium channels in smooth muscle and release of vasoactive proteins. This depletes ATP, causing ischaemia and eventually cortical necrosis.

■ *Hydrocephalus* – estimated to occur in around 20–30% of patients with SAH. It is classified as acute within 3 days, subacute 4–14 days and chronic beyond 14 days. It can be obstructive or communicating.

> The neurointensive care consultant performs transcranial Doppler (TCD) which shows increased mean velocity in both middle cerebral arteries (approximately 180 cm/s). You also take Debbie for a CT head which reveals loss of sulci and reduction in ventricular space.

What is the significance of the TCD and CT head report?

The TCD suggests cerebral vasospasm (normal range for MCA blood flow is 50–75 cm/s). The CT head report suggests raised ICP. Raised ICP is often seen alongside cerebral vasospasm. Manage both these problems urgently to prevent cerebral ischaemia.

What other methods are used to diagnose cerebral vasospasm?

Digital subtraction angiography (DSA) is the standard for detecting cerebral vasospasm after SAH. CT angiography is also widely used.

What methods can be used for intracranial pressure monitoring and how do they work?

Clinical signs can be used as an indication of raised ICP. GCS should be assessed regularly and examine for papilloedema. Don't wait to see the Cushing reflex as it is a late sign (bradycardia, widened pulse pressure and abnormal respiratory pattern).

Invasive monitors are more precise but risk infection and haemorrhage:

■ *ICP bolt/subdural screw/intraparenchymal microsensor (e.g. Codman)* – a strain gauge sensor is inserted into the parenchyma or CSF. This allows analysis of pressure waveforms (A waves suggest raised ICP, B waves suggest poor compliance and C waves are a normal finding; Figure 15.5).

■ *Extraventricular drain (EVD)* – a catheter is inserted surgically into the ventricle, facilitating manometry with CSF. This has the added benefits of facilitating sampling of CSF if needed, allowing drainage of CSF if ICP is high, and intrathecal drug administration if required.

■ *Epidural sensor* – a sensor is sited between the skull and dura via a burr hole drilled through the skull.

How do you manage cerebral vasospasm?

The mainstay of treatment is nimodipine. This is usually given orally but adjusted doses can be given intravenously (or intra-arterially under radiological

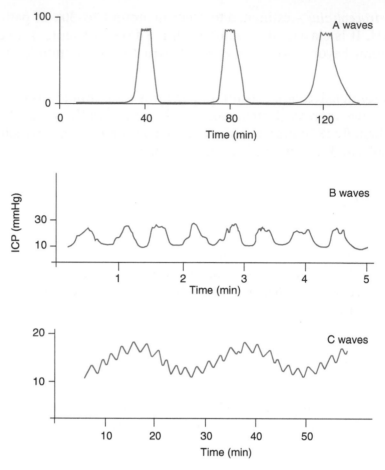

Figure 15.5: Lundberg waves. A waves – last around 5–20 minutes and are described as plateau or vasogenic waves between 50 and 100 mmHg. They compromise cerebral perfusion pressure (CPP). B waves – short-duration elevations in ICP that are smaller in amplitude occurring at a frequency between 1 and 2 minutes. They may be associated with changes in partial pressure of carbon dioxide and oxygen due to respiration. C waves – occur at a frequency of 4–8 minutes and are also of low amplitude. They are products of cardiac and respiratory cycle interactions.

Source: Theophilus Samuels.

guidance). Careful fluid balance to ensure normal circulating volume is indicated. Other treatments such as magnesium and statins have been trialled but there is no good evidence to support routine use.

How do you manage Debbie's blood pressure?

When vasospasm occurs, the patient's blood pressure normally rises in response. Where the aneurysm is secure, many centres aim to maintain hypertension in such cases to promote cerebral circulation against high ICP and increased resistance to flow. Vasopressors may be needed to induce systolic BP > 180 mmHg. Aims may be set higher on an individual basis if GCS is seen to improve with higher systemic blood pressure.

Your management improves Debbie's condition, and she settles over the next 2 days. On day 8, as part of your daily assessment, you discover Debbie's sodium has increased from 142 to 151 mmol/L. Her urine output has also increased and is now over 500 mL per hour.

What do you think is happening and why?

Debbie appears to be developing diabetes insipidus (DI). It usually develops 1–3 days following the initial insult to the brain and is often transient but can persist for several months. Around 15% of SAH patients develop DI and it tends to be associated with a worse prognosis.

Decreased production of arginine vasopressin results in reduced ability to concentrate urine. The patient therefore passes large volumes (>200 mL/h) of dilute urine (<300 mOsm/kg) and plasma sodium concentration increases.

How do you manage this?

Investigations include paired urine and serum osmolality and sodium levels. In non-acute situations, a water deprivation test can be undertaken. Where clinical suspicion is high and there is rapid loss of sodium and water homeostasis, desmopressin (DDAVP) can be given in a divided dose of 0.2–1.2 mg/d.

Of which other sodium regulation disorders is Debbie at risk?

Hyponatraemia after SAH is usually caused by the syndrome of inappropriate antidiuretic hormone (SIADH) but can also be caused by cerebral salt wasting (CSW).

- *SIADH* – due to central overproduction of arginine vasopressin following stimulation of the hypothalamus. The result is low serum sodium and relatively normal urine output. Treatment normally focuses on fluid restriction (<500 mL/d) but this can be challenging to maintain and can predispose to cerebral vasospasm. Alternative therapies include hypertonic saline, fludrocortisone (0.1–0.2 mg/d) and vasopressin receptor antagonists such as conivaptan.
- *CSW* – this is a clinical picture of polyuria with loss of serum sodium. The mechanism for this is unknown but may be related to release of natriuretic peptides (Table 15.1).

You manage Debbie's DI successfully and on day 15 she is well enough to go to the ward. She is discharged home nearly 4 weeks after her initial SAH and hopes to return to work after a period of recovery.

Table 15.1: Sodium disorders with raised ICP.

	Cerebral salt wasting	Diabetes Insipidus	Syndrome of inappropriate antidiuretic hormone
Fluid balance	Decreased	Decreased	Normal or increased
Urine output	Increased	Increased	Decreased
Serum sodium	Decreased	Increased	Decreased
Urine sodium	Increased	Decreased	Increased
Serum osmolality (mOsm/kg)	<280	>290	<280
Urine osmolality (mOsm/kg)	>100	<300	>100

What problems can SAH patients experience during the recovery period?

- Cognitive
  - Inattention
  - Memory deficits
  - Speech and language problems
- Neurological
  - Seizures
  - Headaches
- Psychological
  - Personality change
- Physiological
  - Fatigue
  - Weakness

Further reading

- Macdonald, R. and Schweizer, T. (2017). Spontaneous subarachnoid haemorrhage. *Lancet* 389 (10069): 655–666.
- Lawton, M. and Vates, G. (2017). Subarachnoid haemorrhage. *N. Engl. J. Med.* 377: 257–266. Two useful review articles on pathophysiology and management of subarachnoid haemorrhage.
- Stocchetti, N., Toccone, F., Citerio, G. et al. (2015). Neuroprotection in acute brain injury: an up-to-date review. *Crit. Care* 19 (1): 186. Excellent review article on neuroprotection in critical care.

16 The Patient Who had A Stroke

As the neurointensive care registrar, you receive a call from the neuroanaesthetist who requests a bed for Edward. He is a 63-year-old managing director who developed sudden-onset dense right hemiparesis two hours ago and is now being transferred to your hospital for thrombectomy.

What causes ischaemic stroke?

Ischaemic strokes are embolic or, more commonly, thrombotic:

- *Thrombotic strokes* – usually result where chronic atheroma and plaque development lead to stenosis in large or small cerebral arteries (larger arteries include the carotid or middle cerebral), predisposing them to obstruction with thrombus formation. Thrombus in smaller penetrating arteries gives a pattern of 'lacunar' stroke.
- *Embolic strokes* – secondary to clots that form elsewhere in the body but lodge in the cerebral circulation, impairing distal blood flow. These thrombi tend to develop within the heart secondary to the stagnation of blood that accompanies atrial fibrillation.

What are the risk factors for ischaemic stroke?

Modifiable

- Hypertension
- Smoking
- Diabetes
- Atrial fibrillation
- Hypercholesterolaemia
- Obesity and inactivity
- Carotid artery disease
- Alcohol excess

Clinical Cases in Critical Care, First Edition. Alice Myers and Theophilus Samuels.
© 2023 John Wiley & Sons Ltd. Published 2023 by John Wiley & Sons Ltd.

Non-modifiable

- Increasing age
- Female gender
- Family history of stroke
- African and Caribbean ethnicity
- Previous strokes or transient ischaemic attacks (TIA)

What are the options for managing acute thrombotic stroke?

Refer to NICE guidance (NG 128, 2019). The pathway is different for those with non-disabling TIA.

General measures

- Use FAST (Face, Arm, Speech, Test) prehospital to aid rapid diagnosis.
- Use ROSIER (recognition of stroke in emergency room) or similar tool to aid diagnosis in hospital.
- Exclude hypoglycaemia.
- Immediate non-enhanced CT brain where acute stroke is suspected and any of the following apply:
  - Thrombolysis/thrombectomy could be used.
  - Patient is on anticoagulant therapy or has risk of bleeding.
  - Fluctuating symptoms.
  - Low GCS.
  - Severe headache, neck stiffness or papilloedema.
- If thrombectomy might be an option, a contrast-enhanced CT scan should be performed with CT angiography (CTA) following the initial non-enhanced scan.
- Aspirin 300 mg unless contraindicated (if thrombolysis is to be given, aspirin should be delayed for 24 hours post thrombolysis and should only be administered once repeat CT head has excluded haemorrhagic transformation).

Thrombolysis with alteplase

- Within 4.5 hours of onset of symptoms.
- Haemorrhage must have been excluded.
- This should be discussed with the on-call stroke consultant.

Thrombectomy

- Within 6 hours of onset of symptoms.
- Confirmed occlusion of proximal anterior circulation demonstrated on CTA or magnetic resonance angiography (MRA).
- There should be potential to salvage brain (as assessed by CT or MR imaging).
- The patient was well between 6 and 24 hours prior to the event.
- Pre-stroke modified Rankin score should be <3 and a score of >5 on the National Institutes of Health Stroke Scale.

Where possible, patients should be considered for thrombectomy. In the UK, thrombectomy is currently offered in a limited number of centres and transfer time must be considered when assessing suitability for thrombectomy. Rapidity of diagnosis and management is key to the successful treatment of acute stroke.

> Around 2 hours later, Edward arrives in your neurointensive care. He was intubated for thrombectomy due to being agitated on arrival in the radiology suite. He has now been extubated to facilitate neurological assessment. Following recovery from anaesthesia, he appears confused and has right-sided weakness. The radiologist informs you that it was a difficult procedure and, due to anatomical issues, they could not remove all of the clot.

Review the CT head image (Figure 16.1). What is the diagnosis?

CT head demonstrates extensive left middle cerebral artery (MCA) infarction.

What patterns of neurological deficit can be seen in stroke?

There are subtle differences in the patterns of neurological deficit seen due to the exact point of occlusion of the artery. Grossly, the changes are as follows:

- Anterior cerebral artery (ACA)
  - Contralateral motor/sensory loss
  - Lower more than upper limb

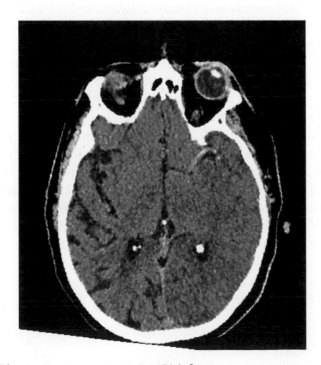

Figure 16.1: CT brain demonstrating left MCA infarct.

- MCA
  - Contralateral motor/sensory loss
  - Greatest in face and upper limb
  - Contralateral homonymous hemianopia
  - Left MCA – aphasia
  - Right MCA – neglect to the left
- Posterior inferior cerebellar artery (PICA) or vertebral artery
  - Wallenburg syndrome – vertigo, ipsilateral Horner syndrome, etc.
  - Various other eponymous syndromes may develop as a result of brainstem lesions – Jackson, Raymond, Fouille, Millard-Gubler, Weber, Claude.

> On day 2, Edward's nurse calls you to say that he has started vomiting and his GCS has dropped to 7 (E1V2M4). On examining his pupils, the ICU nurse also noted that his eyes are deviated to one side.

What do you think may have happened?

- Extension of ischaemic stroke
- Haemorrhage into existing stroke
- Oedema subsequent to original extensive MCA stroke
- Seizure

What are your management priorities?

- *Intubate and neuroprotect* – Edward's GCS is low, he has vomited and is developing pathology for which he requires urgent radiological imaging. Intubate him rapidly, control his gas exchange and haemodynamics, and ensure neuroprotection. Examine Edward and consider treating him for possible seizures but, given the potential differential diagnoses, prioritise urgent imaging of the brain.
- *Imaging* – transfer Edward for urgent CT brain. Discuss with the radiologist, neurosurgeon and intensive care consultant as to the specific modality (i.e. with contrast/focusing on angiography/whether you should perform MRI brain at this point).
- *Call neurosurgeons and ICU consultant* – not only do you need advice regarding the imaging required but you will need senior input as to ongoing management since this could represent significant deterioration.
- *Call next of kin* – Edward's next of kin need to know that he has deteriorated. You may wish to wait to review CT images before calling them in the middle of the night since you are performing the scan urgently and the outcome could be critical to Edward's prognosis.

Review the images in Figure 16.2. What is the diagnosis?

Malignant MCA syndrome.

(a) (b)

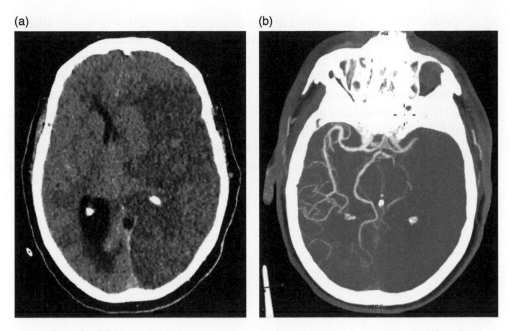

Figure 16.2: (a) Plain CT brain demonstrating malignant MCA with midline shift and associated ACA territory infarction (b) CT angiography of brain demonstrating abrupt left MCA cutoff.

What is the pathophysiology of Edward's deterioration?

Malignant MCA syndrome is a pattern of rapid neurological deterioration following hemispheric infarction. Initially, ischaemic tissue induces cytotoxic oedema. Subsequently, brain tissue swells and vessels are occluded. As tissue necrosis develops, there is a breakdown in the integrity of the blood–brain barrier. Proteins and ischaemia-induced mediators leak into the parenchyma and vasogenic oedema further increases the volume of brain tissue. The oedema which develops as a result can be dramatic, leading to mass effect and, eventually, brainstem compression. Classically, this presents 2–4 days following the initial infarction.

The prognosis for MCA syndrome is generally poor. Up to 80% of patients die within 1 week.

How does information from the CT head influence your management now?

- *Urgent discussion with neurosurgeons regarding whether Edward would be suitable for decompressive hemicraniectomy (DHC)* – pooled analysis has shown that DHC can reduce the risk of major disability in those younger than 60 years of age (Rajwani et al. 2017). Similarly, analysis of several studies shows improved survival for patients like Edward. DHC is included in guidelines for management published in 2015 (Torbey et al.). Removing a large bone flap allows for expansion of the brain which would otherwise continue causing compression as explained by the Monro–Kellie doctrine (see Case 15).
- *Temperature control* – this is a controversial topic and local guidelines should be consulted. Maintaining a core temperature of 33 °C

for 48–72 hours has been shown to reduce mortality in some studies but is not universally accepted as beneficial. In the UK, some centres use evidence-based guidelines recommending targeted temperature management aiming for 36.5–37.5 °C or preventing hyperthermia.

■ *Consider osmotic therapy with mannitol or hypertonic saline* – discuss this with your consultant and the neurosurgeons since beneficial effects are only transient. It is usually used as a 'bridging' therapy to other treatment such as surgery. If the blood–brain barrier lacks integrity, this could propagate further oedema so should not be administered without due consideration.

> Neurosurgeons decide to take Edward straight to theatre for decompressive surgery. They perform a 15 cm craniectomy, leaving Edward with no bone flap over the left temporoparietal region.

How will you manage Edward in neurocritical care at this point?

■ *Consider sedation* – discuss with the team whether to wake Edward immediately or to keep him sedated for a period of time. Many centres would favour a period of sedation where others would immediately stop sedation postoperatively and assess Edward's neurology.

■ *Neuroprotection* – ensure positioning of head and neck to promote venous drainage, optimise gas exchange for cerebral blood flow, optimise blood pressure to improve cerebral perfusion pressure (see Case 15).

■ *Monitoring* – advanced monitoring should include invasive arterial blood pressure monitoring. Neurosurgeons may also have inserted an intracranial bolt or extraventricular drain (EVD) to help monitor intracranial pressure (ICP) and allow drainage of CSF if required.

■ *Blood tests* – frequent measurement of sodium is vital. Rapid changes in sodium, with the associated risks of cerebral oedema, must be avoided. Monitor inflammatory markers as Edward is susceptible to infection following surgery.

■ *Urine output monitoring* – observe for disorders of sodium homeostasis (see Table 15.1).

■ *Daily review of venous thromboembolism (VTE) prophylaxis with a neurosurgeon* – Edward is high risk for devastating intracranial bleeding following surgery. However, he is also high risk for developing deep venous thrombosis and pulmonary embolus. The decision of whether to give or withhold VTE prophylaxis is extremely important and should be considered and documented daily.

■ *Treat seizures to avoid increases in cerebral metabolic rate.*

■ *Document where the bone flap is kept, if it is being kept at all* – traditionally these have been surgically implanted subcutaneously (often on the abdomen) or cryopreserved. Many centres now prefer to craft a titanium plate as a replacement, should the patient survive.

What are the complications of neurosurgery?

- Bleeding
- Infection – systemic, surgical site, intracerebral
- Seizures
- Hydrocephalus
- CSF circulation derangement and hygroma development
- Cognitive, neurological or psychological changes

On day 4 you assess Edward's neurology. The sedation has been off for 24 hours. You are unable to elicit a response from Edward. He remains fully ventilated and has shown no signs of coughing on suction. His pupils are unreactive and 5 mm each.

Why is it important to examine Edward's eyes regularly?

Increased ICP can lead to expansion of the brain towards the foramen magnum and consequent damage to soft tissue structures as they are compressed against the bony base of skull. The observed pattern can reflect the manner or extent of that damage.

Rapid identification of 'false localising signs' can lead to earlier recognition and management of raised ICP. The abducens (VI) nerve (due to its long course and tendency to be stretched over the petrous temporal bone), the trigeminal (V) and the oculomotor (III) nerves are particularly susceptible to early damage from raised ICP.

Describe the clinical presentations of different patterns of brain herniation secondary to raised ICP

- Uncal herniation (transtentorial herniation)
  - Temporal lobe compression leads to damage to the ipsilateral cranial nerve III, resulting in a dilated pupil.
  - This is accompanied by hemiparesis, decerebrate posturing and coma.
- Central tentorial herniation
  - Compression of the diencephalon can lead to small reactive pupils or Parinaud syndrome (paralysis of vertical gaze).
  - The patient will also have decreased consciousness (eventually deep coma) and decorticate rigidity, and may develop Cheyne–Stokes breathing.
- Transcalvarial herniation
  - This type of herniation can occur through a defect in the skull, e.g. via craniotomy site or fractured skull. The eye signs here can be unpredictable.
- Cerebellar tonsil herniation ('coning')
  - Bilateral fixed and dilated pupils.

- Herniation of the tonsils through the foramen magnum compresses the medullary respiratory centre.
- Death is inevitable.

What is your management plan in light of your neurology assessment?

Examination findings could be consistent with damage to Edward's brainstem. Urgent imaging of the brain is indicated. MRI is a superior modality to CT for visualising the posterior fossa.

> You take Edward to the MRI suite and imaging demonstrates that he has 'coned', i.e. he has suffered cerebellar tonsil herniation and irreversible damage to the brainstem.

What other signs might you expect to see?

- Cushing's triad – bradycardia, widening pulse pressure, irregular respiration.
- Papilloedema.
- Headache and vomiting may be seen in early stages but sadly, Edward's case is too far advanced for this now.

What is your assessment of the clinical situation and how will you proceed?

Edward has suffered catastrophic, irreversible brain injury which is not compatible with life. The case must be discussed with the consultant intensivist and the neurosurgeon. Given the information from the nurse (absence of cough reflex, pupils unresponsive to light, no attempt to initiate breaths in the absence of sedation) in conjunction with his brain imaging, Edward may have suffered brainstem death.

Continue supportive measures and speak to his next of kin urgently to explain the situation.

> You have a discussion with Edward's family about his neurological status and the prognosis. You tell them that you would like to test him for brainstem death. In light of his clinical condition and his brain imaging, even if he is not brainstem dead, he will not recover from this event. The family do not object to brainstem death testing and choose not to be present for this.

What preconditions must be met before you commence brainstem testing?

- *Evidence for irreversible brain damage* of known aetiology.
- *Exclusion of reversible causes* of apnoea and coma.

- Absence of sedative drugs (test levels where unsure, e.g. thiopentone must be <5 mg/L, midazolam <10 mcg/L)
- Absence of paralysing agents (test using a nerve stimulator)
- Temperature >34 °C
- Sodium 115–160 mmol/L
- Potassium >2 mmol/L
- Phosphate 0.5–3 mmol/L
- Magnesium 0.5–3 mmol/L
- Glucose 3–20 mmol/L
- Confirm absence of endocrine or metabolic disorder as potential cause for coma
- *Patient should be suitable for testing* – absence of high cervical cord lesion and absence of severe lung disease precluding the apnoea test. Visualise the tympanic membranes via otoscopy to ensure they are clear and intact.

Who can perform brainstem death testing?

In the UK, this requires two qualified doctors who are competent in the procedure. One should be a consultant. Both should have been fully registered with the General Medical Council for at least 5 years. Practice is variable worldwide.

Which nerves are tested in brainstem death testing?

- *Sensory* – cranial nerves II, V, VIII, IX, X
- *Motor* – cranial nerves III, IV, VI, VII, X

Which tests are performed?

Each doctor performs the tests independently. Usually, each observes the other.

1. A bright light is shone into each eye in turn looking for direct and consensual reflexes (II, III). In brainstem death there is absence of pupillary response.
2. Each cornea is brushed with cotton wool or a swab while gently retracting the eyelids enough to allow them to move (V, VII). In brainstem death there is an absence of blinking.
3. 50 mL ice cold saline is instilled into the external auditory meatus over 1 minute (III, IV, VI, VII) while the eyes are observed for response such as nystagmus. This is then repeated with the other ear. Brainstem death causes absence of eye movement.
4. Painful stimulus is applied to the supra-orbital ridge, trapezius and sternum (V, VII). In brainstem death there is an absence of movement in the cranial nerve distribution – however, movement may still be seen in spinally mediated reflexes.
5. A spatula is used to stimulate the pharynx (IX, X). There is an absence of gag reflex in brainstem death.
6. Stimulation of the carina is achieved through insertion of a bronchial catheter (X). In brainstem death there is no cough reflex.
7. Apnoea test.

How do you perform the apnoea test?

- Pre-oxygenate with 100% oxygen.
- Pre-test normocarbia should be confirmed via arterial blood gas with $PaCO_2$ at least 6 kPa (6.5 kPa in chronic CO_2 retention).
- Apnoea is commenced while oxygenation continues (for instance, by inserting a suction catheter into the airways with oxygen flowing or using a Mapleson C breathing circuit with oxygen flow) and the patient is observed for spontaneous respiratory effort.
- At the end of the apnoea test, $PaCO_2$ must have risen at least 0.5 kPa – again confirmed by arterial blood gas.
- The patient must not desaturate as they should not be allowed to develop hypoxia during the test.

What is the definition of death?

In the UK, the Academy of Medical Royal Colleges in 2008 agreed that death is defined as the irreversible loss of the capacity for consciousness and the irreversible loss of the ability to breathe. Therefore, there is irreversible cessation of the integrative function of the brainstem.

Is brainstem death testing a universally accepted process?

No. In places such as the UK, proof of brainstem death, via the tests outlined above, is confirmation of death.

There is variability throughout the world, and elsewhere, such as in the USA, whole brain death must be proven. Ancillary tests (such as EEG, cerebral angiography, transcranial Doppler ultrasound) may be required to demonstrate whole brain death.

> You and your consultant perform the brainstem death tests. Edward shows no response to any of tests 1–6 (as written above) but on the first apnoea test he desaturates rapidly. You try again, but again he desaturates.

What is the significance of this?

Edward may be brainstem dead but, due to his poor gas exchange, it is not possible to complete the tests. This must be explained to his family.

Brainstem death cannot be officially diagnosed but it is strongly suspected to be the case here. The ethical implications of maintaining or withdrawing treatment at this stage must be considered. Since Edward has no chance of recovery, it could be argued that it is not in his best interests to continue life support. However, many people throughout the world hold religious or cultural beliefs which are not compatible with withdrawal of treatment. This topic must be broached with great sensitivity. Be prepared that the family may hold a very different belief system to your own. Offer them the opportunity to discuss what they believe Edward would have wanted in this situation.

You have a candid discussion with Edward's family. They feel strongly that Edward would not want to be kept alive without any chance of a meaningful recovery. The organ donation team contact you to say that Edward was registered as a donor. They have already spoken to his wife and the family would like to explore the possibility of donation before cessation of invasive organ support.

What kind of donation would be possible for Edward?

Had Edward been diagnosed brainstem dead, he could have become a 'DBD' donor – donation after brainstem death. In that case, he could have been taken to theatre with ongoing ventilation and optimisation, allowing for retrieval to be performed with his organs in the best possible condition.

Since you cannot confirm brainstem death, Edward can only donate his organs after circulatory death (DCD). This means he must be taken to theatre where life supportive treatment is stopped. The anaesthetist will wait for his heart to stop before diagnosing circulatory death, at which point organ retrieval can begin. The time from onset of hypotension or desaturation (often agreed to be systolic blood pressure <50 mmHg or oxygen saturations <70%) until organ retrieval or cold perfusion indicates the warm ischaemic time (WIT). A long WIT results in compromised organs.

The Modified Maastricht classification would define this as a category III donation:

- Category I – dead on arrival
- Category II – unsuccessful resuscitation
- Category III – anticipated cardiac arrest
- Category IV – cardiac arrest in brain-dead donor
- Category V – unexpected arrest in ICU patient

What investigations may be done at this stage?

- *Blood tests* – FBC, U&Es, LFTs, clotting, viruses (HIV, hepatitis viruses, EBV, CMV, etc.), immunology, blood typing, etc.
- *Imaging and bedside tests* – chest radiograph, 12-lead ECG, echocardiography, coronary angiogram.
- You may also be asked to perform bronchoscopy and lavage followed by lung recruitment manoeuvres.

What medications and management strategies might you need to employ at this stage?

- Administer methylprednisolone 15 mg/kg.
- Optimise cardiovascular status – use invasive cardiovascular monitoring, correct hypovolaemia, use vasopressin if required, avoid noradrenaline (catecholamines are already high due to the autonomic storm resulting from progressive ischaemia of the brainstem).

- Consider tri-iodothyronine bolus and infusion – circulating thyroid hormone levels are diminished in brainstem-dead patients and supplementation can reduce vasopressor requirements, preventing cardiovascular collapse.
- Maintain temperature >35 °C.
- Treat any infections.
- Lung-protective ventilation.
- Avoid positive fluid balance, avoid hypernatraemia.
- Monitor urine output and if diabetes insipidus develops, administer 1-desamino-8-d-arginine vasopressin (DDAVP).
- Maintain blood glucose 4–8 mmol/L with NG feed or glucose infusion and insulin infusion if required.
- Continue thromboprophylaxis.
- Correct clotting if bleeding and transfuse if necessary.

The organ donation nurse specialist tells you that Edward has been accepted for donation of multiple organs including kidneys, liver and tissues.

Which organs can be donated?

- Kidneys (WIT <120 minutes)
- Liver (WIT <30 minutes)
- Lung (WIT <60 minutes)
- Pancreas (WIT <30 minutes)
- Other tissues (corneas, tendons, etc.) can be retrieved much later
- Heart – previously these could only be from DBD donors, but now suitable DCD donors can also donate their heart

You withdraw life support in the anaesthetic room after Edward's family have said their goodbyes. He dies in 15 minutes and successfully donates his liver, kidneys, pancreas and tissues to multiple recipients.

Further reading

- McGee, A. and Gardiner, D. (2019). Differences in the definition of brain death and their legal impact on intensive care practice. *Anaesthesia.* 74 (5): 569–572. Thought-provoking article on brain death.
- Smith, M., Reddy, U., Robba, C. et al. (2019). Acute ischaemic stroke: challenges for the intensivist. *Intensive Care Med.* 45 (9): 1177–1189. World leading expert review article on current best practice stroke management in ICU in the UK.

17 The Patient with Chest Pain and a Rash

One of your anaesthetic colleagues has intubated a man in the resuscitation department and you are now admitting him to critical care. Sudip, who is 51 years old, called an ambulance because he was short of breath with chest pain. Paramedics administered 300 mg aspirin. The ED team gave piperacillin/tazobactam and gentamicin. They tried delivering oxygen via high-flow nasal cannulae but Sudip became confused and unmanageable. The best oxygen saturations the anaesthetist could achieve prior to intubation were 87%.

Sudip has had a CT head and CTPA on the way to ICU. There is an interesting-looking rash covering his chest and abdomen. Sudip's family are on their way to the hospital. No past medical history is immediately available.

Your colleague has inserted arterial and central venous catheters and stabilised his blood pressure with 0.4 mcg/kg/min noradrenaline. He was paralysed for transfer and is achieving saturations of 93% on FiO_2 0.6, PEEP 10 cmH$_2$O. His temperature is 38.4 °C.

What differential diagnoses are you considering at this point?

- *Sepsis.*
  - Meningococcal meningitis – the presence of a rash in association with agitation and confusion may suggest meningococcal meningitis. Inspect the rash, take cultures and ensure antibiotic choice is appropriate if this is a possible diagnosis.
  - Another source of sepsis – Sudip's chest pain could be pleuritic. Shortness of breath, hypoxia and agitation could fit with chest sepsis. Rapid deterioration and severity of illness could be consistent with gram-negative sepsis, invasive group A *Streptococcus* and *Legionella*. Respiratory infection accompanied by a rash could also represent measles. Ensure personal protective equipment is used when performing droplet-inducing procedures (see Case 24).

Clinical Cases in Critical Care, First Edition. Alice Myers and Theophilus Samuels.
© 2023 John Wiley & Sons Ltd. Published 2023 by John Wiley & Sons Ltd.

- Other infection – certain pathogens are notorious for presenting with a spectrum of symptoms and signs, e.g. tuberculosis (TB), Lyme disease, malaria, human immunodeficiency virus (HIV), etc. Establish whether there is a history of potential exposure.
- *Myocardial infarction (*MI*)* – chest pain and shortness of breath in a man aged 51 could be consistent with MI. The paramedics most probably administered aspirin with this in mind.
- *Pulmonary embolism* – chest pain, hypoxia and fever could be due to pulmonary embolism, but this would not explain his rash.
- *Allergic reaction* – Sudip may have been exposed to allergens causing bronchospasm, leading to chest pain, shortness of breath and hypoxia. An urticarial rash could also be explained by this.
- *Drug reaction* – this could be a type A (predictable or dose-related) or type B (idiosyncratic) reaction to drugs. Establish whether Sudip is taking prescription medications and over-the-counter drugs, or utilises recreational drugs.
- *Pneumothorax* – chest pain, shortness of breath and hypoxia all fit with pneumothorax. This would not explain Sudip's rash, and pneumothorax alone could not account for his symptoms. A pneumothorax may, however, co-exist with other acute pathologies.

What investigations do you need at this point?

Bedside investigations

- *Arterial blood gas* – for rapid quantification of hypoxia and quick assessment of glucose and electrolytes. Determine the lactate and base excess to ascertain the degree of metabolic derangement in Sudip's acid–base status.
- *12-lead ECG* – MI and PE are on your list of differential diagnoses.

Blood

- *Full blood count* – anaemia could induce cardiac chest pain. The white blood count will help assess whether infection is implicated in Sudip's deterioration. Thrombocytopenia may develop rapidly with sepsis and can be a cause of a purpuric rash.
- *Liver function tests* – background medical history for Sudip is currently unavailable. He may have pre-existing liver disease which could complicate his treatment or prognosis. Sudip is at the start of an acute illness. Liver function may become deranged with ongoing sepsis or due to antibiotic use, so baseline function is useful.
- *Urea and electrolytes* – acute kidney injury (AKI) frequently develops with sepsis and critical illness.
- *Clotting with fibrinogen* – disseminated intravascular coagulation (DIC) may accompany sepsis. Lumbar puncture (LP) may be indicated as part of the diagnostic panel but the risk of bleeding should be established before performing this investigation.

■ *Troponin* – it is possible that Sudip could have suffered an MI subsequent to myocardial dysfunction induced by hypoxia and hypotension. Measure troponin now and at 6–12 hours. Further measurements may be indicated if the level is raised. Levels can increase with PE and AKI but the pattern of increase and decrease is different to that seen in acute MI.

Microbiology/virology

■ *Cultures (blood, urine, sputum)* – complete a full septic screen. Swab any wounds or breaches in skin integrity.
■ *Viral throat swab* – consider viral causes of respiratory infection.
■ *Measles and Lyme serology.*
■ *HIV test.*
■ *Urinary antigens* – test for *Pneumococcus* and *Legionella*.
■ *Skin scrapings* – review the rash and try to take samples (skin scrapings or swabs) for viral and bacterial analysis.
■ *Consider sending sputum* for acid-fast bacilli.
■ *Lumbar puncture* to obtain CSF for microscopy culture and sensitivity (once clotting and CT head report are available) and request viral PCR.
■ *Cross-infection swabs.*

Imaging

■ *Plain chest radiograph* – part of the septic screen.
■ *CT head and CTPA reports* – required to assess for intracranial pathology and PE. Signs of raised ICP on CT head would suggest it may be unsafe to perform LP.
■ *Echocardiogram* – there are multiple reasons why cardiac impairment may occur acutely in this context. Use echocardiography to assess fluid status to guide your resuscitation. Formal echocardiography can be performed to assess for:
  ■ Regional wall motion abnormalities as supportive evidence for MI
  ■ Global impairment that can occur in sepsis
  ■ Right ventricular dysfunction in PE.

What is piperacillin/tazobactam ('pip-taz')? What is gentamicin?

■ *'Pip-taz'* – a combination of piperacillin and tazobactam. Piperacillin, a ureidopenicillin, inhibits cell wall synthesis by binding to penicillin-binding proteins (PBPs) inside bacterial cell walls. Tazobactam is a beta-lactamase inhibitor. It has a beta-lactam ring which binds to the beta-lactamase enzyme produced by bacteria. When given in combination, tazobactam prevents the breakdown of piperacillin and hence enhances its actions.
■ *Gentamicin* – this bactericidal aminoglycoside agent inhibits bacterial protein synthesis by binding to the 30S ribosome.

What do you think about this choice of antibiotic regimen?

At the moment, the cause of Sudip's rapid and severe deterioration is not clear. Sepsis is high on the list of differential diagnoses but without knowing the organism, antimicrobials with a broad spectrum of action are required. Most hospitals will have their own protocols for treatment of sepsis of unknown source. This will usually involve 'broad-spectrum cover' using a combination of agents, e.g. co-amoxiclav (which is active against anaerobes, many gram-negative and gram-positive organisms and incorporates a beta-lactamase inhibitor) with an aminoglycoside (this extends activity against gram negatives in particular).

'Pip-taz' has a similar spectrum of activity to co-amoxiclav but is additionally effective against *Pseudomonas*. However, a carbapenem, such as meropenem, would be required to treat the ESCHAPPM organisms (*Enterobacter, Serratia, Citrobacter freundii, Aeromonas, Proteus, Providencia, Morganella morganii*).

What additional antimicrobial agents might you consider?

If central nervous system infection is suspected, an agent with improved penetration of the blood–brain barrier is required, such as ceftriaxone. Additionally, an antiviral agent to treat encephalitis would be useful. Examine Sudip's rash to ascertain whether this looks like meningococcal septicaemia. In patients over 50 years old, or those with immune compromise or heavy alcohol intake, amoxicillin should be added to this regimen in case of infection with *Listeria monocytogenes*.

Sudip is extremely unwell and close liaison with the microbiologist is required. If there is reason to suspect infection with MRSA (methicillin-resistant *Staphylococcus aureus*), the choice of antimicrobials may need to be altered. Although gentamicin does have some activity against MRSA, agents such as vancomycin or linezolid would usually be preferred. PVL-MRSA (Panton-Valentine leukocidin MRSA) is a particularly virulent strain. The PVL toxin forms pores in infected cells. It can cause necrotising haemorrhagic pneumonia and is associated with extremely high mortality.

Gram-negative sepsis and invasive Group A *Streptococcus* infection (iGAS) can both cause rapid, severe deterioration with overwhelming sepsis. Unless there is a resistant organism, the current antimicrobial regimen is a reasonable first choice. If iGAS is implicated, treatment escalation may be required, e.g. meropenem and clindamycin.

Gentamicin and 'pip-taz' are an appropriate empirical choice at this stage. Once a pathogen has been identified, antimicrobial choice can be targeted. If it is impossible to identify a pathogen and Sudip continues to deteriorate, consider escalation of antimicrobials in consultation with the resident microbiologist.

On examination, Sudip has a diffuse macular erythematous rash over his trunk spreading down over his thighs. He also has some darker red/purple papular lesions over his chest which are more discrete and around 2–3 cm in diameter.

He has bilateral axillary lymphadenopathy. On auscultation of Sudip's chest, you hear crepitations throughout both lung fields, worse in the mid to lower zones. He is sedated with 1% propofol 150 mL/h and fentanyl 150 mcg/h (ideal body weight 81 kg, actual body weight 75 kg). His HR is 136 bpm and he remains on the same amount of noradrenaline as earlier.

One of the nurses points out that he has oral candidiasis.

What could be the cause of the dermatological manifestations?

It sounds like there are two distinct rashes:

- The *diffuse erythematous rash* could be urticarial. Spontaneous urticaria (a smooth erythematous papular rash) is common. It is usually caused by the release of histamine from mast cells and, if the patient is conscious, is usually pruritic. There are multiple causes, including exposure to allergens such as food substances or drugs. Assess this rash to establish whether it blanches on pressure. A non-blanching rash could be due to development of petechiae. This is more concerning as it represents intradermal capillary haemorrhage. The causes of this include meningococcaemia, leukaemia, thrombocytopenia and vasculitis. It can also be caused by blunt trauma or raised pressure as seen during straining (e.g. violent vomiting, coughing or strangulation).
- The *darker lesions* could be congenital or acquired. These could be benign naevi, malignant melanoma or lentigo melanoma. Kaposi sarcoma can present as multiple painless papular lesions of various sizes which are red or deep purple and non-blanching. These are usually associated with states of immunocompromise and are caused by human herpes virus 8. Check in Sudip's mouth to see if there are lesions present on the mucosa. Around a third of cases will involve the hard palate or gums.

Pemphigus vulgaris can initially present as erythematous macules which later develop into flaccid blisters. These intraepidermal lesions are caused by IgG deposits between epidermal cells. They do not involve the basement membrane and blisters rupture easily. Bullous pemphigoid tends to form more tense and stable blisters, usually in the flexures. Biopsy reveals C3 deposits along the basement membrane. The mucosa is often involved in pemphigus vulgaris but rarely in bullous pemphigoid.

Take scrapings or swabs where possible for virology and bacteriology and request review by a dermatologist.

What are the causes of lymphadenopathy?

- *Reactive/infective* – bacterial, viral, fungal or parasitic (including mononucleosis/Epstein–Barr virus, HIV, toxoplasma)
- *Inflammatory* – including autoimmune causes such as rheumatoid arthritis or lupus.
- *Malignancy* – cancer, lymphoma, leukaemia
- *Infiltrative* – e.g. amyloid
- *Other* – including follicular hyperplasia, sarcoid, Castleman disease, Kawasaki disease

What is the significance of oral candidiasis?

This is usually due to *Candida albicans* (around 50%) as this forms part of the normal oral microbiome. Other causes are more strongly associated with immunocompromise. These include *Candida tropicalis, glabrata, parapsilosis, krusei, dubliniensis* and *geotrichum*.

- It is often an insignificant, incidental finding. Oral thrush can occur after taking an extended course of antibiotics.
- Steroid treatment can predispose to oral candida. Establish whether Sudip has been taking steroids (systemic or inhaled), and if so, why.
- Immune suppression through viral causes (e.g. HIV), malignancy or drugs (including cancer chemotherapy drugs) can make patients vulnerable to developing oral candida and possibly more invasive candida infection.
- Inspect the oral cavity, including the tongue, lips and back of the throat. Look for angular cheilitis, glossitis and pseudomembranous candidiasis.
- Treatment is usually with nystatin mouthwash. Systemic antifungals may be required for more invasive candidiasis or where the species is resistant to treatment.
- If fungus or yeast is isolated from blood cultures, patients should be referred to ophthalmology for fundoscopy due to the risk of ocular involvement.

Are there any particular elements of the history you would like to know?

Obtain a thorough collateral history for Sudip, including details of his recent symptoms, his premorbid state, travel history, recreational drug use, sexual history (if possible), occupational history (including asbestos exposure) and exposure to potential pathogens, e.g. farming (*Aspergillus* species), birds (*Chlamydia psittaci*), mushrooms (thermophilic actinomycetes), etc.

Sudip's family arrive. His next of kin is his eldest son who is accompanied by Sudip's three adult daughters, his ex-wife, his mother and his flatmate Ben. They are all extremely upset but are able to tell you that Sudip is normally independent, he works in a bank and does not see the doctor for anything in particular. He has been drinking more alcohol lately as work has been stressful but no more than 2–3 glasses of wine in the evening. He has not travelled anywhere recently.

You thank the family for their time and, shortly after you leave the room, Ben comes to find you to speak confidentially. He informs you that Sudip is undergoing treatment for HIV. Following Sudip's divorce, he started a relationship with Ben. All the family, except Sudip's mother, are aware of this and are supportive. Sudip, however, does not want his mother to know that he is in a relationship with a man. None of the family are aware that Sudip is HIV positive and he does not want them to know. Sudip recently started taking antiretroviral drugs. Ben knows nothing more about the HIV treatment as Sudip is a very private man. Ben is HIV negative.

With this new information, will you add any diagnoses to your original list of differentials?

- *Opportunistic infections defining development of acquired immunodeficiency syndrome (AIDS)*
  - Most opportunistic infections occur with CD4$^+$ count <200 cells/µL. If Sudip has oesophageal candidiasis rather than simply oral, this is categorised as an opportunistic infection. Investigate for candida involvement of the trachea, bronchi and more distal respiratory tracts.
  - Other opportunistic infections include the following.
    - Coccidioidomycosis ('valley fever' pneumonia)
    - *Cryptococcus neoformans* (particularly in lung and brain tissue)
    - *Cryptosporidium* (usually causing diarrhoea)
    - Cytomegalovirus (brain, eye, gut and respiratory involvement)
    - Herpes simplex (multisystemic)
    - *Histoplasma capsulatum* (pneumonia)
    - *Mycobacterium* (multisystem disease, especially pneumonia)
    - *Pneumocystis jirovecii* (particularly causing pneumonia; previously *Pneumocystis carinii* or PCP)
    - *Toxoplasma gondii* (particularly lung and brain involvement)
    - *Salmonella*
- *Immune reconstitution inflammatory syndrome (IRIS)*
  - This is a worsening of symptoms following the initiation of antiretroviral treatment (ART). There is restored immunity to a range of infective and non-infective elements. Presentation varies between individuals. The incidence of IRIS is unknown but may be up to 25%. Risk factors include male sex, young age, lower CD4$^+$ count and higher viral RNA load.
  - Diagnostic criteria for IRIS (French et al., AIDS, 2004).
    - Major criteria – opportunistic infections in patients responding to antiretroviral drugs, decrease in plasma HIV RNA by at least 1 $\log_{10}$ copies/mL.

- Minor criteria – increased CD4$^+$ T-cell count after ART, increase in immune response to relevant pathogen or 'delayed-type hypersensitivity', spontaneous resolution of disease without specific treatment and with continuation of antiretroviral therapy.
- *Sudip's confusion may be explained by HIV or AIDS*
  - HIV-related encephalopathy or progressive multifocal leucoencephalopathy (PML). Although most adults have been exposed to JC (John Cunningham) virus, most do not experience problems. In patients with HIV, JC virus infects oligodendrocytes and leads to widespread demyelination in the central nervous system, causing PML.
- *Lymphoma* – can develop during HIV stage 3. This may explain the lymphadenopathy.
- *Kaposi sarcoma* – Sudip's lesions would be consistent with Kaposi sarcoma. This manifestation of infection with human herpes virus 8 would be consistent with a diagnosis of AIDS.
- *Mycobacterium tuberculosis* (TB)
  - TB is the most common pathogen seen in association with IRIS. Presentation often involves fever, respiratory failure and lymphadenopathy.
  - HIV patients are particularly vulnerable to multidrug-resistant TB (MDR-TB). Extensively drug-resistant TB (XDR-TB) has been described in HIV-positive patients and has an extremely high mortality.
  - Consider moving Sudip to a side room if he is not already in one and use an FFP3 mask when performing aerosolising procedures until TB has been ruled out.

How does this information affect your investigations?

Background information is needed regarding Sudip's diagnosis and treatment. When was he diagnosed, when did he start treatment, what treatment did he start? Review relevant clinic letters. Discuss his case with specialists in HIV management, microbiology and infection control.

Request the following additional investigations:

- CD4$^+$ count and CD8$^+$ count.
- RNA viral load.
- Galactomannan and beta-D-glucan to look for invasive fungal infection.
- Serum lactate dehydrogenase (LDH).
- Bronchoscopic washings for MC&S.

If a family member wants to know Sudip's HIV status, what can you tell them?

Ben has stated that Sudip does not want his family to know his HIV status. There is no information to suggest that his family are at risk of having contracted

HIV from him. In the UK, the risk of harm to others must be serious enough to outweigh breaching the patient's right to confidentiality – that does not appear to be the case here. If in doubt, consult your hospital legal team and your medical protection society.

What is HIV?

HIV is a type of lentivirus. This cytopathic retrovirus is known to have two types: HIV-1 (majority of cases) and HIV-2 (usually a milder course and mostly seen in mother-to-child transmission in West Africa). The retrovirus uses reverse transcriptase to transcribe viral RNA into host DNA. $CD4^+$ cells, T-helper cells, are preferentially infected and produce multiple copies of the HIV virus. Eventually this leads to the premature death of the host cell. There is a marked drop in the $CD4^+$ count, leaving the patient susceptible to infection and malignancy.

Primary HIV begins when HIV first enters the body. The HIV life cycle involves six phases:

1. Binding and entry
2. Reverse transcription
3. Integration
4. Replication
5. Budding
6. Maturation

Unchecked, the infection normally progresses through four phases – seroconversion illness, an asymptomatic stage, a symptomatic stage and finally late-stage HIV and AIDS.

The World Health Organization (WHO) classifies infection as follows:

- Stage 1 (HIV infection) – $CD4^+$ count at least 500 cells/μL
- Stage 2 (HIV infection) – $CD4^+$ count 350–499 cells/μL
- Stage 3 (advanced HIV disease, AHD) – $CD4^+$ count 200–349 cells/μL
- Stage 4 (AIDS) – $CD4^+$ count <200 cells/μL

According to UNAIDS/WHO, in 2020 there were approximately 37.7 million people worldwide living with HIV/AIDS. The vast majority of those are in low- or middle-income countries.

What drug treatments are available for HIV?

- Nucleoside analogue reverse transcriptase inhibitors (NRTI), e.g. zidovudine, lamivudine, abacavir
- Non-nucleoside reverse transcriptase inhibitors (NNRTI), e.g. nevirapine and rilpivirine
- Protease inhibitors (PI), e.g. darunavir, ritonavir and indinavir
- Integrase inhibitors, e.g. raltegravir and elvitegravir
- Fusion inhibitors, e.g. maraviroc and enfuvirtide

HAART (highly active ART) or cART (combination ART) is a combination of these drugs designed to decrease viral load and promote the patient's natural immune system. Often the combination will be two NRTIs plus a PI.

Adverse effects from these drugs can be multiple and include neuropathy, myopathy and hepatotoxicity. Ritonavir is a potent cytochrome p450 inhibitor so care must be taken to review polypharmacy and avoid potentially catastrophic drug interactions.

Cabotegravir and rilpivirine can now be delivered via injection every 2 months to qualifying patients.

The CT head reports no abnormality found. The CTPA does not show pulmonary embolus and rules out a pneumothorax. There are widespread pulmonary infiltrates, mediastinal lymphadenopathy and pleural effusions. You get in touch with the HIV specialist centre and find that Sudip was diagnosed with HIV 4 weeks ago. He started ART 3 weeks ago and was also being treated for TB.

Your investigations reveal CD4+ count 37 cells/μL, CD8+ count 321 cells/μL, CD4+/CD8+ ratio is 0.12, HIV RNA 5.3 $\log_{10}$ viral load.

How do you interpret the CD4+/CD8+ ratio and viral load results?

An immunocompetent patient should have a CD4+/CD8+ ratio greater than 1.0 (normally >1.5). In chronic HIV infection, increasing numbers of CD8+ cells with depletion of CD4+ cells result in a falling ratio. Sudip's ratio is extremely low, suggesting immunocompromise.

A CD4+ count below 200 cells/μL leaves a patient vulnerable to opportunistic infections.

A viral load of 5.3 $\log_{10}$ equates to approximately 200 000 copies/mL. A high viral load is generally considered to be greater than 100 000 copies/mL (approximately 5 $\log_{10}$). Undetectably low viral load is less than 20 copies/mL (approximately 1.3 $\log_{10}$).

What treatments are available for TB?

- First-line drugs are rifampicin, isoniazid (often given in combination with rifampicin as Rifinah®), pyrazinamide and ethambutol. A standard course of treatment is all four drugs for 2 months then Rifinah for a further 4 months.
- Second-line drugs include streptomycin, levofloxacin, moxifloxacin, linezolid, carbapenems with clavulanic acid, and cycloserine.
- Regular visual field testing is required with ethambutol, which can limit its use in critical care.

You discuss the case with the HIV specialist doctor who thinks this is IRIS. After discussing the risks and benefits, you decide to start high-dose steroids. She recommends you treat for *Pneumocystis jirovecii* – you commence high-dose co-trimoxazole. After discussion with your resident microbiologist, you also decide to add an antifungal agent.

What antifungal drugs are available and how do they work?

See Figure 17.1.

- *Azoles* – inhibit the conversion of lanosterol to ergosterol, an integral component of fungal cell membranes. These are the triazoles (e.g. fluconazole, itraconazole, voriconazole) and imidazoles (e.g. ketoconazole).
- *Echinocandins* – e.g. caspofungin, anidulafungin, micafungin. They inhibit 1,3-beta-D-glucan synthase. Beta-glucan is essential for production of the cell wall.
- *Polyenes* – such as amphotericin B and nystatin. These bind to ergosterol and increase the permeability of cells, leading to cell death.
- *Allylamines* – such as terbinafine. These inhibit squalene epoxidase which converts squalenc to ergosterol. Squalene, toxic to fungal cells, accumulates and causes cell death.
- *Nucleoside analogues* – for example, flucytosine. This pyrimidine analogue is converted into 5-FU in fungal cells. Through various mechanisms, this inhibits fungal DNA synthesis.

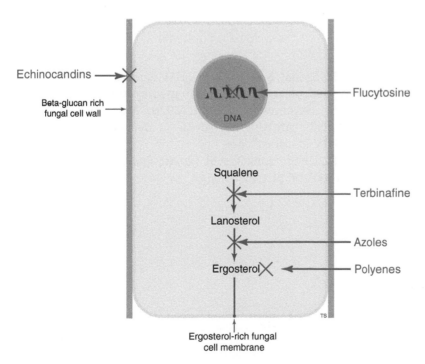

Figure 17.1: Mechanisms of actions of antifungal drugs.

Source: Theophilus Samuels.

Sudip continues to deteriorate over the next 24 hours with worsening gas exchange and renal impairment. You insert bilateral chest drains, commence renal replacement therapy and place him into the prone position. Two further prone positioning sessions are repeated for 16 hours each and Sudip's condition eventually begins to improve. Following discussion with the HIV specialist, you briefly withhold ART while Sudip's condition is precarious. By day 3, he begins to improve.

What is the mortality for patients with HIV?

The Antiretroviral Cohort Collaboration published an article in the *Lancet* in 2017 which showed that survival rates are improving, possibly through a combination of less toxic antiretroviral drugs, better adherence and better management of co-morbidities.

Prognosis continues to improve for those treated early in the course of their disease. Young people in Europe and the developed world who survive the first year of ART are now likely to have near normal life expectancy.

The mortality associated with IRIS is not clearly documented but with mild IRIS, it is extremely low. ART should generally be continued throughout illness except in life-threatening situations.

Sudip is successfully extubated on day 9. Moved by the experience of nearly losing him, Ben proposes marriage to Sudip on day 10. Sudip accepts. He is discharged to the ward on day 11.

Further reading

- Ghosn, J., Taiwo, B., Seedat, S. et al. (2018). HIV. *Lancet* 392: 685–697. Excellent of overview of HIV, particularly with regard to medications.
- Barbier, F., Mer, M., Szychowiak, P. et al. (2020). Management of HIV infected patients in the intensive care unit. *Intensive Care Med.* 46 (2): 329–342. Informative review article on HIV in critical care.
- Ritter, J., Flower, R., Henderson, G. et al. (2020). *Pharmacology*. St Louis: Elsevier. Authoritative textbook on pharmacology.

18 The Young Patient Who Collapses

You attend the resuscitation department following a medical emergency call. An 18-year-old woman has been brought in by ambulance following a collapse at home. Her parents tell you that she 'blacked out' after going running. By the time the ambulance arrived at her home, she had roused. Now, in the ED, she is found to have fluctuating consciousness, at worst GCS 8 (E1V2M5), BP 82/43 mmHg, HR 184 bpm, RR 10 breaths per minute, oxygen saturations 93% on air. She does not appear to have lost cardiac output at any time.

Describe Figure 18.1. What is the diagnosis?

This is an ECG rhythm strip showing a polymorphic ventricular tachycardia, i.e. torsades de pointes.

What are the adverse features of arrhythmias?

According to the Resuscitation Council UK, these are as follows:

- Shock
- Syncope
- Myocardial ischaemia
- Cardiac failure

How do you proceed?

The patient has developed torsades de pointes and is cardiovascularly unstable. Follow the Resuscitation Council Advanced Life Support Guidelines (2021), taking an ABDCE approach.

Clinical Cases in Critical Care, First Edition. Alice Myers and Theophilus Samuels.
© 2023 John Wiley & Sons Ltd. Published 2023 by John Wiley & Sons Ltd.

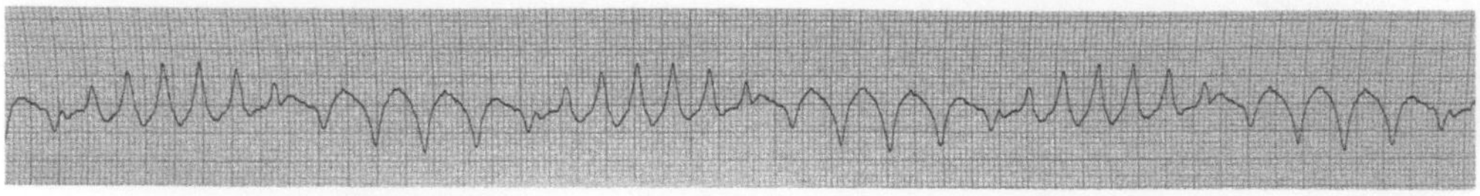

Figure 18.1: ECG rhythm strip

■ Administer oxygen, protecting the airway if required.
■ Obtain intravenous access, send bloods and a blood gas (paying attention to electrolytes and glucose).
■ Ensure full monitoring.
■ Give magnesium 2 g over 10 minutes as the specific treatment for torsades de pointes.

You treat the arrhythmia successfully and the young woman, Belle, stabilises and regains consciousness. You are now able to assess her fully. Belle looks extremely thin. She remains quiet and minimally communicative, saying only that she is cold and wants some water. Her BP is now 90/52 mmHg, HR 125 bpm, RR 22 breaths per minute. She appears dehydrated with poor skin turgor and central capillary refill time of 5 seconds. She has bibasal crepitations on auscultation of the lung fields.

What could be the underlying cause of Belle's arrhythmia?

1. *Congenital* – Belle is only 18 years old. This could represent the first presentation of a congenital cardiac disorder.
   ■ Inherited channelopathy – congenital long QT syndromes include Jervell Lange–Neilsen (associated with deafness) and Romano–Ward. Brugada syndrome may first present as sudden cardiac death in a young person and the arrhythmia produced can resemble torsades.
   ■ *Structural defect* – although it is less likely than many of the acquired causes, it is possible she could have an undiagnosed congenital anomaly such as hypertrophic obstructive cardiomyopathy (HOCM), or valvular or septal defect.
2. *Acquired*
   ■ Electrolyte imbalance – possibly secondary to malabsorption, drug use, metabolic disorders, or eating disorders.
   ■ Thyroid disease.
   ■ Sepsis.
   ■ Drug toxicity – prescription or illicit.
   ■ Coronary artery disease – the most common cause of polymorphic ventricular tachycardia in adults is coronary artery disease. Myocardial infarction (MI), hypertension and acquired valvular defects, while not impossible, are less likely in this young patient.

What are your immediate concerns?

- Cardiac status – she has presented with a malignant arrhythmia and has signs which could be consistent with cardiac failure.
- Nutritional status.

Which key aspects of Belle's medical history do you want to know?

Ideally, obtain a history from Belle herself. However, if she is unwilling or unable to communicate, obtain a collateral history from her GP, family or friends.

Medical notes from any previous admissions should be reviewed for the following:

- Symptoms suggesting cardiac pathology, e.g. fainting, blackouts, seizures or palpitations.
- Symptoms of underlying gastrointestinal disease.
- Past medical history of deafness.
- Family history of long QT syndrome or sudden cardiac death.
- Psychiatric history – in light of a possible eating disorder.
- Drug history – prescribed, over the counter and illicit.

What investigations do you need?

Bedside tests

- *12-lead ECG* – look for evidence of long QTc interval.
- *Pregnancy test* – amenorrhoea and collapse in a young woman of child-bearing age could represent ruptured ectopic pregnancy.

Blood tests

- *Arterial blood gas* – gas exchange may be impaired due to cardiac failure. Metabolic acidosis may have developed due to dehydration and kidney or liver injury. Metabolic alkalosis could have developed due to hypokalaemia. Assess lactate, base deficit and electrolytes.
- *FBC* – malnourishment may lead to anaemia or neutropenia and sepsis could be indicated by raised WBC.
- *U&E* – with malnutrition, it is necessary to measure sodium, potassium, calcium, phosphate and magnesium levels. Review urea and creatinine as Belle is dehydrated.
- *LFTs* – important to review for nutritional status and drug history.
- *Glucose and ketones.*
- *Thyroid function tests* – thyroid disease can cause arrhythmias and changes in weight. In addition, hypothyroidism may develop because of starvation.

Imaging

- *Chest radiograph.*
- *Echocardiogram.*

Belle's parents tell you that she dropped out of university 2 months ago and has been withdrawn, refusing to eat and exercising excessively. They tried encouraging her to seek help but she refused. There is no family history of cardiac disorders. Belle has always been fit (a keen dancer) and is not known to take drugs or drink alcohol. She has never been seen by a psychiatrist although her parents note that the nurse at her secondary school did suggest she should see someone for counselling.

The arterial blood gas (on 3 L/min O_2 via nasal cannulae) reveals pH 7.30, PaO_2 8.1 kPa, $PaCO_2$ 3.2 kPa, base excess –6.7 mmol/L, Na 134 mmol/L, K 2.3 mmol/L, HCO_3 17 mmol/L, Cl 101 mmol/L, lactate 3.4 mmol/L. Urine dip is positive for blood and strongly positive for ketones.

The initial blood tests reveal Hb 114 g/L, WBC 3.9×10^9/L, plats 117×10^9/L, urea 8 mmol/L, creatinine 125 μmol/L, magnesium 0.5 mmol/L, phosphate 0.3 mmol/L, Ca 0.98 mmol/L, ALP 93 U/L, bilirubin 6 μmol/L. Blood ketones are high. CRP result is pending. ECG demonstrates long QTc interval.

Focused ultrasonography demonstrates a small hyperdynamic left ventricle, with visual evidence of hypertrophy. No significant valvular regurgitant lesions are seen. Lung US demonstrates multiple bilateral B-lines throughout.

What is Belle's anion gap?

$$Anion\,gap = \left(Na^+ + K^+\right) - \left(Cl^- + HCO_3^-\right)$$

Belle's anion gap is $(134 + 2.3) - (101 + 17) = 18.3$ mmol/L. The normal anion gap is between 4 and 12 mmol/L. A raised anion gap suggests the presence of unmeasured anions. Note, that even with omitting K^+ (see Case 4), the anion gap is still above normal.

What are the most likely causes of Belle's raised anion gap?

The main causes to remember are lactate, ketones, toxins and renal failure (see Case 4).

In Belle's case, she may have taken an overdose so it would be appropriate to add paracetamol and salicylate levels to her blood tests and a toxicology screen.

Belle's raised anion gap is most likely to be due to ketosis.

Patients with eating disorders can present with different patterns in acid–base derangement. Metabolic alkalosis is common secondary to vomiting or diuretic misuse. Acidosis can arise following laxative misuse. Belle's case is complicated through presentation with cardiovascular instability and renal impairment.

What are the main clinical concerns and where would you like Belle to be managed?

- Severe electrolyte disturbance.
- Clinical presentation and ultrasound evidence which could be consistent with cardiac failure and associated pulmonary oedema.
- Long QTc interval on ECG.
- Dehydration and renal impairment (even modestly increased levels could suggest significant renal injury in patients with extremely low body weight).
- Possible starvation ketosis.
- Low body mass index (BMI) and possible psychiatric disorder.

Belle should be admitted to a high-dependency facility where she can be carefully monitored and managed.

Which other healthcare professionals should you involve in Belle's care?

- Cardiologist
- Dietitian
- Psychiatrist
- General physician
- The full critical care MDT

You ask the liaison psychiatrist to review Belle urgently. They attend to review her in the resuscitation department, and, after thorough review, they tell you that their working diagnosis is anorexia nervosa or anorexia nervosa with bulimic subtype. She has not taken an overdose on this occasion, but the psychiatrist believes that Belle is at risk of harm to herself if she were to be allowed to go home now.

What is anorexia?

Anorexia means loss of appetite and is seen in organic disorders (e.g. cancer) and psychological problems (e.g. depression).

Anorexia nervosa is a specific psychiatric diagnosis according to the ICD-11 (International Statistical Classification of Diseases and Related Health Problems version 11) and DSM-5 (Diagnostic and Statistical Manual of Mental Disorders). Signs and symptoms include a distorted perception of body shape or weight, behavioural issues regarding food and control of calorie intake, as well as other psychological and physical issues, most notably low BMI.

Diagnosis involves the following (as per ICD-11):

1. BMI <18.5 kg/m² or rapid weight loss more than 20% total body weight in 6 months
2. Restriction of calorie intake and extreme fear of weight gain often associated with the following behaviours:

- Purging
- Vomiting
- Excessive exercise
- Use of appetite suppressants, diuretics or laxatives
3. Distorted body image and/or excessive pre-occupation with body weight or shape.

There may be amenorrhoea and/or loss of libido in adults.

What are the cardiovascular complications of anorexia and starvation?

- Bradycardia and long QTc interval.
- Severe autonomic dysfunction leading to tachycardia.
- Orthostatic hypotension secondary to severe dehydration.
- Hypotension, even in sitting position.
- Adaptive vagal hyperactivity in chronic states.
- Loss of cardiac muscle mass over time (up to 50% decrease in LV mass) which can lead to overall decrease in cardiac output.
- Mitral valve prolapse, pericardial effusions and cardiomyopathies have been documented.

The precise pathophysiology of cardiac failure in anorexia and starvation is not clearly elucidated. There is a risk of cardiac failure with aggressive correction of dehydration.

> You explain your findings to Belle. You tell her that she is very unwell and that you would like to move her to the critical care unit for ongoing management. She refuses.

How do you proceed?

This is a difficult situation. Proceeding to admit to critical care depends on whether Belle has capacity or not (see Case 19). Persuading her to stay is the ideal option. Belle has just been treated for a life-threatening arrhythmia which could re-develop at any time. She has a metabolic acidosis secondary to starvation ketosis and severely deranged electrolytes as a result of malnutrition. In addition, the psychiatrist believes she would be a risk to herself if she were allowed to go home.

Given her malnutrition and unstable clinical state, it is likely that she does not possess the capacity to make this decision. Best interests principles outlined in the Mental Capacity Act 2005 and DoLS (Deprivation of Liberty Safeguards) may be required to treat her life-threatening medical problems (including treatment for malnutrition). A compulsory treatment order using section 2 of the Mental Health Act 2007 (England) allows assessment and treatment for up to 28 days (the law varies in different parts of the UK and throughout the world). Consider discussing whether a patient should be treated against their will with the hospital's legal team.

Belle should be encouraged at every opportunity to engage with her treatment as she is likely to require medical and psychiatric support for many months/years.

Do you know any guidelines for the management of critically unwell patients with anorexia?

MEED (**Me**dical **E**mergencies in **E**ating **D**isorders) was published in 2022. This document replaces MARSIPAN and Junior MARSIPAN for those aged under 18 years (**Ma**nagement of **R**eally **Si**ck **P**atients with **A**norexia **N**ervosa). This extensive document includes advice on nutritional, psychiatric and medical management. It provides a risk assessment framework using a 'traffic lights' system.

NICE also publishes guidelines on managing patients with eating disorders (NG69, updated 2020).

> Fortunately, after discussion with her parents, Belle agrees to be admitted to the HDU. She tolerates the insertion of invasive monitoring, a nasogastric tube and a urinary catheter. Her weight is measured as 41 kg and her height is 178 cm.

What is Belle's BMI?

BMI (kg/m^2) is used as a rough guide to measure whether a person is a 'healthy weight'.

$$BMI = \frac{Weight\ in\ kg}{\left(Height\ in\ m\right)^2}$$

The NHS recommended range for most adults is 18.5–24.9 kg/m^2.

Criticisms of BMI calculation include the fact it does not reflect percentage body fat or muscle mass. A falsely high BMI will be recorded in the presence of oedema or fluid overload. Recommended healthy ranges consider neither ethnic variability regarding risk of diabetes nor the true nutritional status of the patient. However, BMI can be useful as a quick guide to whether the patient is under- or overweight.

Belle's calculation:

$$\frac{41}{1.78^2} = 12.9$$

A healthy weight range for an 18-year-old woman of this height would be 58.6–78.9 kg.

According to MEED, patients over 18 years old with BMI <13 have high impending risk to life (BMI > 15 have a low impending risk to life).

What other features can be used to categorise risk in patients with anorexia nervosa?

Physical examination

- Reduced muscle power
- Low score on sit-up-squat-stand test (two or less)
- Postural hypotension
- Hypothermia (<35 °C)

Blood tests

- Hyponatraemia (<130 mmol/l)
- Hypokalaemia (<3.0 mmol/l)
- Raised transaminases
- Hypoglycaemia (<3 mmol/l)
- Raised urea or creatinine outside the typical range

ECG

- Bradycardia (<40 bpm)
- Prolonged QTc interval (>450 ms)
- Non-specific T-wave changes
- Signs of hypokalaemia

What are the stages of starvation?

Starvation is an adaptive state where the human body eventually becomes hypometabolic to preserve glucose for brain use (Table 18.1). It is worth noting that the brain is also adept at using ketones as a source of energy.

Table 18.1: Phases of starvation.

Phase	Comments
Phase 1 (up to 6 h)	Increase in catecholamines and cortisol. Decrease in insulin. Hepatic glycogenolysis and gluconeogenesis. Blood glucose levels are maintained.
Phase 2 (6–72 h, but may be up to weeks)	Once glycogen stores depleted gluconeogenesis continues using lactate, with glutamine and alanine from body proteins. Glutamine derived almost entirely from gut protein content. Lipolysis releases glycerol, the carbon from which can be used with carbon from muscle protein hydrolysis for de novo glucose synthesis. Proteolysis in skeletal muscle releases amino acids.
Phase 3 (72 h to 2 wks)	Increased hepatic synthesis of ketone bodies by day 3 attempts to minimise loss of body protein. Body attempts to conserve proteins but with prolonged fasting, amino acids from skeletal muscle are used in gluconeogenesis. Brain uses ketones metabolised from free fatty acids (acetoacetate and beta-hydroxybutyrate). By 4 days into starvation, 70% of the brain's energy is derived from ketones. Cardiac muscle can use ketones as a fuel source. Note that in the presence of sepsis, ketone production is impaired, resulting in significantly greater loss of lean body mass in the first week as proteins are mobilised and specific amino acids released are utilised for gluconeogenesis.
Phase 4 (beyond 2 wks)	Fat stores depleted. Proteolysis becomes only means of generating energy. Loss of lean body mass and organ tissue reduces resting energy expenditure. Eventually, chronically reduced basal metabolic rate (BMR) with reduced body weight.

Do you start full nasogastric feed immediately? Justify your answer.

No. From the history and physical examination, there is suspicion that Belle is in a state of starvation. Care must be taken to avoid inducing potentially fatal refeeding syndrome.

Belle's basal metabolic rate (BMR) will probably have reduced by up to 25% and her body has adapted to utilising fat and protein for energy rather than carbohydrate. Her brain will have switched to using ketones as its main energy source.

What is refeeding syndrome?

Prolonged starvation reduces overall cell mass, along with intracellular mineral content (serum levels may well be maintained). When sugars are reintroduced suddenly, glycaemia leads to increased insulin and decreased glucagon levels. This stimulates synthesis of proteins, fats and glycogen. These synthetic processes would consume Belle's modest plasma stores of intracellular ions (potassium, phosphate and magnesium). Provision of carbohydrate generates a specific demand for B group vitamins involved in metabolism, specifically thiamine.

Refeeding syndrome results in massive fluid shifts and mineral depletion, particularly hypophosphataemia. Other clinical features include hypokalaemia, hypomagnesaemia, hyperglycaemia, arrhythmias, pulmonary oedema and cardiac failure.

Which other patients are particularly at risk of refeeding syndrome?

NICE Guidance was published in 2006 (CG32) to help identify those at risk. Refeeding syndrome should be considered a risk where the patient has **one** or more of these factors:

- BMI <16 kg/m^2
- Unintentional weight loss >15% during preceding 3–6 months
- Minimal nutritional intake for >10 days
- Low levels of potassium, phosphate or magnesium before commencement of feeding

Or **two** or more of the following:

- BMI <18.5 kg/m^2
- Unintentional weight loss >10% during preceding 3–6 months
- Minimal nutritional intake for >5 days
- History of alcohol or drug misuse

Belle meets the first criteria with her BMI <16 kg/m^2. From the collateral history, she has probably also had minimal nutritional intake for more than 10 days. She already has low potassium, magnesium and phosphate.

Other patient groups who should be assessed for risk of refeeding syndrome include the following:

- Patients with cancer.
- Those with malabsorption or maldigestion, e.g. inflammatory bowel disease, pancreatitis, short bowel syndrome, etc. Note that food provision will not increase the risk of refeeding in this group if feed is not absorbed. Review feed options with the dietitian, e.g. hydrolysed NG formula or parenteral nutrition.
- Frail patients.
- Uncontrolled diabetes mellitus.
- Postoperative patients – particularly those undergoing bowel surgery or surgery for conditions which reduce the ability to eat, e.g. head and neck cancers, etc.
- Chronic alcoholism.
- Morbidly obese patients.
- Those with increased losses – potassium and magnesium losses with loop diuretics, magnesium losses with high-output ileostomies.
- Patients with substantial confirmed weight loss commencing enteral or parenteral nutrition.

How will you manage Belle to avoid refeeding syndrome?

This strategy is best undertaken with the advice of a dietitian and based on NICE guidance.

- Identify Belle as being at risk.
- Check her potassium, calcium, phosphate and magnesium.
- Administer thiamine 200–300 mg orally, high-potency vitamin B tablets three times daily, and a trace element supplement once daily before feeding commences, as per NICE guidance. Check with the ICU pharmacist as to whether typical doses need adjustment for low body weight.
- Start feed at a low rate and slowly increase over the following week.
- Rehydrate carefully with electrolyte supplements, monitoring fluid balance closely and physical symptoms of fluid overload.
- Closely monitor and replace electrolytes as required for the first 2 weeks in conjunction with advancing nutritional intake.
- If oral/enteral phosphate and magnesium fail to correct levels, measure vitamin D and PTH status. Vitamin D deficiency can compromise calcium, phosphate and magnesium uptake. If vitamin D levels are low, supplement carefully to avoid hypervitaminosis D due to lack of adipose tissue and liver mass to store excess.

Would you use parenteral nutrition to feed Belle?

There is no indication in Belle's case for parenteral nutrition since there is no evidence of gut failure, although gut morphology will have adapted due to the absence of food and glutamine provision for gluconeogenesis. There are multiple complications secondary to parenteral nutrition, so it is to be avoided where possible in favour of the enteral route.

What are the risks associated with parenteral nutrition?

- Risks associated with insertion or presence of the intravenous catheter
  - Infection
  - Vascular injury
  - Air embolus
  - Bleeding
  - Extravasation
  - Thrombosis
- Risks associated with TPN (total parenteral nutrition)
  - Electrolyte imbalance
  - Hyper/hypoglycaemia
  - Micronutrient deficiencies
  - Liver dysfunction/hyperammonaemia
  - Volume overload
  - Cholecystitis
  - Metabolic bone disease can develop with long term use

You ask the critical care dietitian to design a nutritional plan for Belle.

What are Belle's daily nutritional requirements?

There are various methods of calculating a patient's nutritional requirements.

The Harris–Benedict formula calculates BMR using height, weight, sex, age and general level of activity. The calculation is best applied to healthy individuals. BMR is increased in fever (by 10% per 1 °C above 37 °C), and in burns, sepsis and surgery to varying degrees.

Belle's case is extremely challenging due to her chronic malnutrition and will require frequent liaison with an experienced dietitian.

Nutrition provides macronutrients and micronutrients and the following is a rough estimate for established enteral feeding but which would be calculated and adjusted for each individual.

Current enteral feeds provide a full profile of vitamins, minerals and trace elements. After the first week or two of stabilisation, the goal for weight gain is 0.5–1.0 kg per week. This is achieved by gradual increase in enteral nutrition provision. It is not uncommon for those with a high-risk BMI to require 50–90 kcal/kg/d of actual body weight before weight gain becomes consistent (Table 18.2).

You notice Belle has an erythematous rash. The dietitian suggests this could be due to zinc deficiency.

Zinc deficiency can manifest as skin rash typical of the condition acrodermatitis enteropathica. Once hydration and nutrition are established, consider empirical zinc supplement for 3 days. Note that zinc excess competitively inhibits iron, calcium and magnesium uptake across the gut.

Table 18.2: Nutritional requirements for adults.

Energy	25–35 kcal/kg/d is usual approximate requirement for healthy adult. No absolute recommendation. 20 kcal/kg/d is a good starting point for younger adults Intake should be increased 200 kcal/d until weight gain of 0.5–1.0 kg/wk is achieved. If hypophosphataemia occurs, this should be corrected before feed is advanced further.
Protein	1.5 g/kg/d
Fats	Approximately a third of daily calorie intake should come from fats. Standard enteral feed is approximately 55% carbohydrate and 35% fat
Carbohydrates	2–7 g/kg/d (depending on health and exercise)
Water	25–35 ml/kg/d
Sodium	0.9–1.2 mmol/kg/d
Potassium	1–2 mmol/kg/d
Calcium	0.25 mmol/kg/d
Phosphate	0.3–0.6 mmol/kg/d
Magnesium	0.2–0.4 mmol/kg/d
Other additives	Zinc, copper, iron, chromium, manganese, selenium, molybdenum. May also need to supplement vitamins A, B, C, D, E and K, folate and niacin, etc.

What are the non-cardiac complications of severe malnutrition?

- Anaemia is common – related to iron deficiency and vitamin B12/folate deficiency.
- Immune suppression.
- Oedema in the lower limbs and abdomen.
- Flaky skin.
- Apathy.
- Listlessness.
- Eventually, marasmus (more usually in infants) and kwashiorkor (more usual in children) may develop.

After 13 days in critical care, you manage to correct Belle's electrolyte imbalances and establish her on enteral feed. She has remained stable from a cardiac point of view and is now safe to be discharged to a medical ward.

What are the possible outcomes for Belle now?

Mortality risk in anorexia is approximately 6%. With appropriate treatment and follow-up, Belle could be part of the 50% who make a full recovery. Approximately 20% will suffer relapses in their lifetime. Belle is likely to require long-term follow-up with psychiatric and nutritional support.

Further reading

- Royal Colleges of Psychiatrists (2022). *College Report* CR233. The MEED guidance is essential reading for anyone with an interest in the management of anorexia nervosa.
- Steinhauser, M., Olenchock, B., O'Keefe, J. et al. (2018). The circulating metabolome of human starvation. *JCI Insight* 3 (16): e121434. Fascinating research article on the metabolic effects of starvation.

19 The Patient Who has Taken an Overdose

The medical registrar calls you about Sarah, a 21-year-old student who has been brought into hospital by ambulance having been found vomiting by her housemates. She was surrounded by empty containers of paracetamol, aspirin, zopiclone, amitriptyline and propranolol. Her housemates also found two empty bottles of wine. She is known to suffer from mental health problems, including depression and anxiety. She had a loud argument with her boyfriend earlier in the evening and a similar one a couple of nights ago. Her GCS is 11 (E3V3M5). She is confused, agitated and unmanageable and is now vomiting a mixture of bile and blood-stained fluid.

What are your concerns regarding her airway?

Sarah appears to have taken a potentially life-threatening deliberate overdose of multiple agents. As yet, it is not clear how much of each she has taken or how long ago. Although her conscious level is not so low that she requires intubation for airway protection, she is combative and it is impossible to manage her. In addition, a decreased GCS in combination with frequent vomiting increases her risk of aspiration. She needs investigation and treatment. She may need sedation and intubation to gain control of the situation and make her safe.

What are the medico-legal and ethical implications of attempting to save this woman's life?

In most cases, information is scarce when such patients arrive into hospital. Often, their conscious level or lucidity is compromised by their overdose. In most cases, the obvious course of action is to treat to save life. This is usually the appropriate course of action.

Rarely, you may need to consult the hospital legal team for advice in advance of intervention. In 2007, a 26-year-old woman died in the UK following ingestion of anti-freeze. She arrived in hospital with a letter clearly stating that she

Clinical Cases in Critical Care, First Edition. Alice Myers and Theophilus Samuels.
© 2023 John Wiley & Sons Ltd. Published 2023 by John Wiley & Sons Ltd.

understood the consequences of her actions and wanted no attempts at resuscitation, only comfort measures. She was fully conscious and was deemed to have capacity. The doctors managing her in the emergency department did not treat her because she was accompanied by this 'living will' or 'advance decision'. At the inquest in 2009, the coroner supported their decision. There is ongoing debate regarding the ethical implications of this case.

Doctors are guided by the principles of:

- Autonomy
- Non-maleficence
- Beneficence
- Justice.

Any patient with reduced consciousness cannot have capacity. In many cases, the veracity of an accompanying suicide letter will be difficult to ascertain in the acute event. Where there is doubt as to the chain of events and the capacity of the patient, doctors will treat to save life. If in doubt, and time allows, you should consult the hospital's on-call legal advisor.

In our case, Sarah is not accompanied by an advance decision. She may have been intoxicated with, and compromised by, alcohol at the time of overdose. There are many unknown factors here and the priority is to administer life-saving treatment.

What is capacity?

Capacity is a legal term related to the ability to make an informed decision. The UK Mental Capacity Act 2005 asserts the following:

- A person is unable to make a decision for themselves if they are unable to:
  - Understand the information relevant to the decision
  - Retain that information
  - Use or weigh that information as part of the process of making the decision, or
  - Communicate their decision (whether by talking, using sign language or any other means).

The principles of the Mental Capacity Act are as follows:
- A person must be assumed to have capacity unless it is established that they lack capacity.
- A person is not to be treated as unable to make a decision unless all practicable steps to help them to do so have been taken without success.
- A person is not to be treated as unable to make a decision merely because they make an unwise decision.
- An act done, or decision made, under this Act for or on behalf of a person who lacks capacity must be done, or made, in their best interests.
- Before the act is done, or the decision is made, regard must be had as to whether the purpose for which it is needed can be as effectively achieved in a way that is less restrictive of the person's rights and freedom of action.

While you are assessing her, Sarah's GCS drops to 7 (E1V2M4) and her respiratory rate drops from 30 to 8 breaths per minute.

What could be the cause of Sarah's decreased GCS?

- *Intoxication* – the history suggests overdose of multiple agents, including several with the capacity to induce sedation, i.e. alcohol, the tricyclic antidepressant (TCA) amitriptyline, and zopiclone (a cyclopyrrolone which acts via GABA receptors and has a similar pharmacological profile to benzodiazepines). In addition, Sarah may have had access to other CNS depressants. Attention should be given to establishing whether there is evidence of a staggered overdose, particularly with paracetamol as this will induce more prolonged deterioration in acute liver failure.
- *Hypoglycaemia* – don't ever forget glucose! Many substances taken in excess can cause hypoglycaemia. Sarah's medical background is unknown. She may have a history of alcohol excess, liver injury or diabetes.
- *Decreased cardiac output* – beta-blockers cause decreased heart rate and blood pressure. In overdose, this can lead to decreased cardiac output, decreased end-organ perfusion (including to the brain) and even cardiovascular collapse.
- *Renal failure* – many substances in overdose can cause renal impairment and hence accumulation of urea in the blood. Uraemic encephalopathy can develop in acute or chronic renal failure and may manifest as tremor, delirium, seizures or coma. Acidaemia may also play a role.
- *Hyperammonaemia* – ammonia is a gut-derived neurotoxin which may accumulate secondary to overproduction or reduced metabolism, i.e. liver failure. Among the substances likely to have been ingested by Sarah, paracetamol ingested in excess is notoriously toxic to the liver.
- *Intracranial event* – there is not yet enough evidence to rule out a spontaneous or traumatic brain injury, particularly given the history of a recent altercation and the fact that she may have been at risk of falling while intoxicated. Examine her head for signs of injury but be aware that bruises may hide beneath hair.
- *Meningitis or encephalitis* – CNS infection is low on the list of differential diagnoses given a strong history of overdose. However, this has not yet been ruled out. Look for signs of sepsis.
- *Respiratory depression or postictal state* – there is no available arterial blood gas result. She may have had a seizure and be in a transient state of reduced consciousness.

What is your management plan at this point?

Emergency management

- *Advanced Life Support ABCDE approach* – the situation has changed, and Sarah should be reassessed, managing problems simultaneously. Give oxygen and call for help if needed.
- *Gain IV access and secure the airway* – her conscious level has reduced sufficiently that she cannot protect her own airway. Sarah has been vomiting

and may have aspirated already. She may have a stomach full of alcohol and will need a modified rapid-sequence intubation (see Introduction Part 2).

- *Consult TOXBASE* – this is the national poisons information service commissioned by Public Health England. It is an invaluable resource for clinicians needing to find information regarding the diagnosis and management of substance exposure (see Case 6).
- *Consider giving naloxone* – if Sarah may have ingested opioids, this reversal agent could be used. Usually, a test dose is given to assess response. Due to the short half-life of the drug, an infusion will be required for ongoing management. Use naloxone with caution as it may lower seizure threshold. Time the administration carefully if paralysing drugs have recently been administered to facilitate intubation.
- *Start an infusion of N-acetylcysteine (NAC)* given the likelihood of paracetamol overdose.

Monitoring

- *Basic monitoring* – ECG, pulse oximetry, HR, end-tidal CO_2 monitoring, non-invasive BP.
- *Establish intra-arterial BP monitoring.*
- *Urine output.*

Bedside tests

- *Point-of-care blood glucose level.*
- *Arterial blood gas sample* to review gas exchange (to aid in setting the ventilator), acid–base derangement, lactate, and calculate the anion gap (see Case 4).
- *12-lead ECG* – amitriptyline can cause sinus tachycardia secondary to muscarinic blockade. Broad QRS (interventricular conduction delay) and right axis deviation may be due to sodium channel blockade.
- *Urine pregnancy test.*

Lab tests

- *FBC, LFTs, clotting, fibrinogen, U&Es.*
- *Request paracetamol, salicylate and alcohol levels.*
- *Urine toxicology screen.*
- *Blood culture* since you do not yet know whether there is an infective element.
- *Ammonia level.*
- *CRP.*

Imaging

- *Chest radiograph* – review the position of your endotracheal tube. This is also part of your septic screen.
- *CT head* – rule out intracranial abnormalities as a cause of decreased consciousness.

Transfer Sarah to critical care for ongoing management

■ *Insert an NG tube and a urinary catheter.*
■ *Contact next of kin.*
■ *Request old medical notes (hospital, psychiatric and general practitioner)* – this will be vital in planning her ongoing care and support needs. A significant history of self-harm may affect her suitability for transplant if required.

> You transfer Sarah safely to critical care, having secured her airway uneventfully. You site an arterial and central venous catheter and a VasCath™. The lab calls you to say that the paracetamol level is 260 mg/L, salicylate level is 34 mg/dL. And the alcohol level is still pending. They also tell you the INR is 1.8. The remaining blood tests are outstanding.

What is the pathophysiology of paracetamol overdose?

Paracetamol is normally metabolised in the liver by glucuronidation (approximately 70%) and sulfation (approximately 30%). A small amount is excreted unchanged renally. When these pathways are saturated, paracetamol is metabolised by CYP450 (mainly 2E1) in Phase 1 biotransformation to NAPQI, which is cytotoxic. In Phase 2, NAPQI reacts with glutathione to form an inactive metabolite. In overdose, glutathione stores are depleted through overloading of this oxidation pathway and NAPQI will then bind covalently to sulfhydryl groups and hepatocellular death ensues (Figure 19.1).

What are the stages of paracetamol hepatotoxicity?

■ *Stage 1* – 0–24 hours, general malaise, abdominal pain.
■ *Stage 2* – 24–72 hours, AST and ALT begin to rise. Right upper quadrant pain.
■ *Stage 3* – 72–96 hours, hepatic failure with jaundice, coagulopathy and encephalopathy and lactic acidosis.
■ *Stage 4* – beyond 96 hours, resolution of hepatotoxicity or multiorgan failure and death.

What treatments are available for paracetamol toxicity and resultant acute liver failure?

Initial management of significant paracetamol overdose

■ NAC can be given at any time following ingestion. If it is given enterally, its effectiveness will be reduced by activated charcoal. The paracetamol overdose treatment graph (which can be found in the

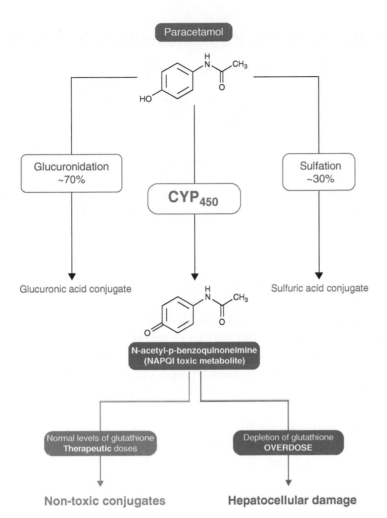

Figure 19.1: Paracetamol hepatic metabolism. Main hepatic metabolic pathways after administration of toxic or therapeutic doses of paracetamol.

Source: Theophilus Samuels.

British National Formulary, BNF) is used to guide treatment with NAC. Blood paracetamol levels measured at or after 4 hours following ingestion are plotted on the graph. If the level is below the line for hepatotoxicity, treatment can be stopped. However, it should be noted that it is difficult to apply the graph where the overdose was staggered or overdose time is unknown. Normal practice would be to treat pre-emptively with NAC.

■ If the patient is stable and arrives into hospital within the first 4 hours of their paracetamol overdose, 50 g oral activated charcoal can be considered to reduce absorption. However, in clinical practice this is rarely used now since often timing of overdose is unknown, the overdose is staggered or presentation is delayed.

■ MARS (molecular adsorbent recirculating system) allows selective removal of albumin-bound toxins in the blood and has been used as a bridge to transplant. This is an expensive therapy with limited availability in specialist centres only. High-quality evidence to prove benefit is lacking and its effectiveness is still under investigation.

Coagulopathy arising from subsequent liver impairment

- Correction of coagulopathy is only indicated if there is active haemorrhage.
- Thromboelastography and similar methods are a useful guide to assessing and managing coagulopathy and transfusion requirements.

Management of hepatic encephalopathy

A major concern with hepatic encephalopathy is that, in up to a third of cases, cerebral oedema secondary to ammonia causes raised intracranial pressure (ICP). Consult local protocols to ensure neuroprotection.

- Keep well sedated.
- Neutral neck position, avoid ligatures which prevent jugular venous drainage, maintain 20–30° head-up tilt.
- Frequent monitoring with neurological observations.
- Blood sampling for coagulation, pH, lactate, glucose (aim 5–10 mmol/L), AST, renal function, phosphate, potassium and ammonia.
- Assess cerebral oxygen delivery and uptake using central venous saturations, arterial venous saturations and reverse jugular saturations (aim 65–70%).
- Minimise stimulation from suction.
- Aim $PaCO_2$ 4.5–5.0 kPa, PaO_2 >13 kPa, saturations >94%, tidal volumes 4–6 mL/kg ideal body weight (IBW).
- Aim cerebral perfusion pressure 55–70 mmHg (see Case 15).
- Aim sodium 145–150 mmol/L.

Drug treatments to consider for encephalopathy

- Lactulose, a non-absorbable disaccharide, acidifies the gut lumen, promoting conversion of ammonia to ammonium which is poorly absorbed. Ammonium is excreted and plasma ammonia reduced. In addition, the acidic environment inhibits ammoniagenic bacteria in the gut.
- Rifaximin is a non-absorbable derivative of rifamycin. Rifaximin is used to prevent hepatic encephalopathy by decreasing the presence of urease-producing flora in the gastrointestinal tract. Under normal physiological conditions, ammonia generated by gut flora enters the systemic circulation via the portal vein and is metabolised by the liver. However, in liver failure, a combination of decreased hepatic metabolism and portosystemic shunting leads to blood bypassing the liver, or passing through the liver without metabolism, causing an increase in serum ammonia concentrations and hepatic encephalopathy. Adding rifaximin to lactulose therapy may result in significant reductions in hepatic encephalopathy recurrence and hospitalisations.
- Neomycin reduces the presence of ammoniagenic bacteria. It is usually given following commencement of lactulose.
- In discussion with experienced members of the team, mannitol and hypertonic saline may be used with ICP monitoring.
- L-ornithine L-aspartate (LOLA).

General ICU care

- Fluid resuscitation.
- Renal replacement therapy may be required. Exchange rates up to 90 mL/kg/h can be used where ammonia levels are extremely high.
- Gastric ulcer prophylaxis.
- Ensure nutrition is ongoing.
- Antimicrobial prophylaxis.
- High-volume plasma exchange has been shown to improve outcomes in acute liver failure.
- Ultimately liver transplant may be required.

How is LOLA believed to work?

LOLA treats hepatic encephalopathy by stimulating the urea cycle. Both salts are substrates for glutamate which reacts with ammonia to form glutamine, thereby reducing ammonia levels.

How does NAC work?

NAC is a precursor for glutathione. By replenishing glutathione stores, NAC reduces the presence of hepatotoxic NAPQI. In addition, NAC may decrease the saturation of the glucuronidation and sulfation pathways, promote oxygen delivery and improve hepatic microcirculation.

What are the risk factors for increased likelihood of toxicity in paracetamol overdose?

- Pre-existing hepatic impairment.
- States of reduced glutathione stores, e.g. malnutrition, anorexia, HIV, chronic alcohol excess.
- Enzyme-inducing states, e.g. use of certain drugs such as the oral contraceptive pill, phenytoin, rifampicin, carbamazepine.
- Staggered overdose.

What are the criteria for referral to a liver transplant centre?

The King's College Criteria (KCC) were originally described in 1989 by O'Grady et al. The criteria are widely used internationally as an early predictor of the need for liver transplant. Meta-analysis by Bailey et al. in 2003 showed that in paracetamol toxicity, mortality prediction using the KCC had a specificity >90% and a sensitivity 69%.

In cases of paracetamol toxicity

- Arterial pH <7.30.

OR, in a 24-hour period all three of:

- INR >6.5 or prothrombin time >100 seconds
- creatinine >300 μmol/L or 3.4 mg/dL
- grade III or IV hepatic encephalopathy.

The *modified* KCC includes:

- Arterial lactate >3.5 mmol/L following fluid resuscitation
- pH <7.30 OR lactate >3.5 mmol/L following fluid resuscitation 12 hours after admission.

In non-paracetamol toxicity

- INR >6.5 or PT >100 seconds.
OR three of the following five:
- Age <10 or >40 years
- Bilirubin >300 μmol/L or >18 mg/dL
- Time from onset of jaundice to coma >7 days
- INR >3.5 or PT >50 seconds
- Idiosyncratic drug reaction, seronegative, or non-A or B hepatitis.

NB: phosphate >1.2 mmol/L beyond 48 hours is a predictor of a poor prognosis.

Following fluid resuscitation, the arterial blood gas reveals pH 7.12, $PaCO_2$ 4.6 kPa, PaO_2 11.6 kPa (FiO_2 0.45), base excess −12.2 mmol/L, lactate 5.3 mmol/L. The ECG shows sinus tachycardia but is otherwise normal. The blood glucose is 3.2 mmol/L.

What is the pathophysiology of aspirin (salicylate) toxicity and how do you interpret Sarah's level of 34 mg/dL?

Salicylates uncouple oxidative phosphorylation, thereby impairing cellular respiration. Dual actions may mask acid–base disturbances in the early phases of toxicity as salicylates stimulate the medullary respiratory centre, causing a respiratory alkalosis, while metabolic acidosis develops due to mitochondrial damage. Eventually, the metabolic acidosis becomes the predominant feature as circulating salicylates decrease.

Sarah's salicylate level is slightly above the therapeutic range (15–30 mg/dL). Levels above 60 mg/dL should prompt concern and >100 mg/dL at 6 hours post ingestion may be life-threatening and certainly warrants renal replacement therapy. Her metabolic acidosis may be secondary to multiorgan failure developing as a result of a cocktail of toxins, including a large concentration of hepatotoxic paracetamol. Given her current clinical condition, it would be highly advisable to commence haemofiltration as soon as possible. It should also be borne in mind that you still do not know the timing of the overdose, whether it was staggered, or whether there is any element of chronicity.

Treatment of salicylate toxicity is generally supportive with good hydration to avoid rhabdomyolysis, correction of glucose and electrolyte imbalance, and treatment of seizures with benzodiazepines. Other options include activated charcoal (within 1–3 hours of ingestion) and, controversially, urinary alkalinisation aiming for pH >8 to enhance elimination.

What are the options for management of tricyclic antidepressant (TCA) overdose?

Ingestion of more than 10 mg/kg TCA may cause life-threatening dysrhythmias, seizures and coma. Usually doses >20 mg/kg are required for adverse signs and symptoms to develop and >30 mg/kg results in severe toxicity.

- Gastric lavage is only useful within the first hour (so rarely performed).
- Volume resuscitation, airway protection and avoidance of drugs which prolong depolarisation are important steps.
- Since TCAs are weak bases, an alkalinised environment will increase protein binding and decrease the free fraction, i.e. reduce the concentration of active drug available to cause dysrhythmias. Sodium bicarbonate can be used to achieve an arterial pH of 7.45–7.55.
- In haemodynamically unstable patients, intravenous lipid emulsion therapy has been used but the supporting evidence is weak.

> You discuss the case with the regional liver transplant centre. They would like you to transfer Sarah to their unit as she warrants consideration for an urgent liver transplant.

In which ways can drugs cause liver injury?

The majority are idiosyncratic drug reactions. Drug-induced hepatitis can also result from dose-dependant and predictable injury. Drug-induced liver injury can cause hepatocellular, cholestatic or mixed damage. Drugs causing hepatocellular damage include ciprofloxacin, amiodarone and diclofenac. Drugs causing cholestatic injury include co-amoxiclav, azathioprine and carbamazepine.

Recreational drugs causing liver injury include cocaine and alcohol. Drugs administered in critical care can also induce liver damage. Idiosyncratic reactions to propofol have been described.

How is liver failure categorised?

Acute liver failure

This is the rapid onset of failure of hepatic synthetic and metabolic function. There are various categorisation systems that stratify according to the time in which encephalopathy develops after the onset of jaundice in patients without previous liver impairment:

- The O'Grady or King's College classification (1993)
  - Hyperacute: <7 days
  - Acute: 8–28 days
  - Subacute: 4–12 weeks
- Bernau system
  - Fulminant: <2 weeks
  - Subfulminant: 2–12 weeks
- Japanese system
  - Fulminant
    - Acute: <10 days
    - Subacute: 10 days–8 weeks
  - Subfulminant: 8–12 weeks
  - Late onset: >8 weeks

Chronic liver disease

Progressive deterioration of hepatic function over >6 months. Unchecked, this results in liver fibrosis and cirrhosis.

Acute on chronic liver failure

Acute hepatic decompensation (i.e. hepatic encephalopathy, variceal haemorrhage, jaundice, ascites usually developing over less than 4 weeks) and organ failure in a patient with chronic liver failure. Short-term mortality is high.

What are the causes of acute or fulminant hepatic failure?

- *Viral* – hepatitis A–E, cytomegalovirus (CMV), herpes simplex virus (HSV), Epstein–Barr virus (EBV), varicella zoster virus (VZV), human herpes virus (HHV), parvovirus B19, yellow fever, parainfluenza virus.
- *Drugs and toxins* – paracetamol, ethanol, phenytoin, rifampicin, carbamazepine, valproate, coumarins, volatile anaesthetics, penicillin, sulfonamides, herbal drugs, psilocybin. Also idiosyncratic drug reactions.
- *Metabolic causes* – Wilson's disease, alpha-1 antitrypsin deficiency, galactosaemia, Reye's syndrome.
- *Vascular* – Budd–Chiari syndrome, shock, heart failure, veno-occlusive disease.
- *Pregnancy-related causes* – acute fatty liver of pregnancy, HELLP syndrome.
- *Autoimmune* – autoimmune hepatitis.
- *Sepsis*.
- *Malignancy*.
- *Hyperthermia*.

What are the causes of chronic liver disease?

- *Alcohol* misuse.
- *Hepatitis* B, C and D.
- *Non-alcoholic-related steatohepatitis (NASH)* – this important cause of cirrhosis and liver cancer is becoming increasingly common and is

associated with obesity, diabetes and dyslipidaemia as a progression from non-alcoholic fatty liver disease (NAFLD). NICE guidance (2016) stated that the prevalence of NAFLD in the general population is 20–30% and NASH is 2–3%.
- *Autoimmune disease* – Primary sclerosing cholangitis, primary biliary cholangitis, autoimmune hepatitis.
- *Secondary sclerosing cholangitis.*
- *Haemochromatosis.*
- *Alpha-1 antitrypsin deficiency.*
- Other causes are the same as those which cause fulminant liver disease (listed above).

How many solid organ transplants occur each year?

The NHS Blood and Transplant service manages donation, storage and transplantation of blood, organs, tissues, bone marrow and stem cells. In the UK in 2017–18:

- >5000 transplants were performed (approximately 800 liver transplants per year)
- 955 donations after brain death
- 619 donations after circulatory death

You transfer Sarah to the liver intensive care unit. One week later she has developed grade IV hepatic encephalopathy. Her urea rises to 24 mmol/L and creatinine to 256 μmol/L. Her ammonia rises to 171 μmol/L and she is placed on the super-urgent transplant list.

What scoring systems are used in the assessment of liver failure?

- *MELD* (Model for End-stage Liver Disease) – this composite score uses bilirubin, INR and creatinine to prognosticate 3-month survival following transjugular intrahepatic portosystemic shunt (TIPS) in patients with cirrhosis. A modified version is also used to prioritise patients awaiting liver transplantation. Revised MELD, or MELD-Na, incorporates serum sodium.
- *PELD* – paediatric version of MELD (used for children under 12 years old).
- *Child–Pugh* – 1–3 points are allocated for the degree of derangement in each of five categories (bilirubin, albumin, INR, ascites, encephalopathy). A composite score is used to predict mortality in cirrhotic patients: grade A (10%), B (30%) or C (70–80%).
- *UKELD (UK model for End-stage Liver Disease)* – this scoring system, used to prognosticate for patients with end-stage liver disease, is derived

from MELD and incorporates sodium. It is used to prioritise patients for liver transplantation.

■ *Transplant Benefit Score (TBS)* – this score supersedes UKELD as a method of organ allocation in the National Liver Offering Scheme (UK). It allows for patient matching by taking seven donor characteristics and 21 recipient characteristics and allocating a score to identify which individual will benefit most from a specific organ.

What are the West Haven grades of severity of encephalopathy?

1. Change in behaviour but minimal change in consciousness.
2. Inappropriate behaviour, gross disorientation, drowsiness.
3. Somnolent but rousable, marked confusion, incoherent speech.
4. Unresponsive, comatose. May be decerebrate or decorticate posturing.

Does Sarah have hepatorenal syndrome? Explain your answer.

Although she has renal and liver impairment, Sarah's case does not fit the diagnostic criteria for hepatorenal syndrome (HRS). HRS is acute kidney injury (AKI) in the context of cirrhotic liver failure. The diagnostic criteria have changed over time and are now in line with the KDIGO (Kidney Disease Improving Global Outcomes) criteria for AKI.

Diagnostic criteria for HRS (International Ascites Club)

■ Cirrhosis and ascites.
■ Diagnosis of AKI.
■ Absence of shock.
■ No response after two consecutive days of diuretic withdrawal and plasma volume expansion with albumin (1 g/kg of body weight).
■ No current or recent use of nephrotoxic drugs.
■ No macroscopic signs of structural kidney injury (i.e. absence of proteinuria [>500 mg/d], absence of microhaematuria [>50 RBCs per high-power field], normal findings on renal ultrasonography).

Categorisation

■ HRS-AKI (hepatorenal syndrome acute kidney injury)
■ HRS-AKD (hepatorenal syndrome acute kidney disease)
■ HRS-CKD (hepatorenal syndrome chronic kidney disease)

Hepatorenal system is associated with significantly increased mortality. A possible pathophysiological mechanism is renal vasoconstriction which develops with the multisystemic effects of cirrhotic liver disease.

What is the likely outcome for Sarah now she is on the transplant list?

- In 2018, median waiting time to adult liver transplant in the UK was approximately 56 days (blood type AB), 78 days (type A), 173 days (type B) and 208 days (type O).
- Approximately 11% of adult transplants in 2017–18 were super-urgent. Patients are placed on the super-urgent list if they require an organ as soon as possible due to the rapid failure of their native organ. These patients are prioritised above the other 'elective' transplant candidates and their waiting time is approximately 72 hours. They are allocated organs in order of date of listing and compatible blood group.
- In 2017–18, >400 patients died while awaiting a transplant (all transplants) and 755 were removed from the transplant list mainly due to deteriorating condition. Around 4% of patients registered on the transplant list in 2017–18 died while awaiting liver transplant.
- 1059 liver transplants were performed in the UK in 2017–18.

Fortunately, on day 4 after being placed on the super-urgent transplant list, Sarah receives a DBD liver transplant.

What is 'DBD' donation? How does this compare with 'DCD' donation?

DBD is donation after brainstem death. Following confirmation of brainstem death (see Case 16), continued physiological optimisation of the donor means that perfusion can be better maintained and organ retrieval can be scheduled. This improves the likelihood of successful transplantation compared with donation after circulatory death (DCD).

Donation after circulatory death is possible where a ventilated patient is to have life support withdrawn and they die within a limited time (usually 1 hour) following cessation of artificial ventilation. The time to death is critical since this dictates the warm ischaemic time (WIT). A longer WIT results in poor organ quality and worse outcomes for the recipient.

New technology such as OrganOx is transforming the way in which transplantation is managed. Following retrieval, the OrganOx machine perfuses the donor liver with oxygenated blood and bile production can be maintained. This decreases graft dysfunction and also allows scheduling of transplantation, even in DCD cases.

How should Sarah be managed post transplant?

- The team – initially she will be managed by the liver critical care MDT with hepatologists, liver transplant surgeons and transplant co-ordinators.
- Aims of management
  - Early extubation and enteral nutrition are ideal if possible.

- Meticulous supportive care with judicious fluids and blood pressure management to optimise perfusion but avoid hepatic congestion will increase chances of graft survival.
- Additional monitoring
  - Regular liver function, lactate, glucose, coagulation and drug levels.
  - Bile production should be monitored (via the T drain).
  - In acute liver failure, some patients continue to have invasive ICP monitoring postoperatively.
  - Renal function should be monitored, and replacement therapy used if required.

What medication will Sarah require following her transplant?

- *Venous thromboprophylaxis*
- *Immunosuppressive medication* – required to minimise graft rejection.
  - Tacrolimus requires careful titration and monitoring, especially in the context of new medications or acute illness.
  - Steroids – initially high dose. Three doses of methylprednisolone are given postoperatively. Taper steroids over 3 months.
- *Ulcer prophylaxis* – while taking steroids.
- *Prophylactic anti-infective medication*
  - Antibiotics
  - Antivirals and antifungals may be required

What complications can occur following transplant?

Early

- Coagulopathy, haemorrhage, hypothermia, electrolyte disturbance, hypoglycaemia (in the context of new graft failure).
- Sepsis (fungal, viral, bacterial).
- Small for size syndrome – hyperbilirubinemia, graft dysfunction, ascites, portal hypertension. Usually resolves as liver volume increases.
- Graft failure.
- Biliary leakage.
- Hepatic encephalopathy or central pontine myelinolysis.
- Biliary stricture.
- Hepatic artery thrombosis (0–21 days post transplant and would be relisted super-urgently).
- Rejection – acute or hyperacute.
- Graft-versus-host disease.
- Primary non-function.

Delayed

- Rejection – chronic.
- Hypertension.
- Diabetes mellitus.

- Renal failure.
- Post-transplant lymphoproliferative disease.
- Disease recurrence, e.g. hepatocellular carcinoma or autoimmune disease.
- Dyslipidaemia.
- Liver abscesses.
- Late hepatic artery thrombosis.

What are the complications related to long-term immunosuppression?

The potential complications are multisystemic and include:

- Renal failure
- Diabetes
- Hypertension
- Increased susceptibility to infection
- Hyperlipidaemia
- Osteoporosis
- Anaemia
- Thrombocytopenia
- Malignancy (e.g. basal cell carcinoma, vulval and Kaposi sarcoma)
- Obesity.

Fortunately, Sarah makes a full recovery post transplant. She accepts psychiatric and psychological support and goes on to live a meaningful and fulfilling life.

Further reading

- Bernal, W. and Wendon, J. (2013). Acute liver failure. *N. Engl. J. Med.* 369: 2525–2534. Excellent review article by world-leading experts.
- NICE. Guideline NG108 Decision Making and Mental Capacity. (2018).
- Mental Capacity Act (2005) and Amendment (2019). UK guidance and law regarding capacity.
- Rotundo, L. and Pyrsopoulos, N. (2020). Liver injury induced by paracetamol and challenges associated with intentional and unintentional use. *World J. Hepatol.* 12 (4): 125–136. Excellent overview of paracetamol toxicity.
- The NHS Blood and Transplant website (www.nhsbt.nhs.uk) publishes up-to-date reports on UK organ donation figures.

20 The Unwell Obstetric Patient

I t is a slow day on call for intensive care until your bleep alerts you to a cardiac arrest in the obstetric department. You run to labour ward to find two midwives attending to an unconscious woman whose abdomen appears distended consistent with term pregnancy. One midwife is administering oxygen using a bag-valve-mask, the other is performing chest compressions. In this scenario, you have the most experience in resuscitation, so you take the lead – you announce who you are and that you are in charge.

What immediate actions do you take?

The arrest call has already been initiated so the rest of the team should soon be on their way. Confirm cardiac arrest and proceed to manage the case according to the Resuscitation Council (UK) guidelines, with the caveat that the patient is either in left lateral tilt (often difficult to achieve in the emergency) or that there is leftward manual displacement of the gravid uterus.

Cardiac arrest in the pregnant patient is a stressful situation. Management may appear more complicated since there are two patients – the mother and the foetus. However, in England, although the foetus is recognised as a unique organism, it is not viewed as a person in the eyes of the law. Therefore, if there is a conflict between preserving the best interests of the mother versus the best interests of the foetus, the mother's life takes precedence. The law varies throughout the world and in some countries the right to life begins at conception.

How can cardiopulmonary resuscitation (CPR) be adapted for the pregnant patient?

According to the Royal College of Obstetricians and Gynaecologists (Green Top Guideline No. 56, 2019):

Clinical Cases in Critical Care, First Edition. Alice Myers and Theophilus Samuels.
© 2023 John Wiley & Sons Ltd. Published 2023 by John Wiley & Sons Ltd.

- Use a 15° tilt in patients more than 20 weeks pregnant
- Protect the airway as soon as possible with a cuffed endotracheal tube (performed by an experienced anaesthetist)
- In the absence of breathing, chest compressions should be commenced immediately
- Insert two wide-bore IV cannulae
- Abdominal ultrasound should be used, if available, to assess for concealed haemorrhage
- If ROSC (return of spontaneous circulation) is not achieved within 4 minutes of correctly performed CPR, the foetus should be delivered. Peri-mortem caesarean section should be performed in situ and not delayed by transferring to the operating theatre.

Why do you need to tilt the patient or manually displace the gravid uterus?

In the supine position, the third-trimester uterus compresses the inferior vena cava and part of the aorta. This can reduce venous return to the heart and decrease cardiac output, thereby impairing the effectiveness of cardiac compressions. Uteroplacental and maternal renal blood flow are also impaired through compression of the aorta. Pressure effects on major vessels must be alleviated to facilitate effective resuscitation.

How common is cardiac arrest in pregnancy?

UKOSS, the UK obstetric surveillance system, reports that cardiac arrest affects approximately 1 in 30 000 women in pregnancy.

How common is maternal death?

According to the World Health Organization (WHO), the maternal death rate is 239 per 100 000 in developing countries and 12 per 100 000 in the developed world. The leading causes of maternal death worldwide are haemorrhage, sepsis and hypertension (eclampsia/pre-eclampsia).

MBRRACE (Mothers and Babies: Reducing Risk through Audits and Confidential Enquiries across the UK) is a collaboration which provides national information on maternal and newborn health. It reports that in the UK in 2014–2016, 9.8 women per 100 000 died during pregnancy or up to 42 days post partum.

Which co-morbidities are implicated in obstetric mortality?

The MBBRACE report for 2018 found that cardiac disease is the overall leading cause of maternal death in the UK. The leading direct cause of death was thrombosis and thromboembolism. Maternal suicide, haemorrhage and sepsis are other important causes.

What are the '4Hs and 4Ts' (RCUK) and how may these reversible causes be particularly pertinent in the obstetric patient?

- *Hypovolaemia* – blood loss is common in the peripartum period. This can be massive and loss can be occult depending upon the cause, for instance abruption.
- *Hypoxia* – a woman able to carry a foetus to term will usually have reasonable lung function. However, there may be underlying lung disease. Alternatively, aspiration of gastric contents can occur and could lead to hypoxia from the resulting chemical pneumonitis.
- An important pregnancy-specific condition which can lead to acute hypoxia and cardiovascular collapse is *amniotic fluid embolism*. Estimates of incidence are variable (1 in 8000 to 1 in 80 000 pregnancies). It usually occurs at the time of delivery or during procedural interventions in late pregnancy.
- *Hypothermia* – less likely without a history of environmental exposure.
- *Hyper/hypokalaemia and other biochemical abnormalities* – pre-eclampsia and HELLP syndrome (haemolysis, elevated liver enzymes, low platelets) can be complicated by acute kidney injury. In addition, pre-existing renal disease can deteriorate in pregnancy. Excessive vomiting may result in hypokalaemia.
- *Thrombosis* – pulmonary thrombosis should be high on the list of differential diagnoses. Pregnancy significantly increases the risk of deep vein thrombosis (occurring in 1–2 in 1000) with the subsequent potential for catastrophic PE. Coronary thrombosis and stroke are less likely but not impossible, particularly if the patient has underlying ischaemic heart or vascular disease.
- *Tension pneumothorax* – pregnancy is not an independent risk factor for tension pneumothorax.
- *Toxins* – consider the possibility of local anaesthetic toxicity; find out whether the woman has an epidural in situ and establish the last dose, time and route of drug administration. Establish whether she may have self-administered any drugs or whether pethidine or other opioids, e.g. remifentanil for pain, have been administered.
- *Tamponade* – pregnancy is not an independent risk factor for tamponade.

You successfully intubate the patient and there is ROSC after one round of good CPR. You are given a brief history from the senior midwife. Oksana was admitted to labour ward only 2 hours ago. They think she is in the UK visiting family and did not bring any antenatal notes with her. She is 33 weeks pregnant with a single foetus. She reported her pregnancy was uncomplicated but came to the hospital as she started having headaches, couldn't see properly and was feeling unwell. The midwives put out an arrest call when Oksana vomited, had a seizure and stopped breathing. The cardiac arrest rhythm was recorded as pulseless electrical activity.

What could be the possible causes for Oksana's presentation?

- *Eclampsia* – there is a history of headaches, visual disturbance and seizures in a previously uncomplicated third trimester pregnancy. Pre-eclampsia is a multisystem disorder specific to pregnancy occurring between 20 weeks gestation and 3 months post delivery. There is abnormal trophoblast invasion and differentiation with involvement of the spiral arteries. The result is hypertension (>140/90 mmHg) and end-organ dysfunction characterised by proteinuria, neurological, haematological or hepatic derangement, or intrauterine foetal growth restriction. Eclampsia is the development of otherwise unexplained generalised seizures in a woman with pre-eclampsia. Oksana's visual symptoms and seizure could indicate progression to eclampsia. Determine blood pressure, urine protein levels and blood urate level.
- *Seizure disorder* – Oksana's previous medical history is unknown and she may have a diagnosed seizure disorder. She may have breakthrough seizures regularly, or she might have stopped taking antiseizure medication for fear of teratogenicity. Aspiration during a seizure could lead to hypoxia and subsequent cardiorespiratory arrest.
- *Embolus* – pulmonary venous or amniotic embolism. There is insufficient information to rule this out.
- *Stroke (haemorrhagic or ischaemic)* – Oksana may have a medical condition which increases her risk of stroke.
- *Drugs/toxins* – Oksana may have taken an accidental or deliberate overdose or have suffered an adverse reaction to a drug. She could also have developed liver or renal impairment during pregnancy (e.g. acute fatty liver of pregnancy) so ammonia and urea levels should be obtained.
- *Sepsis* – systemic or CNS infection is possible. Since Oksana has had a seizure, meningitis and encephalitis should be considered. If she has travelled abroad, the diagnostic net should include malaria, tuberculosis and viral haemorrhagic fever.

What are your management priorities?

1. *Discuss the case* with a consultant obstetrician urgently. If clinical suspicion of eclampsia is sufficiently high, delivery of the foetus should be expedited.
2. *Postarrest stabilisation* – transfer Oksana to an environment where she can be managed safely. This may be an anaesthetic room or operating theatre. Optimise gas exchange and blood pressure, and facilitate investigation and ongoing management. Institute invasive monitoring.
3. *Prevent further seizures* – administer magnesium 4 g intravenously over 5–15 minutes. This is appropriate treatment if Oksana has eclampsia. It will also be useful to help prevent further seizures secondary to many other causes. Consider administering antihypertensive medications if this is eclampsia.
4. *Investigations*

- Assess Oksana's blood pressure.
- Take blood tests
  - FBC – paying particular attention to platelets
  - LFTs – in case of HELLP or acute fatty liver of pregnancy
  - U&Es – in case of acute kidney injury
  - Urate – raised in pre-eclampsia
  - MC&S – in case of bloodstream infection
  - Clotting and fibrinogen
  - Group & save
- Consider CTPA (to rule out pulmonary embolism) and CT head (in case of acute intracranial pathology including stroke). However, acquiring CT imaging now will be associated with the risks of transferring an unstable patient and exposure to ionising radiation, and it will delay any surgical intervention (including delivery of the baby), should this be required. It is unadvisable to do this right now.
- Focused echocardiography allows assessment of right heart dysfunction and may even reveal evidence of thrombus where a clot is large or extending into the chambers of the heart. If pulmonary embolus is present consider thrombolysis – but this would be an extremely high-risk strategy in this patient.

What cardiovascular changes occur during pregnancy?

- Blood volume increases by up to 50%.
- Peripheral vascular resistance decreases.
- Stroke volume increases by up to 30%.
- Heart rate increases by up to 25%.
- Cardiac output increases by up to 50%.
- ECG changes may occur secondary to relative myocardial hypertrophy and mechanical displacement of the heart by the gravid uterus (left axis deviation, T-wave flattening in lead III, ST segment depression).
- Lower limb oedema can result from mechanical compression of the lymphatic drainage system.
- Haematological changes impacting the cardiovascular system
  - Red cell mass increases by up to 20%.
  - Haematocrit decreases.
  - Factors VII, VIII and X, fibrinogen and von Willebrand factor increase disproportionately to the rise in thromboxane and prostacyclin, leading to hypercoagulability and an increased risk of deep vein thrombosis

What are the non-cardiovascular changes of pregnancy and how do they affect your management of Oksana?

Respiratory

- FRC falls by approximately 20%.
- Oxygen demand increases by up to 40%.
- RR increases by up to 15%.
- Tidal volume increases by up to 40%.
- Respiratory alkalosis results from increased minute ventilation and is compensated for by a decrease in serum bicarbonate.

- PaO_2 rises during the third trimester but falls at term through increased oxygen consumption.
- Chest wall compliance falls while lung compliance is preserved.
- Progesterone-mediated smooth muscle relaxation reduces airway resistance.
  - *Impact* – decreased FRC and increased oxygen demand mean the pregnant patient is quick to desaturate when compromised. Intubation should be preceded by meticulous preoxygenation where possible. There is likely to be a need to use higher PEEP than in the non-pregnant patient.

Gastrointestinal

- In the later stages of pregnancy, the increased volume of the gravid uterus increases intra-abdominal pressure and displaces intra-abdominal contents upwards.
- Increased progesterone and oestrogen cause relaxation of smooth muscle (leading to reduced gastric motility) and reduced lower oesophageal sphincter tone.
  - *Impact* – these changes increase the risk of aspiration. Intubation should be managed in such a way as to protect against this.

Renal

- GFR increases by up to 50% due to increased renal blood flow.
- Urinary stasis may result from smooth muscle relaxation leading to an increased risk of urinary tract infections.
  - *Impact* – always include urine MC&S in the panel of tests looking for a source of sepsis.

Endocrine

- There are many endocrinological changes in pregnancy and the full details are beyond the scope of this book.
- Diabetes mellitus and thyroid disease are relatively common in pregnancy.
- Relative insulin resistance develops (secondary to human placental lactogen).
- Increased oestrogen leads to increased production of thyroid-binding globulin. The increase in binding sites for T3 and T4 leads to a rise in thyroid-stimulating hormone, stimulating further release of T3 and T4. When balance is maintained, there is increased total T3 and T4 while free circulating levels remain stable.
  - *Impact* – pay close attention to blood glucose levels.
  - *Assess* clinical thyroid status and consult pregnancy-specific reference ranges when interpreting laboratory results.

Who else needs to be involved in Oksana's care?

- Obstetrician
- Anaesthetist
- Neonatologist or paediatrician
- Anaesthetically trained ODP (operating department practitioner) and theatre team

- Midwives
- Haematology
- ICU MDT
- Next of kin/partner

The obstetric team are concerned about both fetal bradycardia and the possibility that this may be eclampsia. You assist the anaesthetist in taking Oksana straight to the operating theatre where emergency caesarean section under general anaesthesia is undertaken. The baby is delivered but the obstetric team are now struggling to achieve haemostasis.

What is the definition of major obstetric haemorrhage?

There is no universally accepted definition of major obstetric haemorrhage. However, individual organisations require clear definition to organise response processes and undertake audit, so many choose to use one of the following suggested definitions.

- The WHO defines postpartum haemorrhage as >500 mL blood loss within 24 hours of delivery
- Other definitions used include:
  - >1500 mL blood loss in 24 hours
  - haemoglobin drop >40 g/L
  - required transfusion of four units packed red cells.

What are the causes of maternal haemorrhage?

Antepartum haemorrhage – between 24 weeks gestation and delivery (approximately 3% of pregnancies)
- Trauma
- Placental abruption
- Placenta praevia
- Uterine rupture

Postpartum haemorrhage (PPH) – primary PPH, within 24 hours of delivery; secondary PPH, up to 6 weeks following delivery
- **T**one – uterine atony (5% of deliveries – accounts for approximately 80% of primary PPH)
- **T**issue – retained products of conception
- **T**hrombin – coagulopathy
- **T**rauma – injury to genital tract

What are the options for management of maternal haemorrhage?

Take an ABCDE approach and be aware that physiological responses may be altered during pregnancy. Management depends upon the cause and severity of blood loss. This will require a co-ordinated team response utilising local emergency protocols for massive haemorrhage or major obstetric haemorrhage.

Medical

- Transfuse blood products (warmed).
- Ensure calcium levels are maintained during massive haemorrhage or transfusion.
- Tranexamic acid.
- Uterotonic drugs including oxytocin, ergometrine, misoprostol and prostaglandin F2 alpha (oxytocin and ergometrine can cause hypertension and should be avoided in pre-eclampsia).

Surgical

- Bimanual uterine compression.
- B-lynch suture.
- Hysterectomy.
- Intrauterine balloon tamponade.
- Arterial ligation of supply to uterus or ovaries, or even internal iliac arteries.

Interventional radiological

Fluoroscopy-guided targeted embolization or intra-arterial balloon occlusion.

General measures

- High-flow oxygen.
- Left lateral position to avoid aortocaval compression.
- Tolerate Hb of 70 g/L where haemostasis has been achieved.
- Use point-of-care haemoglobin measurement or blood gas analysis for rapid assessment of haemoglobin levels.
- Use real-time thromboelastography to assess coagulopathy.
- Pay close attention to visible blood loss but be aware that there may also be large volumes of occult blood loss.

The theatre team eventually manage to stop the bleeding through a combination of mechanical and pharmacological measures, but Oksana has lost approximately 4.3 L in blood and has received seven units PRC, five units FFP and two pools of platelets. Her arterial blood gas on 0.5 FiO$_2$ is as follows: pH 7.20, PaO$_2$ 8.3 kPa, PaCO$_2$ 6.4 kPa, base excess −7.7 mmol/L, lactate 4.6 mmol/L. You decide to keep Oksana sedated, intubated and mechanically ventilated, and transfer her to critical care for ongoing management.

What are your main concerns for Oksana at this point?

- *Gas exchange* – Oksana is hypoxic with a P:F ratio of 124 mmHg or 16.6 kPa.
- *Complications of blood transfusion* – Oksana has suffered a major obstetric haemorrhage and has now received a massive transfusion. She is at risk of developing transfusion-associated lung injury and disseminated intravascular coagulation or dilutional coagulopathy.
- *Postcardiac arrest ischaemia* – she has had an in-hospital cardiac arrest and she may have suffered hypoxic ischaemic injury to her brain or other major organs. Her lactate is high, and she has a significant base deficit. She is at risk of acute kidney and/or liver injury.
- *Fluid management* – she requires further careful fluid resuscitation. Oksana probably requires additional fluid, but urine output will tend to remain low in pre-eclampsia. Care should be taken to avoid excessive fluid administration by targeting an inappropriately high urine output.
- *Other diagnoses* – she is at risk of developing sepsis.

There are still many unknowns in this case. What is known is that she has significant derangement of her physiology and needs to be managed in a critical care environment.

What is your management plan?

- *Admit to ICU to resuscitate, stabilise and assess*
  - Lung-protective ventilation.
  - Fluid resuscitation guided by cardiac output monitoring.
  - Invasive arterial and central venous monitoring.
  - Urinary catheter.
  - Correct electrolytes.
  - Maintain normothermia.
  - Manage blood glucose.
  - Site NG tube.
  - Review surgical drains.
- *Full blood panel* with coagulation screen, urate, U&Es, LFTs and cultures. Transfuse blood products as necessary to correct anaemia and coagulopathy.
- *Oksana should be managed in isolation* since she has travelled abroad recently. Ensure cross-infection screening is performed, looking for carbapenemase-producing organisms.
- *Complications of pre-eclampsia* – these can develop up to 6 weeks following delivery (though most occur within 48 hours); meticulous blood pressure management and ongoing magnesium administration are important. Local hospital protocols may suggest methyldopa, nifedipine or labetalol, to target a blood pressure at the upper end of normal to prevent precipitous drop (e.g. SBP 130–140 mmHg and DBP 80–90 mmHg). Once there is reliable enteral absorption, enteral

antihypertensive agents can be used. However, ileus is very likely to develop in this case.

- *Septic screen* including chest radiograph, urine MC&S, respiratory secretion MC&S, high vaginal swabs, viral screen and urine atypical antibody screen.
- Oksana is likely to be coagulopathic right now but consider performing lumbar puncture later on. If the baby is developing sepsis, Oksana may also be at risk.
- *Imaging* – consider CTPA and CT head now the baby has been delivered and the clinical situation is more stable.
- *Formal echocardiography* to assess for fluid responsiveness and the presence of LV/RV dysfunction.
- When physiologically stable, stop sedation and assess neurology.
- Obtain collateral history and previous medical notes.

Oksana's partner arrives at the hospital. Gemma and Oksana have been married for 1 year and they conceived their baby with a sperm donor via in vitro fertilisation (IVF). Oksana is 39 years old, works as a graphic designer and has a past medical history of mild asthma. She does not smoke and takes no medicines apart from her salbutamol inhaler as required. Gemma is not aware of any relevant family history. Oksana and Gemma have been travelling around Europe but had returned to the UK to wait for the baby to be born. Gemma has been told that their newborn baby, Rufus, is in the special care baby unit receiving CPAP.

What specific issues should you consider when speaking with Gemma?

There is much to explain to Gemma at this point – likely eclampsia, cardiac arrest, surgery, major haemorrhage and critical illness. Your prognosis at this point should be guarded. Gemma can also provide background medical history and contact details for Oksana's general practitioner.

In addition to her concerns about Oksana, Gemma will undoubtedly be worried about Rufus. Gemma will need support during this difficult time since both her wife and baby are at risk of dying and it is as yet unknown whether they have sustained hypoxic brain injury. Gemma may also be worried about the psychological impact of separation between mother and child and that Oksana won't be able to breast feed or bond with Rufus at this crucial time. There are strategies available to help promote bonding, such as using knitted bonding squares worn in turn against mother's skin then baby's skin. The obstetricians and midwives will need to help with these aspects of management.

You stabilise Oksana in critical care. She requires aggressive BP management. On stopping sedation, she starts to have another seizure. You administer levetiracetam and transfer her to CT for brain imaging. The radiologist reports: 'bilateral symmetrical hypodensities involving the white matter in the parieto-occipital regions'. The plain chest radiograph reveals pulmonary infiltrates.

What is the likely cause of these CT findings?

This is consistent with PRES (posterior reversible encephalopathy syndrome). The hypodensities seen on CT reflect vasogenic oedema which tends to develop in the occipital lobe due to impaired autoregulation and increased pressure in the posterior circle of Willis. Ideally, this should be confirmed with magnetic resonance imaging (MRI). It is not a diagnosis specific to pregnancy but it tends to occur in the context of hypertension, autoimmunity or immune suppression.

What is the prognosis for PRES?

Occasionally, the patient may suffer permanent visual or other neurological impairment. Rarely, death can result. More usually, with appropriate supportive management, a full recovery is made.

What could be the cause of Oksana's pulmonary oedema?

Possible causes include the following:

- ARDS secondary to pneumonia
- Pulmonary oedema associated with pre-eclampsia
- Transfusion-related acute lung injury (TRALI)
- Negative-pressure pulmonary oedema sustained during her seizure

You manage Oksana with antihypertensive and antiseizure medication. You continue magnesium to treat pre-eclampsia. On day 3 you can stop sedation and extubate her. On examination, she has no neurological deficit and has no further seizures. You keep her in the HDU for a further 24 hours for observation and blood pressure management.

Rufus has been doing well in the special care baby unit. He is discharged on day 7 and the new family is reunited and eventually able to return home together.

Further reading

- MBRRACE-UK publishes a confidential enquiry into maternal deaths. The version published in 2021 deals with data collected from 2017 to 2019 and is available from www.npeu.ox.ac.uk/mbrrace-uk.
- Patel, S., Estevez, A., Nedeff, N. et al. (2020). ICU management of the obstetric patient. *Trends Anaesth. Crit. Care* 31: 1–7. Informative review article from the USA regarding ICU management of the obstetric patient.

21 The Patient in Cardiac ICU

During your evening ward round on cardiothoracic intensive care, you notice an increase in the noradrenaline requirement for 78-year-old Isaac who underwent 'on-pump' coronary artery bypass grafting (CABG) and aortic valve replacement (AVR) earlier today. He has not yet been extubated. He remains sedated on 100 mg/h propofol and 100 mcg/h fentanyl and his noradrenaline requirement has increased from 0.1 mcg/kg/min to 0.6 mcg/kg/min over the last 2 hours. During this time, there has been minimal output from his chest drains.

What could be the cause of hypotension in Isaac?

- *Tamponade* – while pericardial effusions have been described as being found in up to 85% of patients post cardiac surgery, tamponade is far rarer. Cardiac tamponade is reported as occurring in 0.1–6% of open heart surgery cases. It is more common following valve surgery than in CABG alone. It can be caused by graft failure or as a complication of pacing wires.

  The rapid and dramatic increase in Isaac's vasopressor requirements, together with decreased chest drain output, place tamponade at the top of the list of potential causes. Urgent echocardiography and urgent surgical review should be requested. Transoesophageal echocardiography (TOE) would be ideal in this case since transthoracic views are usually suboptimal in postoperative patients.

- *Hypovolaemia or haemorrhage* – an increase in noradrenaline from 0.1 to 0.6 mcg/kg/min over 2 hours is extreme and is highly unlikely to be caused by hypovolaemia alone. If hypovolaemia is the cause, this would be more likely to indicate haemorrhage – which could be overt or occult.

  Examine Isaac fully, review the arterial blood gas and lactate, and consider administering a fluid challenge.

Clinical Cases in Critical Care, First Edition. Alice Myers and Theophilus Samuels.
© 2023 John Wiley & Sons Ltd. Published 2023 by John Wiley & Sons Ltd.

■ *Postcardiotomy cardiogenic shock* – this diagnosis should be confirmed using echocardiography. Cardiac output monitoring should be instituted (for instance, a pulmonary artery catheter) and inotropic drugs commenced. If this is the cause of Isaac's deterioration, his case should be discussed promptly with the surgical team. If he fails to improve with the measures taken, mechanical circulatory support should be considered.

■ *Acute blockage of a bypass graft/myocardial infarction* – the third universal definition of myocardial infarction identifies MI within 48 hours of CABG as a type 5 MI. It is usually due to graft failure or an event in the remaining native coronary arteries. The indication for Isaac's CABG may have been atherosclerosis secondary to underlying ischaemic heart disease so it is possible he is at risk of further events. Perform a 12-lead ECG, request a troponin, and perform TOE looking for regional wall motion abnormalities. If suspicion is high, further investigation in the catheter laboratory may be indicated or serial ECG, echocardiography and troponins can be carried out.

■ *Artefact* – it is possible that there could be equipment error. Check that the arterial line pressure bag is appropriately inflated and the fluid bag is not empty. Check that the arterial line trace is not overdamped, that there are no clots in the system and the system should be recalibrated. Check NIBP. Review the chest drains to look for evidence of obstruction or clots.

■ *Rarer causes such as left ventricular free wall rupture, ventricular pseudoaneurysm or chordae tendinae rupture* – these differentials are listed for completeness but are unlikely to occur suddenly in ICU without prior suspicion. Free wall rupture, septal rupture and acute mitral valve regurgitation are potentially devastating complications of acute MI. When free wall rupture is contained within the pericardium, a pseudoaneurysm can develop. Chordae tendinae rupture is more likely to occur following mitral valve repair but can also occur following myocardial infarction and CABG.

What does 'on-pump' mean?

The 'pump', in this context, refers to an extracorporeal cardiopulmonary bypass (CPB) circuit. CPB is used intraoperatively to allow cardiac arrest and deflation of the lungs while maintaining systemic circulation of non-pulsatile oxygenated blood. This facilitates an optimal operative field for the cardiac surgeon.

Cardiopulmonary bypass is not without potential complications and some practitioners prefer to operate 'off pump' where possible, particularly for CABG. Beating heart surgery may be more technically challenging but it reduces the risks associated with CPB. Patients may be selected for off-pump surgery because they have a higher risk of complications due to, for example, chronic lung disease, chronic kidney injury or atherosclerosis of the aorta.

There is conflicting data regarding the comparative outcomes for on-pump and off-pump surgery. The choice of technique remains at the discretion of the surgeon performing the procedure.

Describe a cardiopulmonary bypass circuit

See Figure 21.1.

- *Venous cannula* – usually a polyvinylchloride (PVC) cannula with wire reinforcement is inserted into the right atrium. Drainage occurs under gravity, via tubing, into the reservoir.
- *Tubing* – usually PVC, though more modern materials are being developed. Tubing is plain, for quicker cases, or coated for longer use (i.e. ECMO circuits) to prevent thrombin deposition.
- *Reservoir* – this is usually passive but can be vacuum assisted. Open reservoirs must maintain a minimum level to prevent air entrainment into the system. Closed reservoirs have limited capacity but are less proinflammatory than open systems.
- *Pump* – roller pumps and centrifugal pumps are both used. Roller pumps are cheaper but may induce haemolysis. Centrifugal pumps are associated with better neurological outcomes, platelet preservation and renal function.
- *Heat exchanger* – this is usually a large machine connected to the oxygenator via water pipes.

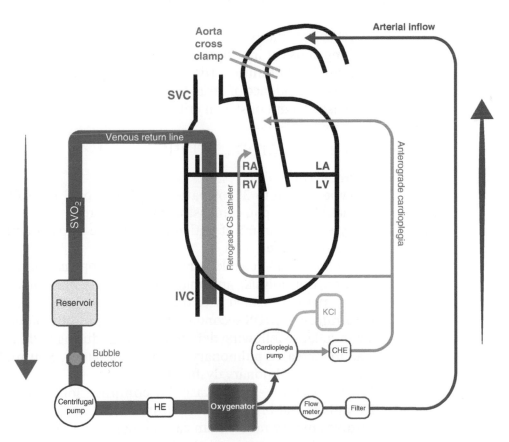

Figure 21.1: Schematic diagram demonstrating a cardiopulmonary bypass circuit. CHE, cardioplegia heat exchanger; CS, coronary sinus; HE, heat exchanger; IVC, inferior vena cava; KCl, potassium chloride; LA, left atrium; LV, left ventricle; RA, right atrium; RV, right ventricle; SVC, superior vena cava; SVO$_2$, central venous oxygen saturations.

Source: Theophilus Samuels.

- *Oxygenator* – membrane oxygenators are made from hollow polypropylene fibres.
- *Cardioplegia* – though this is not strictly part of the CPB circuit, cardioplegia is usually used in association. To protect against cardiac ischaemia following aortic cross-clamping, cardioplegia reduces myocardial oxygen consumption. This mixture may contain potassium, calcium, magnesium, procaine, glucose, glutamate, adenosine, bicarbonate and mannitol. Warm blood cardioplegia (compared with crystalloid cardioplegia) also contains the patient's own blood. The heart is perfused with the solution proximally to the clamp in either anterograde or retrograde fashion.

What is the significance of the aortic cross-clamp time in CABG?

Ruggieri et al. (2018, Heart Lung Circ) showed that prolonged cross-clamp time may be associated with poor early outcome post CABG. This is in keeping with the findings of several other studies (e.g. Al-Sarraf 2011, Int J Surg). The definition of 'prolonged' varies and has been defined as anything from greater than 75 minutes to greater than 300 minutes.

Negative outcomes observed include:

- Increased mortality
- Prolonged use of inotropes
- Increased use of intra-aortic balloon pump (IABP) or ECMO
- Increased incidence of atrial fibrillation
- Increased length of stay in critical care.

What are the complications of CPB?

- *Neurological*
  - Type 1 – up to 3% of patients. Major focal neurological deficits including stupor, coma, stroke and seizures.
  - Type 2 – up to 6% of patients. Cognitive impairment or decreased intellectual function.
- *Haematological* – coagulopathy (thrombocytopenia, platelet dysfunction, dilution, fibrinolysis), anaemia (haemolysis or haemorrhage), haemodilution, risks associated with transfusion (see Case 7).
- *Respiratory* – ARDS secondary to systemic inflammatory response, or lobar collapse following deflation of lungs during CPB. Protamine may lead to increased pulmonary vascular resistance. Neutrophil activation may lead to pulmonary dysfunction.
- *Cardiovascular* – cardiovascular complications such as LV failure, RV failure and biventricular failure, tend to be more associated with cardiac surgery rather than cardiac bypass. However, they can result from inadequate myocardial protection during CPB (e.g. through insufficient cardioplegia). They are also generally associated with longer surgeries and higher risk patients. Other complications include myocardial

ischaemia, myocardial stunning, embolic events and aortic dissection secondary to cannula injury.

- *Renal* – up to 8% of patients develop acute kidney injury.
- *Immunological* – systemic inflammatory response, protamine allergy.
- *Metabolic* – electrolyte disturbance, hyperglycaemia.
- *Gastrointestinal* – gut ischaemia, ischaemic hepatitis, pancreatitis.
- *Cannulation problems* – including bleeding, damage to vessels, dissection, air/particulate embolus.
- *Equipment/operator error.*
- *Other complications* may develop secondary to open heart surgery itself – there are examples of *Mycobacterium chimaera* infections associated with heater-coolers. Although this is rare, the consequences are grave and so it is an important problem. Approximately 1–4% of patients develop mediastinitis or sternal wound infection with an associated mortality of up to 25%, but this is not directly related to CPB.

What do you expect Isaac's coagulation status to be at this point?

Intraoperatively, patients are fully anticoagulated with heparin to achieve an activated coagulation time (ACT) of greater than 400 seconds. Usually, 300 IU/kg heparin is administered prior to cannulation of the atrium. Once the surgery is complete and the patient is separated from CPB, protamine is administered at a dose of 3 mg/kg to reverse the effects of the heparin.

Heparin rebound can occur postoperatively and contribute to ongoing bleeding. This is thought to be due to a proportion of heparin being protein bound and therefore incompletely neutralised by protamine.

Aspirin is recommended within 6 hours of surgery to prevent graft failure. If there are contraindications to aspirin, clopidogrel is usually administered.

On examination, you note that Isaac has wires coming from his chest which are connected to a small control box. What are these and why are they there?

These are temporary epicardial pacing wires which, in many centres, are routinely placed following open cardiac surgery involving CPB (Table 21.1). They are usually maintained until the patient is discharged from critical care because the risk of arrhythmias and heart block is considerable. Arrhythmias can cause haemodynamic compromise in vulnerable postoperative patients.

Epicardial wires can be unipolar or bipolar. Temporary pacing can be dual or single chamber and control is almost as sophisticated as permanent pacing.

The control device usually allows for selection of pacing mode, pacing rate, atrial or ventricular output and sensitivity (mV).

Table 21.1: The revised generic code for antibradycardia pacing, 2002.

I	II	III	IV	V
Chamber(s) paced	Chamber(s) sensed	Response to sensing	Rate modulation	Multisite pacing
0	0	0	0	0
A	A	T	R	A
V	V	I		V
D	D	D		D

Source: North American Society of Pacing and Electrophysiology/British Pacing and Electrophysiology Group (NASPE/BPEG).
0, none; A, atrium; V, ventricle; D, dual; T, triggered; I, inhibited; R, rate modulation. Often, only the first three letters are used, e.g. VVI.

When pacing wires are in place, the pacemaker and controls should be checked daily.

- Are there any pacing spikes visible? Is there capture (i.e. do QRS complexes follow pacing spikes)?
- Set the rate as desired (usually 80–90 beats per minute).
- Gradually turn down the sensitivity number (making pacing more sensitive) until there is capture.

> You rapidly assess Isaac and his invasive arterial monitoring. It appears there is no equipment problem and NIBP agrees with the invasive monitoring. The right internal jugular venous catheter reads central venous pressure of 18 mmHg. You ask the ICU nurse to perform a 12-lead ECG and check an arterial blood gas. You ask a colleague to inform the cardiac surgeon on call and your ICU consultant performs TOE, which demonstrates a large amount of fluid surrounding the heart.

What are your concerns regarding the TOE findings?

Given the clinical presentation of the patient, this is likely to represent tamponade. Real-time echocardiography differentiates simple effusion from cardiac tamponade by, for example, demonstrating diastolic collapse of the right atrium and ventricle and a swinging heart.

The pericardial space may hold up to 50 mL physiological fluid. A pericardial effusion post cardiac surgery is not an uncommon finding (moderate size effusion 100–500 mL; more than 500 mL would constitute a large effusion). Haemodynamic compromise, i.e. obstructive shock, means this is tamponade. Within 72 hours following surgery, this would be described as early tamponade.

How does cardiac tamponade present in postcardiac surgery patients?

Presentation of cardiac tamponade in postsurgical patients can be insidious. The classic signs of Beck's triad (muffled heart sounds, distended neck veins, hypotension) cannot be relied upon in this context. Cardiac tamponade should be considered in a postoperative open heart surgery patient who has decreased cardiac output, tachycardia and hypotension. Reduced output from the surgical drain suggests a clot may be obstructing drainage, leaving the patient at risk of accumulating a larger volume of pericardial fluid. This could result in mechanical impairment of the heart.

There should be a low threshold for performing echocardiography in post-cardiothoracic surgery patients with atypical symptoms.

If Isaac were to arrest, which resuscitation protocol would be the most appropriate to follow?

The Cardiac surgery Advanced Life Support protocol produced by CARE (Cardiac Advanced Resuscitation Education) is accepted by the European Resuscitation Council and also used in the USA. CALS (or CSU-ALS in the USA) is intended for use in ICU patients up to 10 days post sternotomy.

> The cardiac surgeon reviews the drains, attempting to suction and unblock them. This is unsuccessful so you plan with the team to move to theatre for thoracotomy. However, Isaac becomes more unstable and is peri-arrest. The cardiac surgeon performs a rapid scrub, removes the sternotomy clips, opens the chest and drains the pericardial sac manually. Cardiac output immediately improves, as evidenced by an increase in the cardiac output monitor readings.

What are the next steps in management of this patient?

- Identification and definitive management of the bleeding point.
- In order to explore the heart properly, the patient should be moved to a more appropriate environment.
  - Alert the anaesthetic team.
  - Alert theatres to prepare for emergency surgery.
  - The assistance of a perfusionist is likely to be required.
  - Prepare for transfer – assemble appropriate staff, oxygen and equipment, including a ventilator and infusion pumps, etc.
- Ensure blood products are available.
- Call for experienced/senior assistance.
- Aim to optimise Isaac's general condition.
  - Deeply sedate to achieve general anaesthesia.
  - Consider neuromuscular blockade.
  - Optimise gas exchange.
  - Correct electrolytes.
  - Administer antibiotics as per local protocol.
  - Temperature management.
- Inform Isaac's next of kin.

> Isaac is transferred to the operating theatre and you continue with your work in ICU. Two hours later, an operating department practitioner (ODP) comes to critical care with a blood sample, asking you to run thromboelastography

(TEG) and a blood gas. He tells you that CPB was re-established and the surgeon identified a bleeding point at the insertion of one of the coronary artery bypass grafts. The defect was closed with sutures but when they tried to separate from CPB, Isaac became cardiovascularly unstable. He now requires high concentrations of vasopressor and the anaesthetist has noted ST segment elevation in ECG lead II on the intraoperative monitoring. The anaesthetist has said Isaac will probably need levosimendan post-op in ICU.

What could be the cause of this failure to wean from CPB?

- Myocardial infarction.
- Acute myocardial ischaemia as a result of mechanical obstruction of grafts.
- Air embolus.
- Coronary vasospasm.
- Ischaemia reperfusion injury due to the acute inflammatory response associated with the ischaemic period that occurs while CPB is ongoing.

What management options do you expect the team in theatres to be considering?

- Try again, more slowly, to separate from CPB using inotropes or vasodilators as required and checking for patency of bypass grafts.
- If Isaac remains unstable, a bridging device may be required to augment cardiac output in the postoperative recovery stage, e.g.:
  - IABP
  - Venoarterial extracorporeal membrane oxygenation (VA ECMO).

By which mechanisms does levosimendan exert its effects?

There are three main effects:

- *Positive inotrope* – levosimendan binds to cardiac troponin C, increasing its sensitivity to free calcium. This induces an increase in cardiac contractility.
- *Vasodilator* – the mechanism of this effect has not been clearly elucidated but is likely to be due to the opening of potassium channels (including ATP-dependent channels, Ca^{2+} activated channels and voltage-dependent channels).
- *Cardiac cytoprotection* – possibly through the reduction of free radical production and myocardial inflammation.

Compare venoarterial and venovenous (VA/VV) ECMO

See Table 21.2.

Table 21.2: VA and VV ECMO.

VA ECMO	VV ECMO
Used where there is predominantly cardiac failure (respiratory failure may also co-exist)	Aids in supporting patients with severe respiratory failure and no cardiac component
Requires catheterisation of a large central vein. Blood passes via an oxygenator and is then returned to the patient via a cannula into the arterial system	Also drains blood from a large central vein into an oxygenator but then returns that blood to another vein near the right atrium
BOTH: There must be both a reversible problem and a high risk of death	
BOTH: ECMO circuit requires – cannulae, tubing, a pump, heat exchanger, membrane oxygenator and a gas blender	
BOTH: Cannulae are large (15–25 F) and patients must be fully anticoagulated	
BOTH: Carbon dioxide is removed in addition to oxygen being supplied	

What are the complications due to the use of ECMO?

- Cannulation problems, e.g. dissection or gas emboli, and the need for additional cannulae later.
- Coagulation pathway activation (both bleeding and thrombosis).
- Inflammatory response activation.
- Anticoagulation issues.
- Problems specific to VV or VA – in VA ECMO there can be Harlequin syndrome or inadequate unloading of the left ventricle. VV ECMO can lead to recirculation.
- Circuit component issues or system failure leading to cardiac arrest, e.g. failure of oxygenator, kinking of tubing, pump failure, circuit rupture, pulmonary infarction, left ventricular overdistension, 'suck down' vascular collapse due to suction pressure leading to interruption of flow

Would an Impella device or a VAD be useful in this scenario?

A ventricular assist device (VAD) is a mechanical pump used to augment cardiac output in states of refractory cardiogenic shock. These are used as a bridge to transplant or to aid recovery and, as such, have been used in patients who struggle to wean from CPB.

A VAD is placed surgically and can be an R-VAD (supporting the right ventricle by returning blood to the pulmonary artery), an L-VAD (returning blood back to the aorta to support the left side), or a Bi-VAD which supports both ventricles. Usually, a VAD would only be used in severe cases where an IABP was insufficient.

An Impella device pumps blood from the left ventricle into the ascending aorta. This miniature pump needs to be inserted, usually via the femoral artery, under radiological guidance in the cardiac catheter laboratory. Impella devices have been used to augment cardiac output during percutaneous coronary angioplasty where the patient is in shock. They have also been used during cardiac arrest to assist in achieving return of spontaneous circulation.

An Impella device could be an option in this case if the IABP is insufficient or anatomically difficult to insert. However, given Isaac has had his aortic valve replaced, surgeons may be reluctant for an Impella device to be sited.

What is thromboelastography?

Thromboelastography is a point-of-care assay which allows clinicians to assess the global dynamics of whole clot formation (and destruction) in real time. The viscoelastic properties of the clot are reflected in diagrammatic form, the components of which indicate deficiencies or abnormalities in the coagulation cascade.

Traditionally, TEG requires 0.36 mL of whole blood to be placed into a cup and a small pin is suspended within. The cup is rotated to induce clot formation around the pin. Movement of the pin within the blood is impacted as the clot is initiated, propagated and destroyed. A torsion wire attached to the pin transmits those changes in movement to a transducer and a graphical representation of clot dynamics is created in real time (Figure 21.2a).

More modern TEG uses cartridges rather than a pin-in-cup technique. Blood is exposed to resonant frequencies and LED illumination is used to assess clot dynamics.

An alternative point-of-care viscoelastic haemostatic assay is the ROTEM® system, which is based upon similar principles (Figure 21.2b).

Figure 21.3 shows a series of images of abnormal traces and what to do about them.

> Postoperatively, Isaac returns to cardiac ICU, deeply sedated, with an IABP in situ. The AVR appears to be intact and functioning well. The IABP is set to ECG trigger in a 1:1 ratio.

What is the theoretical basis for the use of IABP?

- Counterpulsation aims to augment coronary blood flow during diastole. A balloon is placed in the descending aorta proximal to the renal artery and distal to the origin of the left subclavian artery.
- Helium is used to inflate the balloon due to its low viscosity.
- Inflation occurs at the end of systole (at the dicrotic notch on the arterial blood pressure trace) and deflation at the end of diastole. Ideally, this should decrease left ventricular workload, increase myocardial oxygenation, increase coronary artery perfusion and increase cardiac output.
- The balloon needs to be triggered to inflate and deflate at precisely the right time. This can be synchronised using the ECG, the arterial waveform, pacing spikes (if the patient is paced) or an internal trigger mode if the patient is asystolic. If the balloon inflates at the wrong time, it can cause obstruction to arterial blood flow and lead to decreased cardiac output.

(a)

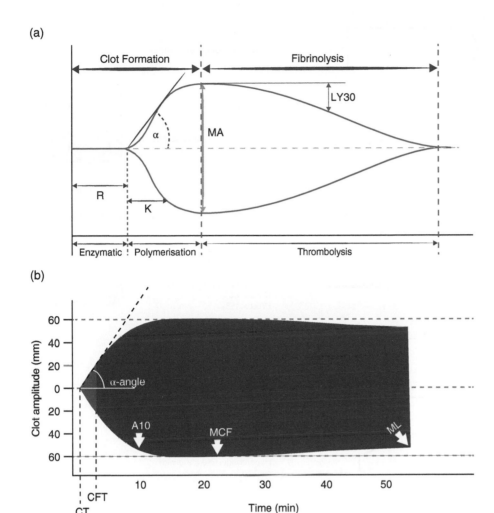

(b)

Figure 21.2: (a) TEG. The R value (reaction time) measures the time taken from the start of the test to the initiation of clot. The K value (kinetics) is the time taken for the clot strength to reach an amplitude of 20 mm. The α-angle assesses the rate of clot formation by measuring the speed at which fibrin build up and cross-linking occurs. The maximum amplitude (MA) represents the ultimate strength of the fibrin clot and overall stability. The LY30 is the percentage decrease in amplitude of the clot at 30 mins. (b) ROTEM example. The clotting time (CT) is the first reported parameter on the tracing and represents the time from the start of the assay to the initiation of clot formation. The clot formation time (CFT) indicates the time from clot initiation until clot firmness has reached an amplitude of 20 mm. The α-angle measures in degrees the tangential line to the clot at an amplitude of 2 mm, allowing for future clot firmness estimates. A10 represents the firmness of the clot at 10 minutes after CT and is an early indicator for coagulopathy. The maximum clot firmness (MCF) provides a measure of clot strength and is dependent upon platelets, fibrin polymerisation and stabilisation with factor XIII. ML represents the maximum lysis of the clot.

Source: Theophilus Samuels.

- If working correctly, the end-diastolic pressure after deflation should be lower than the unaugmented diastolic pressure by approximately 15 mmHg. Augmented systolic pressure will be lower than unassisted pressure by about 5 mmHg.
- Initially, every beat will be augmented (1:1 ratio). As the patient's condition improves, the augmenting ratio can be decreased.

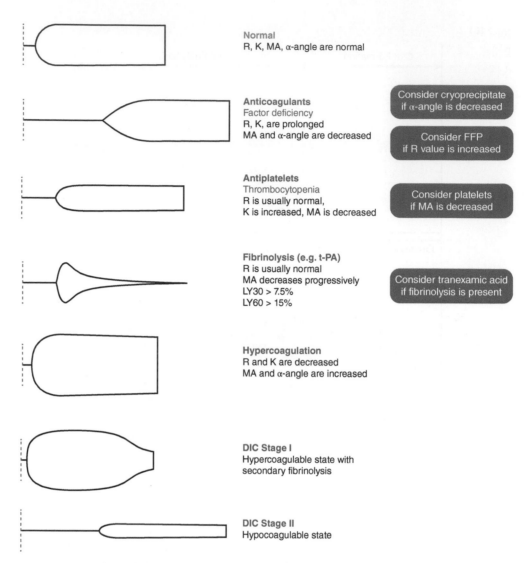

Figure 21.3: Schematic diagram representing normal and abnormal traces observed with TEG. R, R value (reaction time); K, K value (kinetics); MA, maximum amplitude; LY30, percentage decrease in amplitude at 30 minutes post MA; LY60, percentage decrease in amplitude at 60 minutes post MA; DIC, disseminated intravascular coagulation; FFP, fresh frozen plasma; t-PA, tissue plasminogen activator.

Source: Theophilus Samuels.

What is the evidence for the use of IABP?

American College of Cardiology/American Heart Association recommendations maintain class IIA evidence for the use of IABP in cardiogenic shock but the evidence itself is controversial. No improvement has been demonstrated in 30-day mortality (IABP-SHOCK II, Thiele et al, NEJM, 2012) or 12-month mortality for patients with cardiogenic shock post MI. However, meta-analysis by Deppe et al. (J Card Surg, 2017) showed mortality benefit with the use of IABP preoperatively for high-risk CABG.

Since there is conflicting evidence, the use of IABP remains at the discretion of the team managing the patient. Particularly in centres where ECMO is not available, IABP may represent a reasonable, cost-effective, minimally invasive technique to support the patient through an acute episode of myocardial stunning. Intra-aortic balloon counterpulsation is only ever a bridging therapy for a reversible pathology.

What other issues need to be addressed to optimise Isaac's condition in critical care?

- Electrolyte management to avoid arrhythmias:
  - Potassium >4.5 mmol/L.
  - Ionised calcium >1 mmol/L.
  - Magnesium >1 mmol/L.
- Monitor coagulation and correct abnormalities where required.
- Continue cardiac output monitoring aiming to optimise cardiac output. Isaac may have a pulmonary artery catheter.
- Temperature management.
- Avoid shivering.
- Gastric ulcer prophylaxis.
- Blood glucose management.
- Monitor for signs of infection (especially ventilator-associated pneumonia and sternal or mediastinal wound infection) and treat aggressively with antibiotics if suspected.

Isaac weans from the IABP over the course of the next 3 days. On day 4, while you are performing a sedation hold, the nurses call you to say that he has developed fast AF. Isaac is agitated and not waking appropriately.

Why is atrial fibrillation a problem and how will you manage Isaac's AF?

Postoperative atrial fibrillation (AF) usually occurs on day 2 or 3 and has an incidence of approximately 25–40% in patients following CPB and 50–60% following valve surgery.

AF is associated with increased length of stay, increased risk of renal impairment and stroke (up to three times the standard risk).

Atrial contraction is responsible for up to 30% of left ventricle end diastolic volume. AF may, therefore, lead to a decrease in cardiac output and global oxygen delivery.

- Review epicardial pacing.
- Check the wires are still in place, that the box is switched on, and that the wires are connected correctly to the pacing box.
- Check that the wires are not fractured at the insertion site.
- The same principles apply to managing AF in this case as in any other.
  - Rhythm control
    - Have a low threshold for cardioversion but ensure there is no thrombus if AF has been present for more than 24–48 hours.
    - Electrolyte replacement.

- Consider administering a fluid challenge.
- Consider amiodarone.
- Rate control – consider pharmacological treatment, e.g. beta-blockers or amiodarone.
- Anticoagulate if AF persists beyond 24 hours (discuss with surgical team).

What could be the cause of Isaac's agitation and failure to wake appropriately?

- *Drugs* – hangover effect from several days of sedation in critical care. Withdrawal from alcohol and smoking can also be a cause.
- *Delirium* – post-pump delirium or critical care delirium.
- *Stroke* – examine Isaac to try and establish whether there are focal neurological deficits.
- *Infection* – particularly assess for ventilator-associated pneumonia, sternal wound infection and mediastinitis.
- *Communication issues* – take a collateral history to establish whether Isaac is deaf or normally uses hearing aids, or whether there is a language barrier.

You perform CT head which shows no acute abnormalities. You correct Isaac's electrolytes and are able to resolve his AF. His kidney function remains normal throughout. You minimise sedation and perform a CAM-ICU assessment which suggests that Isaac has delirium (see Case 11).

Are there any pharmacological management strategies for delirium?

- Antipsychotics have been used for symptom control, particularly in hyperactive delirium where severe agitation may put the patient or staff at risk. There is no evidence to support that agents such as haloperidol are beneficial in treating delirium itself.
- Dexmedetomidine is a selective agonist of presynaptic alpha-2 adrenoceptors (similar to clonidine but with a more favourable side-effect profile). There are some studies which suggest that the use of dexmedetomidine for sedation can reduce the incidence of delirium in critical care patients.

Over the ensuing 7 days, Isaac recovers sufficiently to be discharged from cardiothoracic intensive care.

What is the prognosis for patients undergoing CABG?

For those patients who survive the first month post surgery, mortality is similar to that of the population in general.

What is the prognosis for patients undergoing aortic valve replacement?

Meta-analysis shows that survival in those under 65 years may be on average 16 years, while for those over 75 years it may be approximately 6 or 7 years. Annual stroke risk is less than 1%. Nearly 50% of grafts continue to function well for up to 20 years and almost all function well for at least 10 years.

What should you include in your handover to the ward team regarding Isaac's ongoing management?

- Isaac should be considered for treatment with the following medications:
  - Ongoing antiplatelet therapy with aspirin or clopidogrel.
  - Statin.
  - Beta-blocker.
  - Antihypertensives (aiming for BP <140/85 mmHg).
- Support to quit smoking and manage obesity if necessary.
- Monitor renal function.
- Structured cardiac rehabilitation is recommended.
- Annual vaccinations are recommended.
- There are high rates of depression following cardiac surgery and patients should be screened for this at follow-up.
- Cardiology and cardiothoracic surgery follow-up.

Further reading

- Mitchell, J., Bogar, L., Burton, N. et al. (2014). Cardiothoracic surgical emergencies in the intensive care unit. *Crit. Care Clin.* 30 (3): 499–525. Important overview of some of the most important emergencies in cardiothoracic ICU.
- Makdisi, J. and Wang, I. (2015). Extracorporeal membrane oxygenation (ECMO): review of a lifesaving technology. *J. Thorac. Dis.* 7 (7): E166–E176. Informative review of ECMO including indications, complications and process.
- Broomhead, R., Myers, A., and Mallett, S. (2016). Clinical aspects of coagulation and haemorrhage. *Anaesthesia Intensive Care Med.* 17 (2): 86–91. Excellent review of the clinical management of haemorrhage.
- Brill, J., Brenner, M., Duchesne, J. et al. (2021). The role of TEG and ROTEM in damage control resuscitation. *Shock* 56 (1S): 52–61. This paper, although centred around trauma-induced coagulopathy, has invaluable explanations regarding interpretation of viscoelastic testing.

22 The Patient Who was in A House Fire

You attend a trauma call in the ED resuscitation area. Philip, a man in his 70s, was extracted from a house fire and has extensive burn injuries to his face, neck, thorax, right arm and right leg. You are told that neighbours reported hearing some sort of explosion before the fire started. Manual inline stabilisation of the cervical spine is ongoing. Philip has a respiratory rate of 45 breaths per minute and you can hear stridor. He has soot around his mouth and nose. He cannot open his eyes due to increasing oedema from burns to the area.

What are your main concerns?

- *Airway* – stridor may indicate the onset of airway swelling. Inhalation of hot gases will result in oedema above the vocal cords. Over the few hours following exposure, this swelling can worsen and may be exacerbated by fluid resuscitation. This means Philip's airway needs prompt attention and it is highly likely that intubation will be required immediately. It should be anticipated to be a difficult airway. A poor view caused by airway oedema may be further impaired by manual inline stabilisation of the cervical spine.
- *Respiratory*
  - There is evidence of inhalational injury, i.e. carbon deposits around the mouth and nose. There may be smoke inhalation injury which could cause bronchospasm and inflammation.
  - The history indicates that an explosion occurred. There may be pneumothoraces. ARDS might develop secondary to blast injury.
  - There are extensive burns to Philip's chest. If this is circumferential, escharotomies may be required to prevent restriction of chest expansion.
- *Cardiovascular* – with extensive burns injuries, Philip will have large insensible fluid losses. Intravenous access may prove to be difficult since cannulae should ideally be inserted through unburnt skin.

Clinical Cases in Critical Care, First Edition. Alice Myers and Theophilus Samuels.
© 2023 John Wiley & Sons Ltd. Published 2023 by John Wiley & Sons Ltd.

- *Trauma* – look for other injuries in addition to Philip's burns. Follow the ATLS (Advanced Trauma Life Support) approach.
- *Extensive burns* – Philip's case should be discussed with a specialist burns centre and he may need to be transferred for ongoing management.
- *Risk of toxins* – house fires carry a significant risk of exposure to carbon monoxide and cyanide. Other potentially toxic chemicals such as ammonia can be released from burning furniture materials. Toxins might be implicated in the aetiology of the fire itself. Inattention caused by intoxication with alcohol or other drugs can lead to fire, or the fire may have been part of a suicide attempt also involving deliberate overdose.

What type of injury can be caused by explosion?

Blast injuries are usually seen in combat situations. Explosions can cause penetrating and blunt injury. Damage is usually more extensive if the blast occurs in a confined space. Broadly, injury is sustained via four mechanisms:

- *Primary* (caused by high-order explosives) – gas-filled structures are most vulnerable as the overpressurised blast wave comes into contact with body surfaces. This causes pulmonary barotrauma, globe rupture, abdominal perforation and middle ear rupture.
- *Secondary* – any part of the body can be affected by flying debris. This usually causes penetrating injury.
- *Tertiary* – the blast wind throws the patient, causing bony fractures or head injuries.
- *Quaternary* – this group includes all the other explosion-related injuries such as burns, crush injury, exacerbation of underlying respiratory illness, smoke inhalation, etc.

The major trauma consultant asks you to secure Philip's airway immediately due to concerns outlined above. The ambulance crew managed to insert a good 20 G IV cannula into the dorsum of Philip's left hand.

How do you secure Philip's airway?

This will need to be a modified rapid-sequence intubation (RSI) – see Introduction Section 2. Specific issues relating to the airway in the burns victim include the following:

- Manual inline stabilisation should be ongoing if C-spine clearance is not possible.
- Difficult airway equipment should be readily available, including video-laryngoscopes.
- Use an uncut endotracheal tube. Over time, orofacial oedema can develop, leading to dislodgement of a short ETT or creating difficulty in accessing the proximal end.

- Have a smaller ETT available in case of supraglottic airway oedema.
- IV access, ideally through unburnt skin, for fluids and drugs. Intraosseous access can be used if it is impossible to secure IV access rapidly.
- Suxamethonium, a depolarizing neuromuscular blocker, is contraindicated beyond 24 hours after burns injuries since these patients are more susceptible to the hyperkalaemic effect of this drug, possibly due to upregulation in nicotinic acetylcholine receptors. In the acute context, it should be safe but emergency clinicians are increasingly using alternative agents such as rocuronium to achieve paralysis due to an improved side-effect profile and the easy availability of reversal agents such as sugammadex.
- Prepare for failed oral intubation. Have a plan for attempting front of neck access if all else fails.
- If Philip's loved ones were close at hand, it would be a good time to invite them to come in and see him quickly prior to intubation. This could be his last opportunity to hear their voices as there is a chance that he may never regain consciousness after this point.
- Don't waste time! The oedema will only increase, making view at laryngoscopy more difficult.

> You secure Philip's airway uneventfully with an uncut cuffed oral endotracheal tube, internal diameter 7.0 mm, secured at 23 cm at the teeth. A colleague has inserted a 14 G IV cannula into the left antecubital fossa. You notice he has very extensive burns which appear to cover his chest and back.

What should you do now regarding immediate management, monitoring and further investigations?

Immediate management

- Administer a high fraction of inspired oxygen in case of toxin exposure. Even if carbon monoxide has been displaced from haemoglobin-binding sites, clearance from protein-binding sites takes longer. Oxygen is also required in case of cyanide poisoning.
- Commence fluid resuscitation.
- Burns assessment – assess the depth, check for circumferential burns, assess distribution and calculate the surface area of burned skin.

Monitoring

- Intra-arterial catheterisation is required for monitoring gas exchange, electrolytes, blood pressure.
- Insert a central venous catheter as vasoactive agents may be needed.

Investigations

- Complete the initial plain radiograph trauma series (chest, pelvis and cervical spine) to assess ABCS (Alignment, Bony Structures, Cartilage and Soft tissues).

- Focused assessment with sonography for trauma (FAST).
- CT head, neck, chest, abdomen and pelvis as part of the trauma sequence.

How do you calculate fluid resuscitation requirements?

The Parkland formula is used to calculate the fluid requirement in the first 24 hours for adults. Half is given over the first 8 hours, the remaining half over the next 16 hours.

$$Fluid\ required\ in\ first\ 24\ hours = 4\ ml/kg \times \%BSAburn$$

(%BSAburn is the percentage burned body surface area)

It is standard to insert a urinary catheter and target fluid resuscitation to aim for urine output of 0.5 mL/kg/h.

How do you assess percentage and depth of burn?

- *Percentage* – the Lund–Browder chart and the Wallace rule of nines are both convenient tools for rapid assessment. The rule of nines is used to calculate percentage BSA. In an adult patient, each of the following accounts for 9% BSA – head, right arm, left arm. Each of the following accounts for 18% BSA – right leg, left leg, chest, back. The final 1% is accounted for by the perineum. In children, the head accounts for 18% and each leg for 13.5%.
- *Burn depth* (degrees) should also be assessed since this affects wound healing, temperature homeostasis, pain and fluid loss:
  - First-degree burns involve the epidermis.
  - Second-degree burns include upper dermis (superficial partial thickness) and lower dermis (deep partial thickness).
  - Third-degree burns are full-thickness burns which involve the lower structures. Deep partial and full-thickness burns result in decreased sensation.

What are the indications for discussion with specialist burns centre?

Remember **BURNS:**

- **B**ody surface area (>3% in adults, >1% in children – varies between trauma networks)
- **U**nder 5 years old or over 60 years old
- High **R**isk burns (full thickness or circumferential)
- i**N**volvement of special areas (face, hands, ears, genitals)
- **S**epsis or **S**pecial causes (chemical, electrical, high-pressure steam, friction burn, inhalational injury, non-burn skin loss, e.g. toxic epidermal necrolysis)

Toxic shock syndrome or burns sepsis syndrome is a medical emergency. Have a low threshold of suspicion in any patient with any size of burn who has any of the following symptoms.

- Malaise
- Anorexia
- Fever (>38 °C)
- Rash
- Diarrhoea
- Tachycardia
- Tachypnoea
- Hypotension
- Oliguria

What is an escharotomy and why may one be performed?

An escharotomy is a surgical technique used to treat circumferential full-thickness burns. The eschar is the tough, inelastic scar-like tissue that remains following destruction of dermis and epidermis. When the eschar is circumferential, rehydration and oedema can lead to increased pressure at the eschar, resulting in compartment syndrome and reduced circulation distal to the eschar. Around the thorax, this can lead to reduced chest expansion. The escharotomy is a surgical incision down to the fatty tissues that is left open and allowed to expand to relieve pressure.

Philip has burns over 46% BSA. Approximately 10% BSA is full thickness. You transfer him to CT for imaging of his brain and whole body. The radiologist is not immediately available, but you cannot see any gross pathology on CT head. The lung parenchyma, however, looks abnormal. You discuss Philip with the ICU consultant and transfer him straight to ICU. You request blood cyanide concentration to be sent.

The first ABG shows:

pH 7.07

PaO_2 11.7 kPa (FiO_2 0.75, PEEP 8 cmH$_2$O)

$PaCO_2$ 12.3 kPa

Base excess −7.3 mmol/L

Lactate 6.5 mmol/l

Carbon monoxide level 35%

What are your concerns regarding cyanide poisoning?

Cyanide leads to cytotoxic hypoxia through inhibiting mitochondrial respiration. Cyanide poisoning can result in severe permanent neurological disability.

Blood cyanide concentration can be tested but, in most centres, results are not acutely available. Early suspicion and management are key with cyanide toxicity so treatment should be administered where the patient has a history of exposure and exhibits signs of neurological impairment, with high serum lactate levels (>8 mmol/L) and soot in the mouth.

100% O_2 should be administered and unconscious patients should have assisted ventilation. Specific treatments include:

- Hydroxycobalamin (vitamin B12)
- Sodium thiosulfate
- Dicobalt edetate.

Methaemoglobin-forming antidotes such as amyl nitrate and sodium nitrate should be avoided in smoke inhalation injury as they can reduce the oxygen-carrying capacity of haemoglobin.

Consult National Poisons Information Services/ToxBase for guidance on therapy.

What is the mechanism for toxicity from carbon monoxide and what is the management?

Carbon monoxide leads to hypoxia through preferential binding to deoxyhaemoglobin (it has 40 times the affinity of oxygen). It also binds to cytochrome p450 enzymes (CYP450).

Carboxyhaemoglobin levels over 25% (normally measured via arterial blood gas analysis) are usually an indication for intubation and ventilation. Severe toxicity may require hyperbaric therapy. NICE guidance is available.

Non-smokers should have a carbon monoxide level <3%. Heavy smokers may have levels up to 15%. Clinical features of toxicity become apparent beyond 15–20% and anyone with a level ≥30% should be considered to have suffered severe exposure.

The clinical features vary according to the degree of toxicity. Brief, low-level exposure may cause dizziness, headache and myalgia whereas higher levels can cause respiratory failure, muscle weakness, myocardial infarction and, ultimately, loss of consciousness and death.

The half-life of carboxyhaemoglobin in air is 320 minutes. This is reduced to 80 minutes in 100% oxygen and should be applied by tight-fitting facemask (or closed breathing circuit). This should be continued until the patient is asymptomatic and, if Philip were awake, repeated neurological examination should be performed to assess this. It is advisable to continue 100% oxygen beyond the time when carboxyhaemoglobin levels are under control since it will take longer for carbon monoxide to clear from CYP450. Do not rely on the pulse oximeter as saturation readings can be misleadingly reassuring.

Hyperbaric oxygen therapy has been shown to be beneficial in cases of severe poisoning. However, it is only available in a limited number of centres and is not routinely offered in the UK.

How do you set the ventilator for Philip?

- Continue 100% oxygen until any carbon monoxide and cyanide toxicity has been treated.
- Philip is at high risk of developing ARDS so ideally opt for a lung-protective strategy such as that supported by ARDSNet (Brower et al., NEJM, 2004). Although the higher pressure end of the PEEP ladder is not universally used (i.e. escalating up to PEEP of 24cmH$_2$O), most other elements of the protocol remain widely accepted as the default strategy for lung protective ventilation.

- $PaO_2 > 8$ kPa.
- pH 7.3–7.45 (many intensivists now tolerate pH > 7.20).
- Increase PEEP to allow reduction of FiO_2.
- Increase respiratory rate to achieve optimal minute ventilation.
- Maintain plateau pressures below 30 cmH$_2$O.
- In addition, since Amato (NEJM, 2015), many intensivists add an aim to minimise driving pressures to <14 cmH$_2$O.
  - However, although gross injury is not immediately obvious on CT brain imaging, Philip is at risk of hypoxic brain injury. So ventilation strategy should be adjusted to facilitate neuroprotective measures where possible. For now, aim for $PaO_2 > 10$ kPa and $PaCO_2$ 4.5–6.0 kPa to maintain optimal cerebral blood flow. Set the ventilator to achieve the neuroprotective measures but aim to keep a lung-protective strategy if possible.

Over the next 24 hours, you keep Philip sedated and ventilate him with a combination of neuro- and lung-protective ventilation. His carbon monoxide level drops to below 15%. You fluid resuscitate him according to your calculations and clinical assessment. The CT performed on admission is reported as showing no acute intracranial abnormality and no bony injury, but it does make note of widespread chronic emphysematous changes in the lungs. You change your ventilatory approach to a purely lung-protective strategy.

On day 2, you note Philip's oxygen requirements increasing, his respiratory pressures increasing and his renal function deteriorating. In addition, it is difficult to control his temperature.

In spite of ongoing analgesia and sedation, Philip appears to be in pain.

The police inform you that the fire may have been related to an oxygen cylinder that was found in Philip's house. The police have informed Philip's two sons that their father is in hospital. They are away on a sailing trip but will be able to come to the hospital tomorrow.

Why might Philip be difficult to ventilate?

- *Inhalational burns injury* – 10–20% of patients with burns injuries suffer inhalational injury. The mechanisms causing subglottic respiratory mucosal damage are complex. Chemical irritants released in house fires cause release of proinflammatory cytokines including substance P, neurokinin A and calcitonin gene-related peptide. This causes bronchoconstriction, chemotaxis and activation of nitric oxide synthase. There is increased vascular permeability, further bronchoconstriction and loss of hypoxic pulmonary vasoconstriction. There is a deterioration in V/Q mismatch, while exudate leads to cast formation and alveolar collapse. Ultimately, mitochondrial dysfunction develops and there is cellular apoptosis.
- *ARDS* – inhalational injury, more than 40% BSA burns or 20% BSA full-thickness burns are risk factors for developing ARDS in association with burns injury. ARDS in this context is associated with extremely high mortality.

- *Pre-existing lung disease* – there was an oxygen cylinder in Philip's house and the CT thorax showed evidence of emphysematous changes. Philip may have been receiving long-term home oxygen therapy, suggesting that his underlying lung function is likely to be poor.
- *Small ETT* – a relatively small internal diameter endotracheal tube has been inserted which will reduce flow according to Hagen–Poiseuille's Law. Any dried secretions within the tube will further impair gas flow. Although 7.0 mm is not ideal in an adult man, it should be possible to ventilate Philip with this. This is unlikely to fully explain the difficulty in ventilation.
- *Pulmonary contusions* – oedema and haematoma alter the natural architecture and elasticity of the lung. These develop over the first 24 hours, making patients increasingly difficult to oxygenate and ventilate.
- *Effusions or pneumothorax* – look for developing pathology. Philip is extremely vulnerable to this given his underlying lung disease, inhalational injury and mechanical ventilation.

Why may it be challenging to control Philip's temperature?

Patients with burns tend to become profoundly hyperthermic with a raised baseline temperature. However, they can also become hypothermic due to exposure and loss of skin integrity which plays an essential role in thermoregulation. Reasons for altered temperature include the following:

- *Hypermetabolism* – severe burns induce a profound catecholamine-induced hypermetabolic state within the first 5 days of injury. Hyperthermia develops as part of the inflammatory response.
- *Skin integrity* – the burned area loses the protective transdermal layer, meaning Philip is more susceptible to evaporative losses. Higher ambient temperatures should be maintained to reduce heat loss by radiation. Patients are particularly at risk of hypothermia during the perioperative period if surgery is required.
- *Infection* – Philip is vulnerable to sepsis, being critically unwell and with a significant breach in his protective skin barrier.

What are the causes of renal failure in burns victims?

- *Intravascular hypovolaemia* – increased vascular permeability, sodium-potassium pump impairment and sodium retention cause generalised oedema and effective intravascular hypovolaemia. Increased free water leads to low plasma tonicity and renal oedema. This is compounded by increased insensible fluid losses.
- *Myocardial depression* – low plasma tonicity, tumour necrosis factor (TNF) and oxygen free radicals all lead to myocardial depression and therefore reduced renal perfusion. Acute tubular necrosis results.

- *Hypoxia* – respiratory injury causing hypoxia reduces oxygen supply to the kidneys.
- *Nephrotoxicity* – antibiotics used in the management of burns patients can be nephrotoxic (e.g. aminoglycosides).
- *Inflammation* – inflammatory mediators (TNF, interleukins, thromboxanes, leukotrienes, platelet activating factor, prostaglandins) released following burns injuries are implicated in both increased vascular permeability and disseminated intravascular coagulation (DIC) causing microthrombi in renal capillary beds.
- *Pigmenturia* – thermal injury can cause breakdown of red blood cells. Large amounts of free haemoglobin pass through the renal glomeruli and can form casts or occlude renal tubules. Further tubular damage can also be caused through oxygen free radicals generated by iron ions as haem is released following the reabsorption and denaturing of haemoglobin.
- *Rhabdomyolysis* – thermal injury, crush injury and electrical injury can cause rhabdomyolysis via several mechanisms, mainly involving capillary leakage leading to decreased perfusion, ischaemia and tissue necrosis.

Why is Philip likely to be in pain?

Philip has many potential sources of pain. Although areas of full-thickness burns may not be intrinsically painful due to loss of nerve endings in the dermis and epidermis, neighbouring areas of partial-thickness burn may still be extremely sensitive. Dressings changes, mobilisation, physiotherapy and surgery or debridement can be exquisitely painful. Other sources of pain and discomfort include the presence of the endotracheal tube, procedure-related pain (e.g. chest drain insertion) and pre-existing pain sources such as arthritis.

Pain can be nociceptive or neuropathic. Initially, A delta (fast) and C (slow) fibres transmit pain stimuli to the dorsal horn of the spinal cord. Neurons travel in the spinothalamic tracts and are distributed to thalamic and cortical areas, particularly the cingulate cortex. Mediators include histamine, bradykinin, leukotrienes, prostaglandin E2 and substance P.

Pre-emptive multimodal analgesia is advisable. Regular paracetamol should be combined with opioids and consideration given to atypical agents, e.g. gabapentin, pregabalin, amitriptyline. Philip is receiving an opioid infusion but this may require supplementation. His needs may exceed usual ICU requirements. Regional techniques can be considered but are limited in terms of duration of effect.

> Philip becomes difficult to ventilate, with reduced compliance and thick black respiratory secretions. You decide to perform bronchoalveolar lavage.

What are the risks and benefits of performing bronchoscopy in cases of inhalational injury?

Benefits

Fibreoptic bronchoscopy can be useful in both the diagnosis and management of inhalational injury. The Abbreviated Injury Score (AIS) for Inhalational Injury requires bronchoscopy to grade severity. Findings correlate with mortality.

There is contradictory evidence regarding the clinical value of daily bronchoscopy and lavage. There are case reports which demonstrate that carbonaceous plugs and casts can be managed effectively in this way.

Risks

Until there is convincing large trial evidence, cases should be assessed individually, particularly where oxygen requirements are high. Risks include:

- Bronchospasm/laryngospasm
- Atelectasis/decruitment/desaturation/increased airway resistance
- Haemorrhage
- Infection
- Perforation of the airways
- Vasovagal stimulation/tachycardia/increased pulmonary arterial pressure/haemodynamic instability
- Raised intracranial pressure.

On day 3, you identify worsening renal function and commence haemofiltration. Philip has stopped absorbing his NG feed and his abdomen is distended. A chest radiograph shows widespread bilateral infiltrates. You diagnose ARDS based on the Berlin criteria. His FiO_2 requirements increase to 0.9 on PEEP 10 cmH$_2$O (giving PaO$_2$ 7.9 kPa). His inflammatory markers are increasing and his temperature is 39.1 °C.

Philip's GP tells you that he is 73 years old and has been on home oxygen for COPD for the last 2 years. The GP suspects that Philip has continued to smoke on occasion. He hasn't reviewed Philip personally for 6 months but on his last home assessment, Philip was living mostly in one room, unable to climb stairs due to shortness of breath, with carers helping him four times per day.

What grade of severity is Philip's ARDS?

According to the Berlin criteria, Philip has severe ARDS with a P:F ratio 8.8 kPa (PaO$_2$/FiO$_2$ i.e. 7.9/0.9 = 8.8).

How would you assess Philip's premorbid status and frailty?

Philip has severe irreversible underlying lung disease and extremely limited physiological reserve. According to the Rockwood Frailty Scale, Philip would score 7 for being severely frail and dependent for his activities of daily living. Increased frailty has been shown to be associated with increased mortality in patients admitted to intensive care.

What scoring systems could you use to grade the severity of Philip's organ dysfunction?

- *MODS (multiple organ dysfunction score)*
  - Awards points in six areas (P:F ratio, platelet count, bilirubin level, pressure-adjusted heart rate, GCS, creatinine).

- The composite score can be used to predict risk of ICU mortality, hospital mortality and ICU length of stay.
- *Injury Severity Score (ISS)*
    - Commonly used in trauma cases; most applicable to blunt injury following road traffic accidents.
    - Awards points for the worst injury to six body areas (head/neck, face, chest, abdomen, extremity, external).
    - The three highest scoring areas are squared and added together to reach a total out of 75 points.
    - This score is generally used as a research tool.
- *Abbreviated Injury Score (AIS) for Inhalation Injury*
    - Can be used to predict in-hospital mortality for patients with inhalational injury as evaluated at bronchoscopy.
    - Grades 0–1 predict 84% in-hospital survival while grades 2–4 predict only 57% survival.

Why is gut failure a significant problem for Philip?

Additional organ failure is a sign of Philip's worsening deterioration. Nutritional requirements increase in patients suffering burns injury due to catabolism and a dramatically increased metabolic rate. Where there is more than 40% BSA burns the resting energy expenditure can be up to twice the normal level. Failure to meet nutritional requirements can contribute to poor wound healing, immune failure and multiple organ dysfunction.

If Philip fails to absorb enteral feed, parenteral nutrition should be considered but this is associated with considerable risk. In patients with burns, damaged skin can make it challenging to site central venous catheters and very difficult to keep them clean. The risk of infection must be considered.

On day 4, despite being on haemofiltration, Philip's renal function continues to deteriorate. He has evidence of lower respiratory tract infection and his gas exchange is extremely poor. He has rising noradrenaline requirements (now 0.7 mcg/kg/min). The doctors overnight used cardiac output monitoring and focused echocardiography to guide fluid therapy and the titrated addition of vasopressin and dobutamine. Philip's lactate has started to rise (now 5.1 mmol/L) and he requires an ongoing infusion of 10% glucose to prevent hypoglycaemia. His clotting is deranged – INR 6.3, platelets 47×10^9/L, fibrinogen 0.8 g/L. Philip's sons, his next of kin, have just arrived in the hospital.

Comment on the clotting derangement

This is DIC. Tissue damage from burns injuries leads to an increase in circulating debris and tissue factor. This activates coagulation pathways. A generalised inflammatory response also activates the complement cascade. The result is a potentially deadly combination of the consumption of coagulation factors, activation of fibrinolytic pathways and reduction in regulatory proteins leading to microthrombi formation throughout the circulation, causing microangiopathy.

Why is Philip hypoglycaemic?

Refractory hypoglycaemia and deranged INR suggest hepatic failure has developed. This may be secondary to hypoperfusion or hypoxic ischaemic hepatic injury. This is a very bad sign in terms of Philip's progression into multiple organ failure.

> Philip's sons tell you their father has been deteriorating over the last 2 years and has not been coping at home. He is unable to leave the house and has spent almost all the last 6 months sitting in a chair. He has been told to stop smoking but his friends still visit with beer and cigarettes twice a week. They say their dad didn't want resuscitation and wouldn't want any of this life support machinery.
>
> You tell them that Philip is dying despite what you are doing and that the kindest thing you can do now is to prioritise his comfort and dignity and allow him to die peacefully. His sons agree that this is the right thing to do.

What are the outcomes for burns patients?

Although survival rates for burns victims are improving due to better care, adult patients with greater than 40% BSA burns have a high risk of suffering complications and death. Elderly patients are highly likely to die secondary to major burns.

Mortality rate for burns patients with inhalational injury is up to 20%. For those with subsequent respiratory tract infections, this is up to 40%. Isolated inhalational injury (i.e. without burns) is associated with much better outcomes.

What problems are faced by survivors with burns injuries?

Physical problems include:
- Pain
- Reduced mobility or dexterity due to scar tissue
- Pruritus.

Psychosocial sequelae include:
- Depression
- Sleep disorders
- Generalised anxiety
- Post-traumatic stress disorder
- Many patients suffer problems with their body image and sexual function
- Difficulty returning to work.

Support networks are important to avoid social isolation. Cognitive behavioural therapy and grief counselling can also be useful.

You withdraw organ support and start end-of-life care later that day when Philip's friends and family are around him. He dies comfortably within minutes of stopping support.

Further reading

- Bishop, S. and Maguire, S. (2012). Anaesthesia and intensive care for major burns. *Cont. Educ. Anaesth. Crit. Care Pain* 12 (3): 118–122. Educational review article on burns management.
- Griffiths, M., McAuley, D., Perkins, G. et al. (2019). Guidelines on the management of acute respiratory distress syndrome. *BMJ Open Respir. Res.* 6: e000420. Invaluable guideline on the management of ARDS according to the Faculty of Intensive Care Medicine and Intensive Care Society, with support from the British Thoracic Society.
- Vincent, J. and Monero, R. (2010). Clinical review: scoring systems in the critically ill. *Crit. Care* 14: 207. Educational review article of critical care scoring systems.

23

The Patient with Low Platelets

As you start your night shift on critical care, you are asked to review blood results for Jackie, a 44-year-old woman who was admitted from your acute medical care unit (AMU) late in the evening. She was brought to hospital by her husband 1 day before, following a witnessed seizure. The medical team have started her on empirical treatment for presumed meningoencephalitis. On AMU, she subsequently developed further seizures, which necessitated sedation and mechanical ventilation. A post-intubation CT head did not report any intracranial pathology. She remains haemodynamically stable and her test results on admission to AMU and post admission to ICU are shown in Table 23.1.

How would you interpret these results?

The white blood cell count and CRP are all within normal limits, which is not in keeping with an infective process. The AST and ALT are within normal limits, but the serum bilirubin level is pending. The normal INR and aPTT suggest that her coagulation is currently within normal limits. Her urea and creatinine levels are mildly raised above normal, suggesting renal impairment. Her haemoglobin level is also lower than normal, but the most striking abnormality appears to be thrombocytopenia.

Define thrombocytopenia

In adults, thrombocytopenia is defined as a platelet count below the lower limit of normal ($<150 \times 10^9$/L) and can be further classified as:

- Mild: $100–149 \times 10^9$/L
- Moderate: $50–99 \times 10^9$/L
- Severe: $< 50 \times 10^9$/L

Jackie appears to have a severe thrombocytopenia as she has a platelet count of 28×10^9/L.

Clinical Cases in Critical Care, First Edition. Alice Myers and Theophilus Samuels.
© 2023 John Wiley & Sons Ltd. Published 2023 by John Wiley & Sons Ltd.

Table 23.1: Blood results.

	Admission to AMU	Admission to ICU
FBC		
Hb (g/L)	98	91
MCV (fl)	80	81
WBC (×10⁹/L)	11	11
Neut (×10⁹/L)	5.5	5.6
Plt (×10⁹/L)	27	28
INR	1.1	1.1
aPTT (sec)	27	28
Blood film	-	Pending
LFT		
ALT (U/L)	-	43
AST (U/L)	-	42
Bili (μmol/L)	-	Pending
U&E		
Na (mmol/L)	136	137
K (mmol/L)	4.8	5.0
Ur (mmol/L)	7.4	7.8
Cr (μmol/L)	121	125
CRP (mg/L)	<5	<5

ALT, alanine aminotransferase; AMU, acute medical unit; aPTT, activated partial thromboplastin time; AST, aspartate aminotransferase; Bili, bilirubin; Cr, creatinine; CRP, C-reactive protein; FBC, full blood count; Hb, haemoglobin; ICU, intensive care unit; INR, international normalised ratio; K, potassium; LFT, liver function test; MCV, mean corpuscular volume; Na, sodium; Neut, neutrophil; Plt, platelet; U&E, urea and electrolytes; Ur, urea; WBC, white blood cell.

What are the risks of thrombocytopenia?

The risk with a low platelet count is usually bleeding. However, the functional quality of platelets (the ability to form clot) can also affect the risk of bleeding. Therefore, a patient with a normal platelet count but dysfunctional platelets has a higher bleeding risk than one with thrombocytopenia and normally functioning platelets. Nevertheless, in the absence of a qualitative defect, a platelet count:

- $<50 \times 10^9$/L may be associated with excessive bleeding post trauma or surgery
- $<20 \times 10^9$/L may be associated with spontaneous bleeding
- $5–10 \times 10^9$/L places a patient at high risk of spontaneous, life-threatening haemorrhage.

In critical care patients, thrombocytopenia is associated with an increased risk of dying. However, this increased risk is not due to bleeding but to thrombocytopenia acting as a marker of severe morbidity.

What would be your platelet count threshold for performing a lumbar puncture (LP)?

Generally, patients without haematological malignancies should ideally have platelet counts greater than 40×10^9/L in the absence of a coagulopathy. However, consult local guidance and policies regarding the acceptable cut-off level in your institution. Additionally, a platelet transfusion may help negate some of the risk associated with the LP but remember that a platelet transfusion will also expose the patient to several additional complications (e.g. infection, transfusion-related acute lung injury, alloimmunization, allergic and anaphylactic reactions). This should only be performed if deemed necessary for guiding treatment, etc. In this case, with such a low platelet count and no clear evidence yet that this is an infective process, the risk of performing an LP and giving a platelet transfusion may outweigh the benefit.

How are platelets made in the body?

Megakaryocytic progenitor cells within the bone marrow divide to form megakaryoblasts. Only nuclei of these cells then undergo division, while the cell itself does not, a process known as 'endomitotic reduplication'. Once this process is completed, mature megakaryocytes are formed, which are large cells with several nuclei and cytoplasm containing platelet granules. Large numbers of nucleus-free platelets then fragment off from these cells and enter the circulation.

Thrombopoietin (TPO) stimulates the formation and maturation of megakaryocytes. It is made within liver and marrow stromal cells. Interestingly, when TPO is released into the circulation, it binds to specific receptors on platelets and is effectively removed. The free and active level therefore possesses an inverse relationship to platelet count.

What is the normal lifespan of platelets?

Normally, the average lifespan is between 7 and 10 days before they are removed from the circulation and destroyed by the reticuloendothelial system of the liver and spleen.

How common is thrombocytopenia in critical care?

Thrombocytopenia is a common finding (25–55%) in critically unwell patients.

What are the mechanisms of thrombocytopenia?

Within critical care, the two most important causes for thrombocytopenia are sepsis and heparin-induced thrombocytopenia (HIT). However, the mechanisms for causing thrombocytopenia can be divided into three main categories:

- Decreased production of platelets
- Increased destruction of platelets
- Sequestration of platelets

What can lead to a decreased production of platelets?

- Bone marrow diseases e.g. myeloma, acute leukaemia, aplastic anaemia, metastatic carcinoma, myelofibrosis
- Chemotherapy
- Radiation therapy-induced myelosuppression
- Viral infections e.g. HIV, EBV, CMV
- Alcohol
- Myelodysplasia (impaired megakaryocyte proliferation)

In these situations, concurrent reduction in other cell lines (e.g. red and white blood cells) would also tend to occur, which can be readily identified on a blood smear. Bleeding associated with these causes usually requires platelet transfusion.

What can lead to an increased destruction of platelets? Non-immune mechanisms

- Sepsis
- Disseminated intravascular dissemination (DIC)
- Haemolytic-uraemic syndrome (HUS)
- Thrombotic thrombocytopenic purpura (TTP)
- Heparin-induced thrombocytopenia (HIT)
- Pre-eclampsia or eclampsia
- Extracorporeal circulation e.g. cardiopulmonary bypass or hae-mofiltration

Platelet transfusions in these circumstances are rarely needed if the underlying problem is identified and treated accordingly. TTP, HUS or HIT are also more likely to be associated with microvascular thrombosis and occlusion rather than bleeding, which again makes platelet transfusions rarely necessary for their management.

There is a risk that clinical deterioration may occur in patients with HIT or TTP following platelet transfusion.

Immune-mediated mechanisms

- Drugs, e.g. beta-lactam antibiotics, vancomycin, quinine, quinidine, sulfonamides, procainamide
- Autoimmune disease
- Alloimmune sensitization

Even though stopping the offending drugs will aid in restoring platelet levels to normal, severe thrombocytopenia may warrant platelet transfusions.

How does platelet sequestration lead to thrombocytopenia?

The spleen normally sequesters approximately 30–40% of the circulating platelet mass, with this proportion increasing in the presence of an enlarged spleen (e.g. due to portal hypertension). Bleeding that occurs in the presence of hypersplenism alone is unusual and platelet counts rarely fall below $40–50 \times 10^9/L$.

What is heparin-induced thrombocytopenia (HIT)?

Heparin-induced thrombocytopenia is a potentially life-threatening complication following exposure to unfractionated or low molecular weight heparin that is independent of the dose, timing or route of administration. It is estimated that HIT occurs in 0.5–1.0% of patients in critical care. Two types of HIT have been described:

- *Type I* (HIT I) is not clinically significant, tends to occur within the first 48 hours of heparin exposure and is thought to be due to non-immune-mediated platelet aggregation. The platelet count rarely falls below $100 \times 10^9/L$ and it typically returns to normal levels despite continued heparin administration. Thrombosis does not occur with HIT I and heparin administration does not need to be stopped.
- *Type II* (HIT II) or heparin-induced thrombocytopenia and thrombosis (HITT) describes a clinically significant syndrome where thrombocytopenia is associated with thrombosis. The risk of thrombotic complications persists until both heparin is discontinued and a non-heparin anticoagulant is started.

What causes HITT and how is it diagnosed?

HITT is caused by a heparin-platelet factor 4 (PF4) immunoglobin G (IgG) antibody that binds to and activates platelets, leading to a prothrombotic effect. Anti-PF4 antibodies can occur in up to 50% of patients in critical care. The most used assay for their detection has a low specificity for diagnosing HITT. Therefore, HITT remains a mainly clinical diagnosis and discussion with an expert familiar with HITT is essential. To reduce the risk of overdiagnosis and from the side-effect profile of alternative anticoagulants that would need to be prescribed, patients should only be tested for these antibodies when the pretest probability using the 4T score (**T**hrombocytopenia, **T**iming of platelet count fall, **T**hrombosis and other causes of thrombocytopenia not evident) is intermediate (e.g. between 4 and 5; Table 23.2).

When does HIT usually occur?

Typical HIT tends to occur between 5 and 10 days after starting heparin. However, a rapid-onset HIT can also develop within hours and up to 1–2 days after starting heparin in individuals who have been previously exposed in the last 100 days, hence the need to take a clear medical history and scrutinise previous drug prescriptions. Rarely, delayed-onset HIT can occur several days after heparin is discontinued and presents with thrombotic complications.

Table 23.2: Pretest probability score: 6–8, high; 4–5, intermediate; 0–3, low.

	Points (0, 1 or 2 for each of the four parameters; maximum points = 8)		
	2	**1**	**0**
Thrombocytopenia (acute)	>50% platelet count fall AND platelet nadir ≥20×10⁹/L	30–50% platelet count fall OR platelet nadir 10–19×10⁹/L	<30% platelet count fall OR platelet nadir ≤10×10⁹/L
Timing of fall in platelet count or other sequelae	Onset day 5–10 OR <1 day (if heparin exposure within 30 days)	>Day 10, timing unclear, OR <day 1 with recent heparin 31–100 days	Platelet count fall <day 4 (without recent heparin exposure)
Thrombosis or other sequelae	New thrombosis OR skin necrosis; post-heparin bolus acute systemic reaction	Progressive OR recurrent thrombosis; erythematous skin lesions; suspected thrombosis – not confirmed	None
Other cause for thrombocytopenia	None apparent	Possible	Definite

What is the mortality rate associated with HITT?

Left untreated, HITT has a mortality rate as high as 20%. However, with early diagnosis and appropriate management, these rates can fall to less than 2%.

When can heparin be given after an acute episode of HITT?

Usually after approximately 100 days following an acute episode, the patient can be re-exposed to heparin in certain circumstances (e.g. cardiovascular surgery) as enough time should have been given for the antibodies to disappear.

Jackie remains haemodynamically stable, sedated and mechanically ventilated with good gas exchange and is receiving empirical treatment for presumed meningoencephalitis. The nurse at the bedside asks you whether you think the platelets are low due to sepsis.

By what mechanisms does sepsis cause thrombocytopenia?

In the presence of sepsis, the platelet count can be reduced:

- By bone marrow suppression
- As part of DIC
- By an increase in platelet destruction
- By platelet consumption not related to DIC.

Effectively managing and treating the cause of sepsis will permit the thrombocytopenia to resolve.

What is DIC?

DIC is a relatively common entity that occurs in up to 19% of ICU patients, usually because of sepsis. It is also known as consumptive coagulopathy and defibrination. It is a systemic process that can potentially cause both thrombosis and haemorrhage. Identifying and correctly treating the underlying cause are essential in the management of DIC as it never occurs in isolation. The basic pathophysiological mechanism involves the release of procoagulant substances (e.g. tissue factor) into the circulation that then trigger the systemic activation of the coagulation system and platelets.

What are the laboratory abnormalities that can occur in DIC?

The basic principles behind these coagulation abnormalities are that in an acute, untreated DIC, coagulation factors are consumed faster than the liver can replace them, and platelets are also consumed at a faster rate than the bone marrow megakaryocytes can release them. This results in:

- Prolonged prothrombin (PT) time/increased international normalised ratio (INR)
- Prolonged activated partial thromboplastin time (aPTT)
- Prolonged thrombin time (TT)
- Thrombocytopenia
- Increased fibrin degradation products (FDPs) from the increased activity of plasmin digesting fibrin (and fibrinogen), which can be measured using a D-dimer assay
- Hypofibrinogenaemia
- Microangiopathic haemolytic anaemia (MAHA) as evidenced by observing schistocytes (fragmented red blood cells) on a peripheral blood smear.

Jackie is low risk for HIT using the 4T score (she has had no heparin exposure in the last 100 days), so testing for anti-PR4 antibodies is not warranted at this point. You ring the laboratory technician to ask about the blood film that is pending, and they inform you that it shows schistocytes. The technician has also run a pre-emptive indirect bilirubin test that comes back at 41 µmol/L.

What other blood tests could be run on the samples already sent at this point?

Request a lactate dehydrogenase (LDH) to be added, along with a Coombs test, fibrinogen level and D-dimer assay. In this case, the blood film has suggested the presence of a MAHA given the presence of fragmented RBCs in the form of schistocytes.

What does the indirect bilirubin result represent?

The liver is responsible for the metabolism of bilirubin and the production of bile. Most of the bilirubin within the blood is formed from the breakdown of haem and is mostly in the unconjugated form. This unconjugated or 'indirect' form is non-water soluble, and so is bound to albumin in the blood and is not excreted in the urine. Therefore, any increase in the breakdown of haem and rise in the indirect form of bilirubin (as evidenced by this result) may point to causes such as haemolysis.

What is the purpose behind ordering a Coombs test?

Immune-mediated destruction of red blood cells is one of the most common causes of acquired haemolytic anaemia. The antibodies responsible for these reactions are divided into *warm* agglutinins (IgG antibodies that can react at body temperature) and *cold* agglutinins (IgM antibodies that react at temperatures below that of the core body temperature). The test can be subdivided into a direct and indirect test as follows:

- *Direct Coombs test or direct antiglobulin test (DAT)* is used to detect the presence of warm agglutinins. Patient RBCs are prepared and directly exposed to antiserum or monoclonal antibodies against various immunoglobulins. When performed correctly, over 99% of patients with warm agglutinin autoimmune haemolytic anaemia will be identified.
- *Indirect Coombs test or indirect antiglobulin test (IAT)* determines if circulating antibodies are present by incubating patient serum with normal RBCs. This test tends to be used when testing blood compatibility for transfusion or for the detection of antibodies with low affinity, e.g. screening in pregnancy for antibodies that may cause haemolytic disease of the newborn.

> The laboratory technician informs you just before morning handover that the direct Coombs test is negative, D-dimer assay is <200 µg/mL, fibrinogen 3.5 g/L, and LDH 510 U/L.

How do you interpret these results?

Discussion with a haematologist would be prudent at this point. However, the negative Coombs test suggests that an autoimmune process is not present. The normal D-dimer assay suggests that FDPs are not present at pathological levels, and therefore in conjunction with her normal coagulation profile and fibrinogen level, this makes the likelihood of DIC very low. This level of LDH is very high and most probably points to haemolysis in this patient.

Considering the haematology results, what are the most likely causes for her thrombocytopenia?

The severe thrombocytopenia, evidence for MAHA, negative Coombs test, elevated LDH, organ dysfunction (e.g. renal impairment) and normal coagulation profile strongly suggest that a thrombotic microangiopathy (TMA) is present.

What is thrombotic microangiopathy?

TMA is a group of disorders characterised by:

- Thrombocytopenia
- MAHA
- Evidence of haemolysis and microvascular thrombosis

They include:

- Thrombotic thrombocytopenic purpura (acquired or hereditary)
- Shiga toxin-mediated HUS
- Drug-induced TMA (e.g. quinine, tacrolimus)
- Syndromes complicating bone marrow transplantation, vasculitis and pregnancy

What is HUS?

This syndrome most commonly affects children and older adults and is usually the result of a preceding infection by *E. coli* O157:H7, which itself can cause severe disease. *E. coli* containing the genes encoding for Shiga toxins 1 and/or 2 are important human pathogens. Referred to as Shiga toxin-producing *E. coli* (STEC), those strains that produce Shiga toxin 2 are considered more virulent than those producing Shiga toxin 1, with the former much more likely to be associated with HUS and painful diarrhoea that becomes bloody.

HUS usually occurs between 5 and 13 days after the onset of diarrhoea and is characterised by:

- Acute renal failure
- MAHA
- Thrombocytopenia.

If these features are present, then a high index of suspicion is needed because STEC can cause severe illness. However, the absence of abdominal pain, greater than 1 week presentation of bloody diarrhoea, microcytic anaemia, weight loss and a fever (>38.5 °C measured in hospital) are some of the features that *decrease* the likelihood for STEC infection.

An atypical HUS (aHUS) can also occur and is due to genetic defects that result in antibodies directed against complement regulatory proteins or chronic complement activation. Managing these cases is challenging and requires specialist intervention.

How is HUS treated?

There is no specific treatment for HUS and it largely remains primarily supportive. ADAMTS13 levels (discussed later in this case) are reported to be normal in HUS and plasma exchange or infusion has not been shown to improve outcome. Patients with HUS may require renal supportive therapy at some point. However, these is no evidence that early dialysis affects clinical outcome. In aHUS, the use of eculizumab (a monoclonal antibody that inhibits terminal complement activation at the C5 protein) has efficacy in resolving aHUS and preserving or improving renal function. It is also used in patients presenting with severe CNS involvement.

> After reviewing the admission clerking and notes from the medical team, you conclude that Jackie had no preceding symptoms of severe abdominal pain or diarrhoea, thus suggesting that STEC is unlikely.

What is thrombotic thrombocytopenic purpura?

Thrombotic thrombocytopenic purpura is a very rare disorder, with an estimated incidence of 6 cases per million in the overall population. Due to the use of plasma exchange, patients rarely progress to present with the complete classic 'pentad' of:

- MAHA
- Thrombocytopenia
- Acute renal failure
- Fever
- Severe neurological symptoms.

Most patients today tend to present with only haemolytic anaemia and thrombocytopenia. Commencing treatment with plasma exchange is urgent. With this modern therapy, the mortality from TTP is approximately 10–20%. However, left untreated, TTP has a mortality of 90% within 3 months.

What causes TTP?

Both the inherited and acquired forms of TTP result from deficiencies or antibodies to a metalloproteinase identified as ADAMTS13 (**a d**isintegrin-like **and m**etalloprotease with **t**hrombo**s**pondin type 1 motif, member 13). The purpose of ADAMTS13 is to cleave the 'ultra-large' multimers of von Willebrand factor (vWF) produced by endothelial cells. If these 'ultra-large' multimers of vWF persist then they can promote platelet aggregation and adhesion. The level of ADAMTS13 and antibodies against it can be detected using assays. ADAMTS13 levels that are less than 5–10% are associated with TTP. Basing the diagnosis solely on the result of an ADAMTS13 activity level is *not* recommended as this test and its results may not be readily or immediately available, especially if the samples need to be sent to other centres to be completed.

What scoring systems do you know that can predict the likelihood of ADAMTS13 activity of less than 10%?

The PLASMIC score is used in hospitalised adult patients with suspected TTP who might benefit from early initiation of plasma exchange while ADAMTS13 activity results are pending (Table 23.3). It should not, however, be used in patients who have already undergone plasma exchange.

Table 23.3: PLASMIC score.

		0 points	1 point
Platelet count	<30×10⁹/L	No	Yes
Haemo**L**ysis	Reticulocyte count >2.5%, haptoglobin undetectable, or indirect bilirubin >34.2 µmol/L	No	Yes
Active cancer	Treated for cancer within the past 12 months	Yes	No
History of **S**olid-organ or stem cell transplant	–	Yes	No
MCV	<9.0 × 10⁻¹⁴ L (<90 fL)	No	Yes
INR	<1.5	No	Yes
Creatinine	<176.8 µmol/L	No	Yes

INR, international normalised ratio; MCV, mean corpuscular volume.

A high PLASMIC score (6–7) is 91% sensitive for predicting ADAMTS13 activity of less than 10% and is superior to clinical judgement. Furthermore, a low score (0–4) suggests that ADAMTS13 activity is not less than 10% with a specificity approaching 99% and an alternative diagnosis should be considered.

Jackie has a PLASMIC score of 7, placing her at high risk for an ADAMTS13 activity of less than 10%. With this score, expert consultation should be obtained, and treatment begun for TTP.

Briefly describe the treatment for TTP

The mainstay of treatment for TTP is plasma exchange (PEX) in an environment with expertise in its management. The best response is seen in TTP associated with antibodies against ADAMTS13. Treatment is continued until platelet counts return to normal levels or an alternative diagnosis is established. In addition, glucocorticoids and rituximab (a monoclonal antibody directed against CD20) should be given to patients with a presumptive diagnosis of TTP. The anti-vWF antibody caplacizumab should also be considered for patients who present with severe features of TTP (e.g. seizures, confusion, coma, encephalopathy). These treatment decisions will fall under the remit of an expert familiar with the management of TTP.

Briefly describe plasma exchange therapy (PEX)

As the name suggests, plasma exchange involves removing, separating and then replacing the patient's plasma with the required replacement solution to treat the underlying problem. Plasma exchange using filtration methods can be found on renal dialysis machines that utilise a semipermeable membrane with pores up to 0.2 µm in diameter. This allows for substances up to 3×10^6 Da to be exchanged, such as immune complexes, complement factors and immunoglobulins. Venous

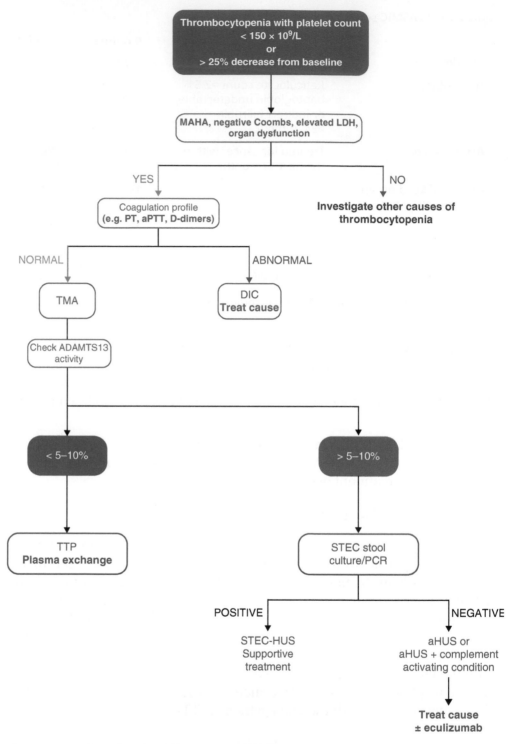

Figure 23.1: Algorithm for differentiating DIC from TTP and HUS in critical care.

Source: Vincent, J.-L. et al. 2018/Springer Nature/Public Domain CC BY 4.0.

access for the procedure would ideally be central, such as a VasCath™ or a tunnelled line (e.g. permacath or Hickman® line). Regional anticoagulation for the circuit is like that for haemofiltration methods, such as the use of citrate, with similar problems that need monitoring. In the case of TTP, the replacement fluid should obviously contain the ADAMTS13 enzyme and functional vWF.

At morning handover, you inform the team that Jackie has remained stable, and you present the results of the tests you carried out overnight and suggest the diagnosis of TTP and consideration for requesting an ADAMTS13 assay (as outlined in Figure 23.1). On returning in the evening to start your last night shift, the day consultant tells you that Jackie was transferred to a specialist centre to begin plasma exchange for the presumptive diagnosis of TTP and congratulates you on a 'great pick-up'. Later, in the night shift, you're called to review one of the other patients on the unit who also has thrombocytopenia, and you smile inwardly to yourself.

Further reading

- Thachil, J. and Warkentin, T. (2016). How do we approach thrombocytopenia in critically ill patients? *Br. J. Haematol.* 177: 27–38. Comprehensive review that provides practical pointers and discusses the mechanisms of thrombocytopenia in critical care.
- Brocklebank, V., Wood, K., and Kavanagh, D. (2018). Thrombotic microangiopathy and the kidney. *Clin. J. Am. Soc. Nephrol.* 13: 300–317. In-depth review of thrombotic microangiopathies and a pragmatic approach to its diagnosis and management.

24 The Patient with COVID-19

The writing of this book was interrupted by the SARS-CoV-2 (COVID-19) pandemic. It was arguably the most challenging period for intensive care in living memory and this book would feel incomplete without including a case dealing with the issues raised.

This case is set at a time towards the latter half of 2021, when the pandemic was well established and far from over – it is likely that further developments will have occurred in both public health management strategies and research into COVID-19 by the time this book is published.

Various terminology developed locally around the time of the pandemic. One example is the naming of infected or quarantine areas. For instance, many centres used a colour coding system (e.g. red, green, blue). For the purposes of this book, a 'hot' area is a zone where patients with definite or suspected COVID-19 are being managed. A 'cold' area is a zone where the likelihood of COVID infection is minimal.

You are the registrar on call for intensive care when you asked to review a 45-year-old man with respiratory distress in 'hot' resus in the ED. The patient, Jonathan, is obese and takes amlodipine for hypertension but is otherwise fit. He works full time as a bouncer at a night club and has a wife and two small children. When you arrive, the nurse in resus directs you to the personal protective equipment (PPE) with a selection of facemasks and hoods. Jonathan's rapid PCR test for COVID-19 is positive.

What is PPE and what are its main characteristics?

PPE is equipment that is used to prevent or minimise exposure to biological, chemical, radiological, electrical and mechanical hazards (e.g. masks, respirators, gowns, coveralls, goggles, faceshields, visors, boots). In the absence of PPE, exposure to these hazards could lead to injuries and illnesses. PPE protects healthcare workers from radiation and biological agents (e.g. viruses, bacteria). The main characteristics of PPE are described in Table 24.1.

Clinical Cases in Critical Care, First Edition. Alice Myers and Theophilus Samuels.
© 2023 John Wiley & Sons Ltd. Published 2023 by John Wiley & Sons Ltd.

Table 24.1: Characteristics of personal protective equipment (PPE).

Category	Characteristic
Design feature	Protect mucous membranes Minimise the number of PPE element junctions Provide unobstructed range of vision Enable communication capability Use human factors design for size and comfort
Material performance	Able to protect for the duration of the work period Able to withstand repeated disinfection Manufacture packaging to withstand tropical climate exposure
Use desirability	Standardise donning and doffing protocol with minimum steps Dispose PPE in non-toxic and environmentally friendly manner

What is meant by the term 'air-borne disease' and what methods can be used to reduce transmission?

The World Health Organization (WHO) defines air-borne particles as aerosols ($<5\,\mu$m diameter) and droplets ($>5\,\mu$m diameter).

- Aerosols can remain suspended in air and travel longer distances than droplets.
- Droplets are typically confined to around 1 m from the source and cannot remain suspended in air.

Methods used to reduce air-borne transmission include the following:

- Social distancing, quarantine and isolation.
- Hand hygiene to reduce contamination secondary to droplet spread (WHO 5 moments of hand hygiene).
- Medical gloves.
- Surgical masks – these are defined as 'masks that are flat or pleated and are affixed to the head with straps'.
- Respirators – these can be divided into either air supplying or air purifying, with the latter being further subdivided into powered (powered air-purifying respirators or PAPR) or non-powered. Since air-supplying and air-purifying respirators are expensive, limited and require appropriate training in wearing, it is non-powered respirators that are recommended for use in healthcare. N95 is a non-powered respirator that has a filtration efficiency of ≥95%. FFP2 and FFP3 are non-powered respirators that have filtration efficiencies of ≥94% and ≥99% respectively. The FFP2 mask is a standard respirator and the FFP3 mask is used where high filtration is required.
- Vaccination programmes.

You choose an FFP3 mask and don your PPE. On review, Jonathan has a respiratory rate of 45 breaths per minute, oxygen saturations of 88% on 15 L O_2 via a non-rebreathe mask and a blood pressure of 155/85 mmHg. He looks scared but can speak to you in full sentences. He tells you that he has not been vaccinated against COVID-19 as he didn't get round to it when the vaccine was offered. Arterial blood gas shows PaO_2 8.5 kPa, $PaCO_2$ 3.5 kPa, pH 7.40, lactate 0.5 mmol/L, base excess −1.5 mmol/L. The ED team are already setting up high-flow nasal oxygen.

Can you summarise your main concerns?

Severe respiratory distress in a young, unvaccinated person with risk factors and confirmed COVID-19. Jonathan is at high risk of deterioration and respiratory arrest.

What is COVID-19?

COVID-19 is the third documented spillover to humans of an animal coronavirus in only two decades. It was first described in Wuhan, China. The Coronaviridae Study Group (CSG) of the International Committee on Taxonomy of Viruses recognised the virus causing COVID-19 as sharing a common viral ancestor with that which caused the SARS pandemic in 2002. They designated this virus as SARS-CoV-2. In virology terms, SARS-CoV-2 is a sister clade to the prototype human and bat severe acute respiratory syndrome viruses (SARS-CoVs) of the species severe acute respiratory syndrome-related coronavirus.

At the time of writing, most individuals infected with SARS-CoV-2 will experience mild to moderate respiratory illness and recover without the need for hospitalisation or specialist treatment. Patients with underlying medical conditions (e.g. cardiac disease, respiratory disease, diabetes, cancer, immunosuppression) are more likely to develop serious disease. However, any individual, at any age, can become seriously ill and die from COVID-19.

Do you want the ED registrar to continue setting up high-flow nasal oxygen (HFNO)?

Yes. The use of HFNO over conventional oxygen therapy is widely recommended for acute hypoxaemic respiratory failure in patients with COVID-19 (weak recommendation). There is still ongoing debate regarding which non-invasive technique is optimal. HFNO or NIV devices such as BIPAP, facemask CPAP or even helmet CPAP (H-CPAP) can all be considered at this stage. H-CPAP has the least amount of particle dispersion and air contamination of those listed, but challenges to its use include noise, possible claustrophobia experienced by the patient, armpit and neck skin breakdown, and availability of equipment and education in its proper use and set-up. HFNO has the benefits of being easily set up and well tolerated by the patient.

What other management strategies should you be considering at this stage to improve his oxygenation?

A recent systematic review suggested that awake prone positioning (APP), i.e. lying on your front, was associated with an improvement of oxygenation but did not reduce the rate of intubation in patients developing acute respiratory failure due to COVID-19. Unfortunately, APP can be impractical for obese patients needing full facemask CPAP so this relatively simple yet effective manoeuvre is sometimes not possible.

The ED registrar gets Jonathan to wear the HFNO (60 L/min flow rate and 80% O_2) and lie on his front. He seems to be tolerating it well and his oxygen saturations immediately improve to 99%. You decide to give Jonathan an hour or so in this position and see whether he is improving enough to avoid intubation.

What else do you need to consider at this point?

- *Prepare for intubation and ventilation* – begin preparing drugs and ensure your support team is aware and available to assist. This is especially important considering that this may be a part of the hospital that has only recently been converted to receive 'hot' resus patients. The environment may be unfamiliar and the medications and equipment needed may not be immediately available (e.g. a fridge storing muscle relaxants).
- *Bedside imaging* – consider performing focused lung ultrasonography and echocardiography. A chest radiograph would be desirable.
- *Blood tests* – ensure that appropriate tests for a patient severely unwell with COVID-19 have been requested, e.g. FBC, WBC, LFTs, CRP, INR, troponin, procalcitonin, D-dimer, LDH, ferritin, etc. Consult your local hospital policy for guidance.
- *Anticoagulation* – the increased thrombotic risk associated with COVID-19 requires venous thromboembolism (VTE) prophylaxis in all hospitalised patients in the absence of contraindications. At the time of writing, NICE guidance is to use standard prophylactic low molecular weight heparin as soon as possible, and within 14 hours of admission, with the usual adjustments for BMI and other risk factors.
- *Steroids* – the Randomised Evaluation of COVID-19 Therapy Trial (RECOVERY) demonstrated that in patients hospitalised with COVID-19, the use of dexamethasone (6 mg for 10 days) lowered the risk of death at 28 days in patients receiving either invasive mechanical ventilation or oxygen alone, but not in patients receiving no respiratory support.
- *Consultant intensivist discussion* – discussing management and the need to admit the patient to critical care should be done as early as possible with the consultant. During a pandemic, the ICU may be over capacity and therefore unable to take this patient, so escalating early will allow for him to be accommodated locally or potentially transferred to another hospital if necessary.

■ *Respiratory consultant review* – if Jonathan improves with the current management strategy, he may be suitable for ongoing management in a respiratory ward area.

■ *Next of kin* – ask Jonathan if he wants his next of kin informed about his situation and offer him the chance to speak to them himself. It is worth remembering that any conversation with next of kin would most probably take place over the telephone (due to quarantine) and that communicating while wearing PPE can prove difficult. It may be best to doff and leave the 'hot' area to have this discussion.

■ *Trial recruitment* – many clinical trials were rapidly deployed during the pandemic to determine effective treatment and management strategies against COVID-19. Jonathan will most probably be recruitable into one of these trials.

What are the radiological changes in COVID-19?

Chest imaging findings of COVID-19 can mimic or overlap those of other infections and disorders (e.g. SARS, MERS, influenza A, H1N1, drug reactions and connective tissue diseases). In addition, *normal* chest radiography and CT imaging do not reliably exclude COVID-19 in the earliest stages of infection.

■ *Chest radiography* – findings vary and can range from normal in the early stages of the disease to unilateral or bilateral lung opacities, sometimes with a basilar or peripheral distribution. Bilateral lower zone consolidation peaks at 10–12 days from symptom onset.

■ *Chest CT* – typically, CT imaging demonstrates bilateral peripheral ground glass opacities (GGO) with a lower lung distribution, sometimes with areas of consolidation, which may be nodular or mass-like. The peak stage for CT changes occurs between 9 and 13 days and features more extensive consolidation, paralleling the evolution of acute lung injury. Less common CT findings include:
  ■ Lobar or segmental consolidation without GGOs
  ■ Discrete small pulmonary nodules
  ■ Pulmonary cavitation
  ■ Septal thickening
  ■ Pneumothorax
  ■ Pleural effusion.

The incidence of barotrauma has been reported to be higher in patients with COVID-19 compared to patients with other causes of acute respiratory distress syndrome (24% vs 11%) receiving mechanical ventilation.

After 90 minutes in the prone position with HFNO (60 L/min flow, 0.5 FiO$_2$), Jonathan's respiratory rate has reduced to 28–30 breaths per minute and his saturations are 96%. He receives dexamethasone and subcutaneous enoxaparin. After 2 further hours in ED with the same management, it has not been possible to wean the HFNO any further. His respiratory rate is now 25–35 per minute and he is beginning to find lying prone uncomfortable. The ED team ask whether you are going to admit to critical care or not.

What is your decision? Give your reasoning

Although many respiratory wards are excellent and able to manage patients with HFNO, early admission to critical care could be prudent. Jonathan is still requiring significant support from the HFNO and his trajectory is no longer clearly that of improvement (his RR has increased). There are signs that he may not tolerate prone positioning for much longer. He is young and could deteriorate quickly. Also, since he is obese, his airway may be difficult and it would be preferable to manage him in a critical care environment.

> You call the ICU consultant to say you want to admit Jonathan. The unit is currently full, but they can organise an interhospital transfer for a more stable patient to admit Jonathan.

What are the main strategic considerations for pandemic planning in critical care units?

Epidemiology and history tell us that pandemics are a constant threat. Examples include the Spanish flu in 1918, H1N1 in 2009 and COVID-19. A dramatic increase in the number of patients requiring Level 2 or 3 beds can lead to national directives to escalate and expand critical care services with minimal notice. The details of how this is accomplished are beyond the scope of this book. However, an overview of resource management can be considered in three categories as per the US Centers for Disease Control and Prevention (CDC):

- *Space* – opening temporary new critical care units, increasing isolation bay availability and cohorting infected bays of patients. Interhospital transfers may be required to spread the workload intensity across critical care networks. This may be referred to as 'mutual aid'. The most stable patients should be selected for transfer.
- *Staff* – nursing and medical staff may need to work emergency rotas, supplementary staff may be drafted from other specialties, volunteer staff organisation.
- *Stuff* – increased use of consumables (e.g. ventilator tubing, haemofiltration sets, etc.), need for more hardware such as ventilators and monitors, etc., PPE and increased demand for drugs including sedatives, steroids, antibiotics, etc.

What are the impacts of a pandemic on the delivery of routine healthcare?

Staff
- Absences due to burnout and sickness.
- Increased stress associated with overburdened responsibilities at work (e.g. caring for more patients than usual).
- Working in unfamiliar conditions (e.g. ward nurse working in critical care).

Ethical issues

- When to stop elective work to facilitate emergency care demands.
- Decisions related to who is the most deserving (e.g. cancer surgery).
- Triaging patients requiring certain services (e.g. resource-limited critical care units).

You transfer Jonathan to critical care.

What do you do for him in critical care?

Monitoring

- Arterial line.
- Urinary catheter.

Medications

- Analgesia for pain if preventing prone position.
- Regular anticoagulation and steroids as per NICE guidance for COVID-19.

Communication

- Update patient and discuss with next of kin via telephone or video call. Explain quarantine measures and restrictions on visiting.
- Establish a plan with parameters to guide when to consider intubation. This is extremely difficult in practice since patients with COVID-19 often experience 'happy hypoxia' so the signs of respiratory distress can be easily missed in these patients. Consider asking the nurse to request the doctor to review Jonathan if, for example, his RR is greater than 30, his FiO_2 is greater than 0.6 and rising, and his oxygen saturations are less than 92%. There is no strong evidence for when intubation should occur, and clinical judgement is always required.

What other pharmacological treatments may be of use in COVID-19?

At the time of writing, in addition to those already discussed, other pharmacological treatments include the following:

- *Tocilizumab* – a monoclonal antibody that inhibits both membrane-bound and soluble interleukin-6 receptors and is used to treat inflammatory conditions (e.g. rheumatoid arthritis).
- *Sarilumab* – the same class of drug as tocilizumab, this monoclonal antibody is recommended if tocilizumab cannot be used or is unavailable.
- *Casirivimab and imdevimab* – these are two recombinant human IgG1 monoclonal antibodies that bind non-competitively to

non-overlapping epitopes of the spike protein receptor-binding domain of SARS-CoV-2, thereby preventing the entry of the virus into host cells.

■ *Remdesivir* – this is an inhibitor of the viral RNA-dependent, RNA polymerase, that has demonstrated activity against SARS-CoV-2.

After admitting Jonathan to ICU and, at his request, speaking with his wife on the phone, you finish your shift pleased that he looks more stable.

When you return to work in the morning you find that Jonathan was intubated overnight. He refused to lie prone, his respiratory rate increased to greater than 40 breaths per minute and he was desaturating down to 80%, despite HFNO.

Jonathan is now sedated with propofol and fentanyl. He is paralysed with a rocuronium infusion. He was placed in the prone position at 05:00 am. His ventilator is set to deliver 25 breaths/minute, P_{high} 35 cmH$_2$O, $P_{plateau}$ 32 cmH$_2$O, PEEP 14 cmH$_2$O (resulting tidal volume 290 mL) with FiO$_2$ 0.9. His PaO$_2$ is 10.2 kPa, PaCO$_2$ 11.4 kPa, base excess −5 mmol/L, pH 7.08, lactate 3.4 mmol/L. He does not require cardiovascular support. His morning blood test results are not yet available.

Interpret the ventilator flow–time curve labelled A (Figure 24.1)

This flow–time curve demonstrates breath stacking. This is seen when too short an expiratory time has been set, which commonly occurs when an underlying disease prolongs the expiratory time constant, e.g. chronic obstructive pulmonary disease (COPD) and severe asthma. In these patients and others with airflow obstruction, lung emptying is slowed, and expiration is interrupted by the next programmed inspiration before the patient's lungs can reach their static equilibrium volume.

Dynamic pulmonary hyperinflation is affected by expiratory time, resistance and compliance of the lung, and tidal volume. In the presence of dynamic pulmonary hyperinflation, inside the alveoli, the average end-expiratory pressure is higher than the PEEP applied by the ventilator. The difference between the two corresponds to auto-PEEP.

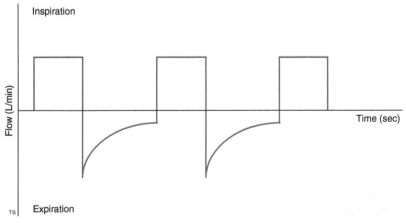

Figure 24.1: Flow-time curve A.

Source: Theophilus Samuels.

What are the potential problems associated with the flow-time curve in Figure 24.1?

Breath stacking can lead to:

- Barotrauma
- Increased work of breathing
- Difficulty triggering the ventilator
- Haemodynamic instability
- Failure to wean from mechanical ventilation.

What driving pressure is being used here? What are your concerns about this?

Driving pressure (DP) is essentially the tidal volume (V_T) normalised to the compliance of the lower respiratory system (C_{RS}). This ratio (V_T:C_{RS}) is used as an index to indicate the functional size of the lung, i.e. the volume of lung available for tidal ventilation. It has been demonstrated to be a better predictor of outcome in patients with ARDS than tidal volume alone. The airway pressure measured when airflow ceases at end-inspiration is referred to as the *plateau* pressure, assuming that the patient is not spontaneously breathing. The driving pressure can therefore be calculated clinically by the difference between the plateau pressure ($P_{plateau}$) and positive end-expiratory pressure (PEEP) *in patients who are not making inspiratory efforts.*

$$\Delta P = P_{plateau} - PEEP$$

In this case, the plateau pressure is measured at 32 cmH$_2$O, which gives DP equal to 32–14 = 18 cmH$_2$O. Amato et al. (2015, NEJM) demonstrated an association between higher driving pressures and increasing mortality so there may be benefit in lowering the DP as tolerated.

> You explain to your junior colleague that you are concerned about the driving pressure and breath stacking.

Draw the compliance curve and mark the lower and upper inflexion points. Use the graph to explain overdistension

Respiratory compliance is the change in respiratory system volume induced by a change in applied pressure (i.e. the inspiratory pressure). It is the mathematical inverse of elastance.

The compliance curve, as shown in Figure 24.2, demonstrates *hysteresis*, which is the difference between inspiratory and expiratory compliance.

The lower inflexion point has been interpreted as the pressure at which underventilated airways or alveoli collapse. It corresponds to the pressure at which 'best PEEP' should be set.

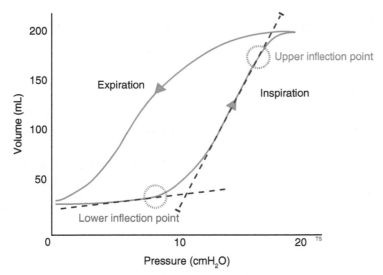

Figure 24.2: Lung compliance curve.

Source: Theophilus Samuels.

The point at which the inspiration curve loses its linearity is referred to as the *upper inflexion point* and represents the highest pressure at which no further lung recruitment occurs. Exceeding this pressure may result in stretching and overdistension. The same driving pressure at a higher PEEP may result in smaller tidal volumes where there is overdistension.

Note that the use of the pressure–ventilation curve and inflexion points in clinical decision making remains the subject of much controversy.

Discuss static respiratory compliance

By imposing a brief inspiratory hold at end-inspiration, *static* respiratory compliance can be measured in patients receiving volume-limited mechanical ventilation. As already discussed, the difference between the plateau pressure and PEEP is taken as the change in pressure (ΔP) required to deliver the tidal volume (V_T). Static system respiratory compliance (C_{RS}) is then determined by:

$$C_{RS} = \frac{V_T}{\Delta P}$$

The C_{RS} also considers the contributions from the chest wall and abdomen, therefore patients with chest wall deformities or morbid obesity have lower lung compliance even in the absence of lung abnormalities. Normal respiratory compliance is in the range of 50–70 mL/cmH$_2$O and is usually less than 30 mL/cmH$_2$O in patients with ARDS. Weaning from mechanical ventilation is often difficult or impossible to achieve when the C_{RS} is less than 20–25 mL/cmH$_2$O, because of the high work of breathing requirements.

After assessing his ventilation, you establish Jonathan on new ventilator settings: PEEP 10 cmH$_2$O, P$_{high}$ 28, RR 25 (but with an increased expiratory period to reduce gas trapping), FiO$_2$ 0.85. You ensure he is fully paralysed. On performing his 09:00 am head turn, Jonathan suddenly desaturates to <65%, he becomes difficult to ventilate, his BP drops to 55/34 and he develops a tachyarrhythmia.

What do you think could have happened?

Taking a systematic ABCDE approach:

- *Airway* – a blocked, kinked or dislodged ET tube would be an immediate concern given that the problem occurred following his head turn.
- *Breathing* – these patients are prone to mucus plugging and/or pneumothorax.
- *Circulation* – vagal stimulation and/or cardiovascular instability (especially if the patient is acidaemic +/− low intravascular volume), acute coronary event and pulmonary embolism may be possible causes.

How would you proceed?

- Call for help and/or pull the emergency bedside alarm.
- Increase FiO_2 to 1.0 (but noting that he was already on FiO_2 0.85!).
- Request the crash trolley is brought to the bedside.
- Begin manual ventilation using a Mapleson C circuit, taking care not to lose the PEEP.
- Assess the ET tube for blockage (are you able to ventilate manually? Can a suction catheter be passed?) and whether both lungs are being ventilated (has endobronchial intubation occurred or could it be a pneumothorax?).
- Ask one of the attending team members to ensure fluids and vasopressors are being given or being prepared.
- Put his head back in the original position where he was stable to see if it improves the situation.
- Get ready to urgently supinate the patient.

You can pass a suction catheter through the ETT and you stabilise his BP with 2 × 250 mL fluid boluses, 10 mL 10% calcium chloride and 1.5 mg metaraminol. You place his head back into the original position but still his saturations do not recover. You rapidly assemble a team and supinate Jonathan. You are now able to see that he has surgical emphysema throughout his anterior chest and up into his neck. The right side of his chest is not moving and the left is moving minimally.

What do you do next?

This is consistent with a tension pneumothorax, and he requires an emergency needle decompression. It is worth remembering that needle decompression may not be successful due to his body habitus and the presence of surgical emphysema and so alternative measures may be required, such as a finger decompression. Following needle or finger decompression, the tension pneumothorax is converted into a simple pneumothorax and subsequent intercostal drain insertion (tube thoracostomy) is mandatory.

You successfully insert a chest drain on the right-hand side and Jonathan's saturations very slowly recover to the mid-80s and he becomes more cardio-stable. His PaO_2 is 8 kPa on FiO_2 1.0, his $PaCO_2$ is 10.5 kPa with ventilator settings as above. Your consultant is reviewing another COVID-19 patient in a different part of the hospital – you phone her at this point.

What would you discuss with your consultant?

- Ask your consultant to return as urgently as possible.
- Explain the situation and inform her of what you have managed to do, but that the patient remains in a precarious situation with no room for further deterioration.
- Discuss making a referral for extracorporeal membrane oxygenation (ECMO), as Jonathan is not stable enough to be placed back into the prone position, and not suitable for APRV due to the pneumothorax.
- Request a chest radiograph.

You refer for ECMO and Jonathan is accepted. The team arrive 2 hours later, stabilise him with ECMO on site and transfer him to their centre for ongoing management. Three weeks later you receive a call to say that Jonathan has progressed well and is ready for transfer back to you.

Further reading

- Amato, M., Meade, M., Slutsky, A. et al. (2015). Driving pressure and survival in the acute respiratory distress syndrome. *N. Engl. J. Med.* 372: 747–755. Landmark paper.
- Randomised Evaluation of COVID-19 Therapy. www.recoverytrial.net. Excellent online resource for the results of the interventions used in the RECOVERY trial.
- A Randomised, Embedded, Multi-factorial, Adaptive Platform Trial for Community-Acquired Pneumonia. www.remapcap.org. Outstanding online resource for the REMAP-CAP platform summarising key findings.
- COVID-19 rapid guideline. www.nice.org.uk/guidance/ng19. Constantly updated NICE UK COVID-19 rapid guideline.

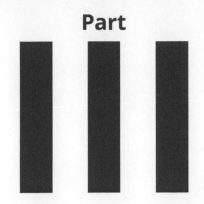

Part III

Test Yourself

MCQs

Multiple Choice Questions

Mark each option (A–E) as true or false

1. **Which of the following are true of drowning?**

   A) Most cases of drowning are described as 'dry drowning'
   B) Pneumonia is common in cases of non-fatal drowning
   C) Salt water, and not fresh water, destroys surfactant
   D) The diving reflex occurs in tropical water and is protective
   E) Cerebral oxygen consumption is reduced by approximately 1% for each reduction of 1 °C in temperature within the range of 37 °C to 20 °C

2. **With regard to myasthenia gravis:**

   A) Osserman grade III disease affects the eyes only
   B) In microelectrode studies, frequency is normal but miniature endplate potential is reduced
   C) The disease is limited to only bulbar muscles in around 15–20%
   D) Insufficient medication can lead to cholinergic crisis
   E) There is loss of the deep tendon reflexes

3. **Regarding 10mg of prednisolone:**

   A) 10 mg of prednisolone is equivalent to 8 mg methylprednisolone
   B) If taken daily for six months, does not require steroid replacement perioperatively for major elective surgery
   C) This is the correct dose to treat myasthenia gravis
   D) This is equivalent to 60 mg hydrocortisone
   E) Was shown to demonstrate no survival benefit to adult patients in severe septic shock in the CORTICUS trial (NEJM 2008)

Clinical Cases in Critical Care, First Edition. Alice Myers and Theophilus Samuels.
© 2023 John Wiley & Sons Ltd. Published 2023 by John Wiley & Sons Ltd.

4. **The following are true of lactate:**

A) Lactate is converted to pyruvate and back to glucose in the Cori cycle
B) Lactate is eliminated via the liver only
C) Type B lactic acidosis is secondary to tissue hypoxia
D) All seizures typically cause a rise in lactate
E) L-lactic acidosis is associated with short bowel syndrome

5. **Regarding an intra-aortic balloon pump (IABP):**

A) It is sited within the aorta in order to improve coronary perfusion during systole
B) A combination of helium and oxygen is used to inflate the balloon
C) It can be triggered using the arterial waveform
D) It should be removed when the ratio of IABP-supported heartbeat to unassisted heartbeat is 1:2
E) Severe mitral stenosis is an absolute contraindication

6. **Haemolytic uraemic syndrome (HUS):**

A) Is defined by the simultaneous occurrence of non-immune haemolytic anaemia, acute renal failure and thrombocytopenia
B) Most cases are associated with viral infections
C) Young children (<5 years) are less likely to develop HUS
D) The presence of neurological symptoms is associated with a worse outcome
E) Atypical HUS (aHUS) is associated with an underlying dysregulation of the alternative complement pathway

7. **Cerebrospinal fluid:**

A) Is produced at a rate of 0.3–0.4 mL/min by the choroid plexus
B) Normally has a protein level of 200–400 mg/L
C) Is absorbed into the arachnoid villi
D) Has high specific gravity
E) CSF production is independent of cerebral perfusion pressure

8. **Glucagon:**

A) Release is stimulated by a rise in blood glucose concentration
B) This hormone is released by the beta cells of the islets of Langerhans
C) In order to raise the blood concentration of glucose by 20 mg/100 mL of blood, 1 mg/kg of glucagon needs to be administered
D) Causes both gluconeogenesis and glycogenolysis
E) Inhibits adipose cell lipase

9. **In water homeostasis:**

   A) Arginine vasopressin (AVP) is produced in the anterior pituitary gland
   B) The most dominating regulating factor affecting water excretion is AVP
   C) AVP binds to vasopressin-2 (V-2) receptors located on the basolateral membranes of the renal epithelial cells lining the ascending loop of Henle
   D) AVP release can be influenced by hypoglycaemia
   E) The normal plasma osmolality is tightly regulated to remain within 275–285 mOsm/L

10. **Regarding the arterial circulation of the brain:**

    A) It utilises approximately 3–5 mL O_2/min per 100 g of tissue
    B) The internal carotid arteries divide into the anterior and middle cerebral arteries (creating the anterior cerebral circulation), and overall provide approximately 30% of the total cerebral circulation
    C) Cerebral perfusion pressure (CPP) can be directly measured easily and accurately
    D) Local myogenic responses of the vessel wall in response to changes in intra-arterial pressure maintain constant blood flow over a wide range of CPP
    E) In patients with chronic hypertension, CPP autoregulation is unaffected

11. **Regarding pacemakers:**

    A) A three-letter code is used to describe the functions of a pacemaker device
    B) The first three letters describe the antibradycardia functions
    C) The fourth letter describes the programmability of rate responsiveness
    D) They can carry one classification (e.g. DDD) and are capable of only one mode of function
    E) The *lower rate-limiting interval* is the time between two consecutive paced beats

12. **Electrolytes:**

    A) Are chemical compounds in solution that dissociate to form ions
    B) Sodium (Na^+) accounts for nearly 85% of the extracellular fluid osmolality
    C) Intracellular Na^+ concentrations can vary between different tissues, and range from 3 to 40 mmol/
    D) Potassium (K^+) is the principal intracellular anion
    E) About 90% of the total body potassium (K^+) is intracellular

13. **The following form part of the management of bradycardia according to the UK Resuscitation Council Guidelines (RCUK):**

A) Syncope and heart failure are life-threatening signs
B) Atropine 500 mcg IV is recommended in the presence of life-threatening signs, repeated up to a maximum of 5 mg
C) Isoprenaline 5 mcg/min IV can be used as an interim measure until expert help is available
D) A ventricular pause of > 5 seconds is a risk factor for asystole
E) Glucagon can be considered in bradycardia associated with beta-blocker overdose

14. **In sepsis:**

A) Pathogen-associated molecular patterns (PAMPs) include bacterial, fungal and viral pathogens such as endotoxin and beta-glucan
B) High mobility group box 1 (HMGB 1) is an intracellular protein that is released upon cell necrosis
C) Pyroptosis refers to the destruction of cells caused by heat
D) Following activation of the innate immune system by PAMPs and DAMPs, transcription of type I interferons and proinflammatory cytokines (e.g. TNF-alpha, interleukin IL-1 and IL-6) is increased
E) The cytokines IL-1-beta and IL-18 can trigger pyroptosis

15. **Regarding stroke:**

A) Diffusion-weighted imaging (DWI) MRI scans cannot be used to detect acute cerebral ischaemia within six hours of symptom onset
B) DWI is not able to discriminate between seizure alone and new stroke in a patient with prior stroke who has had a seizure
C) Magnetic resonance angiography (MRA) is more sensitive than computed tomographic angiography (CTA) in studying intracranial vessels
D) Thrombolysis with alteplase 3–4.5 hours after acute ischaemic stroke significantly improves clinical outcomes
E) Transient ischaemic attacks (TIAs) rarely last for less than one hour

16. **Regarding hepatitis:**

A) Hepatitis is defined as inflammation of the liver, and can be divided into infectious and non-infectious causes
B) A rise in alkaline phosphatase (ALP) is more significant than increases in alkaline aminotransferase (ALT) and aspartate aminotransferase (AST)
C) Hepatitis C is a blood-borne DNA virus
D) Around 70–85% of people infected with hepatitis C will go on to have chronic infection
E) Cirrhotic ascites carries a three-year mortality of 10%

17. **Regarding hepatopulmonary syndrome (HPS):**

    A) HPS is commonly associated with cirrhosis and portal hypertension
    B) HPS-induced shortness of breath is often relieved with the patient standing up
    C) Exhaled nitric oxide (NO) levels are decreased in patients with cirrhosis compared to healthy individuals
    D) Mortality is usually from primary respiratory failure
    E) Liver transplantation is the only effective therapy and improves or resolves HPS in most cases

18. **When performing lung ultrasound, the following are correct:**

    A) B-lines can be a normal finding at the base of the lung
    B) A-lines are usually due to reverberation artefact
    C) The ideal transducer operates at relatively low frequency (1–5 MHz)
    D) The barcode (or stratosphere) sign is a normal finding
    E) Lung sliding is an abnormal finding

19. **Critical illness neuropathy (CIP) and myopathy (CIM):**

    A) Are associated with a prolonged requirement for mechanical ventilation and increased hospital length of stay
    B) Both share the major clinical symptoms of early muscle atrophy, muscle weakness and loss of deep tendon reflexes
    C) Failure to wean a patient from a ventilator may be the first sign of CIP/CIM
    D) CIP carries a better prognosis than CIM
    E) Sepsis and systemic inflammation, severity of disease and low blood sugar concentrations are associated risk factors

20. **Regarding the right ventricle (RV) on echocardiogram, the following are correct:**

    A) A tricuspid annulus plane systolic excursion (TAPSE) of 11 mm suggests normal systolic function
    B) The free wall thickness is normally less than 5 mm
    C) Using visual assessment, its systolic function is best assessed in the parasternal long axis (PLAX) view
    D) Diastolic collapse of the free wall is a finding in cardiac tamponade
    E) The majority of systolic function is derived from radial contraction

21. **Regarding haemophagocytic lymphohistiocytosis (HLH), the following are correct:**

    A) HLH is a group of disorders characterised by activation of macrophages and is rapidly progressive
    B) HLH can be either familial or acquired
    C) Ferritin and triglyceride levels are usually markedly decreased
    D) In <10% of cases of the familial form, there are mutations in the *PRF1* or *UNC13D* genes
    E) Untreated HLH is fatal

22. **Regarding renal replacement therapy (RRT):**

A) RRT utilises diffusion where blood and dialysate flow counter-current on both sides of the semipermeable membrane

B) Small molecules are less efficiently removed using diffusion

C) In the form of haemofiltration, utilises convection to remove solutes and water

D) Involving haemofiltration is more efficient for the removal of water and larger molecules (<60 kDa)

E) Involving haemodiafiltration, exchange of waste products occurs exclusively via diffusion

SBAs

Choose the answer which is the
most correct from the options (A-E)

Question

1. **Formal echocardiography reveals that your 50-year-old patient (IBW 70 kg) with ARDS has severe right heart failure. Currently, you are using a lung-protective strategy with low tidal volume ventilation to achieve PaO_2 9.3 kPa and $PaCO_2$ 10.3 kPa with the ventilator set at PEEP 10 cmH$_2$O, FiO$_2$ 0.5, P_{high} 24 cmH$_2$O, RR 32, V_T 400 mL. Your patient requires noradrenaline 0.3 mcg/kg/min to achieve MAP 65 mmHg. pH 7.1, base excess −3.7 mmol/L, lactate 3.1 mmol/L, urine output 35 mL/h.**
   What should be your first action?

   A) 500 ml intravenous fluid bolus
   B) Abandon low tidal volume ventilation strategy
   C) Call regional ECMO centre
   D) Introduce an additional vasopressor
   E) Commence CVVHF

2. **A patient is intubated and ventilated in ICU for chest sepsis. He is known to have TB, and has received three days of isoniazid and rifampicin, and contact tracing has been undertaken by public health. On day 4, you now discover the patient actually has extensively drug-resistant TB (XDR-TB). Which of the following is the most appropriate first step?**

   A) Add levofloxacin and amikacin to his treatment
   B) Initiate enhanced contact tracing
   C) Ensure you are using a negative-pressure isolation room
   D) Test the patient for HIV
   E) Place the patient in prone position

Clinical Cases in Critical Care, First Edition. Alice Myers and Theophilus Samuels.
© 2023 John Wiley & Sons Ltd. Published 2023 by John Wiley & Sons Ltd.

3. **A 65-year-old male patient is 72 hours post cardiac arrest. He remains comatose and mechanically ventilated with no sedation. CT head confirms loss of grey-white matter differentiation, consistent with hypoxic ischaemic brain injury. Which of the following will have the most robust prognostic value in this patient?**

   A) Presence of myoclonic jerks
   B) Absent pupillary light reflexes
   C) MRI brain
   D) Loss of corneal reflexes
   E) Bilateral absence of N20 (negative peak at 20 ms) somatosensory evoked potentials (SSEPs)

4. **A 47-year-old woman with ARDS is being managed using APRV (airway pressure release ventilation). Ventilator settings are as follows: P_{low} 0 cmH$_2$O, P_{high} 24 cmH$_2$O, T_{high} 5.0 seconds, T_{low} 0.4 seconds, FiO$_2$ 0.35. She is lightly sedated and breathing comfortably in addition to release episodes. Her blood pressure and renal function are unsupported. Arterial blood gas reveals PaO$_2$ 11.4 kPa, PaCO$_2$ 6.5 kPa, pH 7.36, base excess −2 mmol/L, lactate 1.4 mmol/L.**
   What is your best next action?

   A) IV fluid bolus
   B) Change to CPAP with pressure support mode
   C) Increase T_{low} to 3 s
   D) Decrease P_{high} to 22 cmH$_2$O
   E) Decrease T_{high} to 4.5 s

5. **A 53-year-old woman is admitted to ICU with urosepsis. She requires noradrenaline 0.4 mcg/kg/min to achieve mean arterial blood pressure of 65 mmHg. She is drowsy and confused but able to tolerate oxygen via high-flow nasal cannulae (flow rate 60 L/min, FiO$_2$ 0.55, PaO$_2$ 10.2 kPa). Which of the following is the most true in this context?**

   A) Her in-hospital mortality is greater than 10%
   B) SIRS is a more useful scoring system than SOFA
   C) She should be described as having severe sepsis
   D) This patient is likely to have a lower risk of dying through this episode of urosepsis than she would if she had been admitted with an ST-elevation MI rather than sepsis
   E) You are highly unlikely to positively identify the pathogen causing this woman's urosepsis

6. **A 62-year-old man with learning disabilities is intubated on ICU. He has multiorgan failure secondary to severe chest sepsis and his condition is deteriorating (rising oxygen and vasopressor requirements and fully dependent upon renal replacement therapy). He is very frail with an exercise tolerance limited to 5 m with assistance.**

You suspect he will not survive this admission and you would like to change to a palliative approach.

He lives in a care home and has no next of kin.

Which is the most important priority?

A) Sign the 'Not for Resuscitation' order on the patient's ReSPECT form
B) Appoint an IMCA (independent mental capacity advocate)
C) Discuss the case with the learning disabilities nurse specialist
D) Contact the hospital legal team
E) Discuss the patient's wishes with his care home manager

7. A patient is brought to the emergency department by HEMS (helicopter emergency medical service). He has a head injury, multiple rib fractures with a flail segment, an open fracture of his right femur, and may have suffered intra-abdominal injuries. He remains alert, maintaining his own airway, respiratory rate 25–30 breaths per minute, blood pressure 156/95 mmHg, HR 127 bpm. Which is the most appropriate first action?

A) Intubate the patient
B) Perform a full body CT scan
C) Perform a primary survey
D) Place a pelvic binder
E) Splint the fractured leg

8. A 78-year-old male patient with severe COVID pneumonia receiving mechanical ventilation develops a sudden increase in airway pressure (V_T 6 mL/kg, peak airway pressure 40 cmH$_2$O). He remains haemodynamically stable. The left side of his chest is not moving and tracheal deviation to the right is noted on examination. Which of the following lung ultrasonographic findings is most likely to confirm the diagnosis?

A) Presence of A-lines
B) Absence of lung sliding
C) Absence of B-lines
D) Presence of a lung point
E) Absence of lung pulses

9. A 70-year-old male patient presents to the emergency department with acute shortness of breath and chest pain. He appears anxious and is tachycardiac at 130 bpm, BP 130/70 mmHg. An ECG demonstrates electrical alternans and a chest radiograph reveals a globular, enlarged cardiac shadow without pulmonary congestion. On examination, heart sounds are muffled. Which of the following is the most likely aetiology underlying this clinical presentation?

A) Malignancy
B) Acute pericarditis
C) Trauma

D) Uraemia

E) Cardiac failure

10. **A 58-year-old male patient is intubated, paralysed and mechanically ventilated for severe community-acquired pneumonia. After two hours of receiving noradrenaline (current dose is 0.5 mcg/ kg/min), the MAP is between 50 and 55 mmHg. Urine output is <0.5 mL/kg/h and lactate is measured at 3.4 mmol/L. Echocardiography demonstrates a hyperdynamic left ventricle and normal right ventricle systolic function. Stroke volume variation is measured as <5% (with tidal volumes 8 mL/kg). What would be the most appropriate next step in addressing the inadequate MAP?**

A) Give 250 mL bolus balanced crystalloid solution

B) Start hydrocortisone 50 mg QDS

C) Start vasopressin

D) Escalate the dose of noradrenaline

E) Start dobutamine

11. **A 25-year-old man is admitted to intensive care post debridement for type II necrotising fasciitis. Most of his posterior and some of his anterior left leg have been debrided. He is sedated and ventilated, requiring noradrenaline 0.05 mcg/kg/min to achieve MAP >65 mmHg. He has no past medical history and no known allergies. Which of the following is the most correct?**

A) The average mortality for this condition is greater than 60%

B) This can be referred to as Fournier's gangrene

C) He should be treated with high-dose penicillin and clindamycin

D) This is probably due to *Clostridium* infection

E) His CT scan is likely to show subcutaneous gas formation

12. **A 72-year-old female patient is admitted to the acute medical unit with urosepsis. She has received 40 mL/kg fluid resuscitation but remains hypotensive (75/45 mmHg). HR 110 bpm sinus rhythm. Blood gas reveals pH 7.29, PaO_2 12 kPa (4 L/min via nasal cannula oxygen), $PaCO_2$ 4.5 kPa, lactate 3.2 mmol/L, base excess −7 mmol/L, bicarbonate 18 mmol/L. Focused echocardiography demonstrates a left and right ventricle that do not appear significantly impaired or dilated. At present, it will be at least 30 min before the patient can be admitted to the ICU and you will need to remain with this patient. What would be the most appropriate next step in her management?**

A) Further IV crystalloid fluid boluses

B) Commence peripheral vasopressors

C) Site a central venous line

D) Site an arterial line

E) Give albumin fluid boluses

13. A 28-year-old female patient presents to the emergency department with acute shortness of breath. On examination, there is wheeze throughout her chest, a tachycardia (140 bpm sinus rhythm), BP 140/70 mmHg and tachypnoea (RR 40 per minute). There is use of accessory muscles, and she is unable to speak in full sentences or phrases. There is no rash or stridor present. She has only been treated with 15 L/min oxygen therapy prior to your review. Her SpO_2 is 94%. Blood gas on 15 L/min oxygen therapy demonstrates pH 7.49, PaO_2 8.8 kPa, $PaCO_2$ 2.8 kPa, base excess +2 mmol/L, lactate 1.8 mmol/L. Chest radiograph demonstrates hyperinflation with no evidence of infection. Which of the following medications is most appropriate at this point?

A) Intravenous magnesium
B) Intravenous salbutamol
C) Intravenous hydrocortisone
D) Nebulised terbutaline
E) Nebulised adrenaline

14. A 45-year-old male patient with known alcoholic liver disease presents with acute-on-chronic liver failure. He requires intubation and mechanical ventilation for hepatic encephalopathy. He has an ongoing need for fluid resuscitation and requires vasopressor support. Central venous access needs to be obtained. Which of the following tests is most useful in assessing bleeding risk in this patient?

A) International normalised ratio (INR)
B) Platelet count
C) Fibrinogen
D) Viscoelastic test (e.g. thromboelastography, rotational thromboelastometry)
E) Activated partial thromboplastin time (aPTT)

15. A 42-year-old obese woman with no significant past medical history has been admitted to ICU post emergency caesarean section (for foetal distress at 36 weeks of pregnancy). She received general anaesthesia to expedite delivery. Mid-procedure, she became difficult to oxygenate and cardiovascularly unstable. Now in ICU, she remains sedated and ventilated on FiO_2 1.0 for PaO_2 8.4 kPa, noradrenaline is at 0.85 mcg/kg/min to achieve a MAP of 65 mmHg. Haemoglobin is 9 g/L. Which of the following would be the best immediate action?

A) Transfer for computed tomography
B) Perform focused echocardiogram
C) Administer thrombolysis
D) Transfuse packed red cells
E) Replace noradrenaline with dobutamine

16. **A 51-year-old woman is admitted to critical care for postoperative management following pelvic exenteration for ovarian cancer. She requires no organ support but abdominal pain is restricting her recovery. She has a urinary catheter and is passing good volumes of urine. She has an epidural sited at T9–10. Her feet are warm and she has reduced sensation in her legs. She also has mildly reduced power bilaterally symmetrically but can bend both knees. The epidural has been running at 6 mL/h (0.1% levobupivacaine and 2 mcg/mL fentanyl) since her surgery yesterday afternoon. Which of the following is the best first step?**

    A) Request urgent MRI spine to rule out cord compression
    B) Increase the rate of the epidural infusion to 8–10 mL/h
    C) Remove the epidural and prescribe a morphine PCA
    D) Give a cumulative bolus of up to 20 mL local anaesthetic via the epidural
    E) Request urgent surgical review

17. **A 65-year-old male patient has been intubated and mechanically ventilated for seven days. He presented with severe community-acquired pneumonia which has been successfully treated. His Richmond Agitation-Sedation Scale is between −1 and 0. He is currently on spontaneous ventilation, maintaining tidal volumes between 6 and 8 mL/kg, and a PaO_2 between 8 and 10 kPa (FiO_2 0.35). He is haemodynamically stable. Which of the following assessments is most likely to predict successful weaning from mechanical ventilation?**

    A) CORE index (dynamic compliance, oxygenation, rate, effort)
    B) IWI (integrative weaning index)
    C) IEQ (inspiratory effort quotient)
    D) RSBI (rapid shallow breathing index)
    E) Dynamic CROP index (dynamic compliance, respiratory rate, oxygenation, maximum inspiratory pressure index)

18. **A pregnant woman presents at 30 weeks gestation with severe shortness of breath developing over the last two weeks.**
    PaO_2 9 kPa, RR 30, HR 124, temperature 36.5 °C.
    She has recently moved to the UK from India and you do not have access to her previous medical records. She tells you that she has always been well apart from an infection when she was a child. Which investigation is likely to provide the most useful clinical information?

    A) Blood cultures
    B) CTPA
    C) Echocardiogram
    D) D-dimer
    E) Chest X-ray

Answers

MCQs

1.

A) **F** – Dry drowning is a term that is not a medically accepted diagnosis, and many organisations and life-saving institutions around the world discourage the use of this and other similar terms (e.g. 'wet drowning', 'near drowning'). The term arose because it was found that approximately 10–15% of drowning victims had no water found in the lungs at autopsy. The ambiguity of the term may lead to misdiagnosis in cases of sudden death.

B) **F** – Pneumonia is often misdiagnosed initially due to the early radiographical appearance of water in the lungs. In a series of hospitalised non-fatal drowning patients, approximately 1 in 10 required treatment with antibiotics.

C) **F** – Salt water doesn't destroy surfactant; rather, it washes it away and damages the membrane between the alveolus and the capillary blood vessel; the same is true for fresh water.

D) **F** – Young children may have a mammalian diving reflex when drowning occurs in very cold water. On sudden immersion in cold water less than 20 °C, victims can stop breathing, slow their heart rate dramatically and shunt all the blood flow to the heart and brain. Many of these children may be resuscitated and can often return to normal function. Cases of survival have been reported, even after being underwater for an hour.

E) **F** – The rate of cerebral oxygen consumption is reduced by approximately 5%, not 1%.

Clinical Cases in Critical Care, First Edition. Alice Myers and Theophilus Samuels.
© 2023 John Wiley & Sons Ltd. Published 2023 by John Wiley & Sons Ltd.

2.

A) **F** – Myasthenia gravis is graded as follows:
   - Grade I – only eyes affected
   - Grade IIa – mild generalised MG responding well to therapy
   - Grade IIb – moderate generalised MG responding less well
   - Grade III – severe generalised disease
   - Grade IV – myasthenic crisis requiring mechanical ventilation

B) **T** – Suggests neuromuscular transmission defect is secondary to reduced postsynaptic response.

C) **T** – Generalised weakness occurs in around 80%. Diplopia and ptosis occur in most patients and are often early signs.

D) **F** – Insufficient medication will lead to a myasthenic crisis, excessive medication can cause a cholinergic crisis. Both of these crises can have a similar presentation.

E) **F** – There is preservation of deep tendon reflexes, which are lost in Guillain–Barré syndrome.

3.

A) **T**

B) **F** – For major surgery, patients taking 10 mg or more per day of prednisolone should receive steroid replacement perioperatively. An example of a replacement regimen would be: 100 mg hydrocortisone at induction, followed by 50 mg QDS per day for 48–72 hours postoperatively. If the patient has taken steroids for less than a month, they usually do not require additional replacement.

C) **F** – Starting dose should be 15–20 mg per day. This should gradually be increased to 60 mg per day then 60 mg every other day.

D) **F** – 10 mg prednisolone is equivalent to 40 mg hydrocortisone, 1.6 mg dexamethasone, and 8 mg triamcinolone.

E) **F** – It was hydrocortisone at a dose of 50 mg given six hourly which demonstrated no survival benefit in adult patients with severe septic shock.

4.

A) **T**

B) **F** – Kidney as well.

C) **F** – Type A is due to inadequate perfusion of tissues, tissue hypoxia and is classically the result of the various types of shock. Type B occurs in the context of apparently adequate tissue perfusion and oxygenation and is usually due to drugs, poisons and inborn errors of metabolism.

D) **F** – The rapid increase in muscular activity seen in tonic–clonic type seizures leads to a mismatch in oxygen supply and demand and can result in type A lactataemia. This is not seen in absence seizures.

E) **F** – D-lactate is produced by bacteria. Carbohydrate malabsorption can lead to an increase in D-lactate. In humans, lactate is derived from L-lactate. Most routine lactate analysers only measure L-lactate. A rise in D-lactate should be suspected in raised anion gap acidosis.

5.

A) **F** – The IABP is sited within the aorta but is inflated during the diastolic phase of the cardiac cycle. This displaces blood towards the aortic root, which in turn increases flow through patent coronary arteries leading to an increase in diastolic coronary perfusion.

B) **F** – Helium is the sole gas used and is less dense than oxygen at room temperature, which allows for rapid inflation of the balloon under laminar flow (decreases the Reynolds number).

C) **T** – It can be also triggered using the ECG (most common), synchronised with a pacing device or set up in an asynchronous mode.

D) **F** – Weaning from an IABP is usually done over 6–12 hours once the required physiological parameters are sufficiently met. An incremental decrease of the ratio of IABP-supported heartbeat to unassisted heartbeat is performed from the initial ratio of 1:1 to 1:2, 1:4 and 1:8. In the absence of any adverse event from reducing the support, the IABP is removed when the ratio is 1:8 in order to prevent thrombosis.

E) **F** – There are few absolute contraindications to using an IABP. Severe aortic insufficiency and aortic dissection, along with patient refusal, are considered the only absolute contraindications.

6.

A) **T**

B) **F** – The main cause of HUS is Shiga toxin-producing *Escherichia coli* (STEC), also known as enterohaemorrhagic *E. coli* (EHEC), with patients usually presenting with a gastrointestinal prodrome. Viral infections can also cause HUS (e.g. HIV, influenza A and enteroviruses) but are less common.

C) **F** – EHEC-associated HUS occurs primarily in children younger than five years of age and in the elderly.

D) **T** – Neurological symptoms may vary from mild jerks to stroke or severe coma in approximately 30% of cases and are associated with a worse outcome.

E) **T** – The complement abnormality may be a genetic rearrangement, mutation or deletion in a gene encoding a complement factor. aHUS is an ultra-rare disease with an estimated incidence most probably between 0.5 and 2 per million. It is more frequently seen in childhood, particularly under the age of two years.

7.

A) **T**

B) **T**

C) **T**

D) **F** – It has low specific gravity (1.007) which, through buoyancy, serves to effectively reduce the weight of the brain via the Archimedes principle and protect it from acceleration and deceleration forces.

E) **F** – CSF production is reliant on blood flow through the choroid plexus. If cerebral perfusion pressure falls below 70 mmHg, CSF production falls.

8.

A) **F** – Glucagon release is stimulated by a fall in blood glucose concentration. Insulin is released in response to a rise in blood glucose concentration.

B) **F** – Glucagon is released by the alpha cells of the islets of Langerhans, while insulin is released by the beta cells.

C) **F** – It requires only 1 mcg/kg (not 1 mg/kg!) to raise glucose blood concentration by 20 mg/100 mL (a 25% increase) in about 20 minutes. This is the reason why glucagon is called the *hyperglycaemic hormone*.

D) **T** – Gluconeogenesis still occurs in the liver once all of the glycogen stores are depleted. This is due to increased amino acid uptake by liver cells, which then convert these amino acids into glucose by gluconeogenesis.

E) **F** – Glucagon activates adipose cell lipase, thereby making increased quantities of fatty acids available as an energy substrate for the body.

9.

A) **F** – AVP (also called antidiuretic hormone or ADH) is synthesised in the hypothalamus and secreted by the posterior pituitary gland.

B) **T**

C) **F** – Once released, AVP binds to V2 receptors on the basolateral membranes of the renal epithelial cells lining the collecting ducts. Once bound, this results in the insertion of water channels (e.g. aquaporins) into the luminal membrane, permitting passive diffusion of water across the collecting ducts.

D) **T** – Plasma hypertonicity is the major stimulus for AVP release, but its release is also affected by other non-osmotic factors such as hypoglycaemia, effective circulating blood volume and drugs (e.g. thiazide and thiazide-like diuretics, NSAIDs, antipsychotics).

E) **T**

10.

A) **T**

B) **F** – The anterior cerebral circulation provides approximately 70% of the total cerebral circulation and supplies the frontal, temporal and parietal lobes, as well as the basal ganglia and hypothalamus. The remaining 30% of the cerebral circulation arises from the vertebrobasilar system, supplying the brainstem, cerebellum, occipital lobes and thalamus.

C) **F** – CPP is physiologically the difference between the arterial pressure in the feeding arteries as they enter the subarachnoid space and the draining veins before they enter the major dural sinuses; this makes the direct measurement of CPP difficult. Therefore, CPP is estimated by the difference between the systemic mean arterial blood pressure (MAP) and the intracranial pressure (ICP), which is an estimate of the tissue pressure.

D) **T** – In normal individuals, at systemic mean arterial pressures (MAP) between approximately 50 and 150 mmHg, the cerebral vessels are able to change diameter inversely with changing perfusion pressure. Thus, as CPP rises, vessels constrict, and in turn dilate when CPP falls so that blood flow is kept constant.

E) **F** – The autoregulatory range described in part D is affected by age (shifted left in newborns) and by chronic hypertension. In the latter, the range is shifted to the right, so care should be taken in overtreating systolic blood pressure in these patients as there is a risk of cerebral ischaemia at the lower limits of autoregulation.

11.

A) **F** – A five-letter code is used to describe the functions of a pacemaker.

B) **T** – The first three letters describe the antibradycardia functions.
- Position I – chamber paced (A = atria, V = ventricle, D = dual [A + V])
- Position II – chamber sensed (A = atria, V = ventricle, D = dual [A + V])
- Position III – response to sensing (T = triggered, I = inhibited, D = dual [T + I])

C) **T** – The fourth letter is used to describe rate modulation or programmability.
- Position IVR = rate modulation, P = simple programmable (rate or output), M = multiprogrammable, O = none

The fifth and last letter describes the antitachycardia functions.
- Position V – P = pacing, S = shock, D = dual (P + S)

D) **F** – A pacemaker can carry one classification (e.g. DDD) but, depending on how it has been programmed, is capable of several modes of function.

E) **T** – All pacemakers are programmed to fire after a maximum period in which no activity has been detected. This maximum period of time is known as the *lower rate-limiting interval*.

12.

A) **T** – Ions carry an electrical charge, and are termed *cations* if the charge is positive (e.g. Na^+, K^+) and are attracted to a negative electrode or cathode, or *anions* if the charge is negative (e.g. Cl^-) and they are attracted to a positive electrode or anode.

B) **T**

C) **F** – Sodium intracellular concentrations vary between 3 and 20 mmol/.

D) **F** – Potassium is the principal intracellular *cation* (as it is a positively charged ion).

E) **T**

13.

A) **T** – Along with shock and myocardial ischaemia.

B) **F** – Atropine is recommended up to a maximum dose of 3 mg.

C) **T**

D) **F** – A ventricular pause of >3 seconds is a risk factor for asystole.

E) **T** – Glucagon can also be considered in bradycardia associated with calcium channel blocker overdose.

14.

A) **T** – The innate immune system (e.g. macrophages, monocytes, granulocytes, dendritic cells and natural killer cells) has evolved to detect both PAMPs and damage-associated molecular patterns (DAMPs).

B) **T** – HMGB1 intracellular proteins, along with ATP and mitochondrial DNA, are considered DAMPs. HMGB1 is also released upon apoptosis and pyroptosis.

C) **F** – Pyroptosis describes a highly inflammatory programmed cell death process that most probably forms part of the antimicrobial response and occurs most frequently upon infection with intracellular pathogens.

D) **T** – Both PAMPs and DAMPs activate the innate immune system and certain epithelial cells through pattern recognition receptors in the cytosol (e.g. NOD-like receptors) or on the cell surface (e.g. Toll-like receptors). Interestingly, some of these pattern recognition receptors (mainly NOD-like receptors) can assemble into molecular complexes termed *inflammasomes*. It is these inflammasomes that play a key role in the maturation and secretion of IL-1-beta and IL-18.

E) **T** – Both IL-1-beta and IL-18 are very potent cytokines that can trigger pyroptosis by caspase-mediated rapid rupture of the plasma membrane.

15.

A) **F** – DWI MRI can now be used within six hour of symptom onset to detect acute cerebral ischaemia, particularly in doubtful cases. DWI can also reveal silent areas of cerebral ischaemia.

B) **F** – DWI is able to discriminate in this instance.

C) **F** – MRA is notably less sensitive than CTA in this respect.

D) **T** – The ECASS investigators (2008) demonstrated that alteplase given 3-4.5 hour after acute ischaemic stroke significantly improves clinical outcomes. However, it was more frequently associated with symptomatic intracranial haemorrhage. It is recommended for the treatment of acute ischaemic stroke by the National Institute for Health and Care Excellence (NICE) in the UK.

E) **F** – Many TIAs last for less than one hour.

16.

A) **T**

B) **F** – Hepatitis is a process of hepatocellular inflammation and damage that releases intracellular contents into the blood. It therefore results primarily in elevations in AST and ALT, with modest increases seen in alcoholic hepatitis and extreme elevations in acute viral hepatitis. ALP can also be elevated, but elevations are generally less significant.

C) **F** - Hepatitis C is a blood-borne RNA virus primarily transmitted through blood contact with infected individuals. Most acute infections are asymptomatic; 20–30% of infected individuals will have a self-limiting illness.

D) **T** – Chronic infection can lead to cirrhosis and increase the risk of hepatocellular carcinoma.

E) **F** – Cirrhotic ascites is associated with spontaneous bacterial peritonitis and hepatorenal syndrome, and carries a three-years mortality of 50%.

17.

A) **T** – HPS consists of a triad of liver disease, intravascular pulmonary dilation and abnormal pulmonary gas exchange. It commonly presents as dyspnoea or hypoxia in liver disease patients.

B) **F** – The shortness of breath is relieved when the patient is lying down, and is referred to as *platypnoea*. In addition, hypoxia is often worse in the standing position (orthodeoxia), and it can be generally improved with supplemental oxygen.

C) **F** – NO has been implicated as a key vasodilator in HPS, and its levels are correlated with the severity of cirrhosis and gas exchange abnormalities. Exhaled levels are increased in patients with cirrhosis compared to healthy individuals and in HPS patients compared to cirrhotic patients without HPS.

D) **F** – Death is usually due to complications from liver disease, and it is rare for patients to die from primary respiratory failure.

E) **T** – Evaluation for transplant should be pursued in patients with HPS who are symptomatic or have a room air PaO_2 less than 8.0 kPa in seated position.

18.

A) **T** – B-lines (or 'comet tails') are horizontal hyperechoic beams emanating from the inferior margin of the pleural line, which then extend through to the deep edge of the screen. They fan out and move with the motion of the pleural line, removing the ability to visualise A-lines. Due to the lung bases possessing a greater mass of lung tissue, they will often display a B-line pattern, making examination of an upper lung field more informative for the presence of pulmonary oedema.

B) **T** – A-lines are reverberation artefacts originating from the pleural line, and with adequate depth can be seen as parallel lines at regular (equidistant) intervals.

C) **T**

D) **F** – This sign refers to the appearance of parallel horizontal lines that extend through the entire field of view and indicates lack of normal motion in an inflated lung, which can be caused by pneumothorax, atelectasis, apnoea, previous pleurodesis or pleurectomy.

E) **F** – Lung sliding is a dynamic sign, described as shimmering of the parietal and visceral pleura in contact and is part of the normal aeration pattern. Pneumothorax can be effectively ruled out by the presence of lung sliding at the intercostal location under the applied ultrasound probe.

19.

A) **T** – Both CIP and CIM exact a significant economic burden and affect post-ICU quality of life.

B) **F** – They share the major clinical symptoms of early muscle atrophy, muscle weakness. However, loss of deep tendon reflexes and distal loss of sensitivity to light touch, pain, temperature and vibration due to the impairment of sensory nerve fibres are associated with CIP.

C) **T** – In ventilated patients, it can be difficult to carefully evaluate the patient's neurology, therefore failure to wean may be the first sign.

D) **F** – CIM carries the better prognosis, as muscles regenerate faster than nerves.

E) **F** – High, not low, blood glucose concentrations are associated risk factors.

20.

A) **F** – A TAPSE greater than or equal to 17 mm is considered normal. It is an angle-dependent measurement and underestimation can occur when M-mode alignment is not parallel.

B) **T**

C) **F** – Using visual assessment, systolic function is best assessed in the apical four-chamber view (or more specifically, the RV focused view).

D) **T** – This is a late finding in cardiac tamponade; other findings include pericardial effusion, swinging heart, exaggerated respiratory-related changes in RV and LV size (ventricular interdependence), diastolic right atrial collapse, and Doppler inflow velocities and hepatic venous flow pattern change.

E) **F** – Approximately 80% RV systolic function is due to longitudinal contraction.

21.

A) **T** – Histiocytic diseases are divided into five groups:
- L group – these diseases include Langerhans cell histiocytosis (LCH) and Erdheim–Chester disease
- C group – these include non-LCHs that involve the skin and/or mucosal surfaces
- M group – these include the malignant histiocytoses, such as primary malignant histiocytosis and secondary malignant histiocytoses that occur with leukaemias, lymphomas or other haematological neoplasms

- R group – contains the miscellaneous non-cutaneous, non-LCH histiocytoses along with Rosai–Dorfman disease
- H group – contains varieties of HLH and macrophage activation syndromes (MAS)

B) **T**

C) **F** – Ferritin and triglyceride levels form a useful additional clinical test to bone marrow examination. The levels of both are increased, with ferritin potentially being markedly raised (usually in the tens of thousands mcg/L). However, in adults, even though the negative predictive value of a normal ferritin result is high, it is not a discerning marker for adult forms of HLH, as it is also elevated in other chronic inflammatory conditions, haemolytic anaemia and renal failure.

D) **F** – Approximately 50% of cases are found to have mutations in these genes.

E) **T** – HLH is characterised by activation of macrophages, that leads to a progressive and, if left untreated, fatal characteristic presentation of pancytopenia, coagulopathy, deranged liver function and fever.

22.

A) **T** – Diffusion involves the solute concentration gradient driving the movement of solute across the semipermeable membrane, as in haemodialysis.

B) **F** – Diffusion is very efficient at removing small molecules (e.g. potassium, ammonium and creatinine). It is less efficient in removing larger solutes and water.

C) **T** – Solutes and water are transported over a semipermeable membrane by a difference in pressure between both sides of the membrane. The amount of water and solutes transported across the membrane depends upon the permeability coefficient of the membrane and the difference in pressure between both sides of the membrane.

D) **T**

E) **F** – In haemodiafiltration, both convection and diffusion are used.

SBAs

1.

Answer: B

Mild hypercapnia can potentially increase oxygen delivery via an increase in cardiac output (decreased systemic vascular resistance, increased heart rate and increased contractility) and left shift of the oxyhaemoglobin dissociation curve. However, significant hypercapnia can be harmful in patients with right heart failure due to the increase in pulmonary vascular resistance, which is potentiated by acidaemia. The respiratory rate is already very high and you are unlikely to be able to maintain low tidal volumes if you are to reduce the $PaCO_2$ to more acceptable levels.

2.

Answer: C

Strict infection control is vital. Protect staff and other vulnerable patients.

Testing for HIV is useful as it will help prognosticate and initiate appropriate treatment but will not immediately alter management. Discuss with microbiology urgently. The organism may also be resistant to amikacin and levofloxacin as this is XDR-TB. Enhanced contact tracing is important, but is not the most appropriate step at this stage. XDR-TB is transmitted in the same way as normal TB, and is a rare type of multidrug-resistant TB (MDR-TB) that is resistant to rifampicin and isoniazid. Prone position may be useful if the patient deteriorates and clinical state warrants it, but there is no indication for that in the available information.

3.

Answer: E

Bilaterally absent short latency peaks (N20 peaks) are 100% prognostic of poor outcomes at 72 h post ROSC. MRI brain can be used for prognostication two to five days following ROSC. However, the evidence for the use of MRI is prone to selection bias. Absent pupillary light and corneal reflexes at 72 hours are often used as poor prognostic indicators, but strong evidence is lacking and these measurements are operator dependent and qualitative. Myoclonic jerks have little prognostic value.

4.

Answer: D

This patient appears to be progressing well with her APRV and can be weaned. There is no suggestion from the information given that fluid bolus needs to be given right now.

T_{low} should be set according to the time constant of the lung to achieve 75% of peak expiratory flow and is not changed during weaning. T_{low} is usually about 0.5 seconds or less. The $PaCO_2$ is within a good range and the patient is breathing spontaneously so there does not appear to be any indication to increase the frequency of pressure release episodes (E is incorrect).

You could consider changing to CPAP with pressure support but since the patient is progressing well and you are still needing quite high P_{high}, it would be better to continue weaning on APRV. Aim to wean the P_{high} to 12–16 cmH_2O before changing to CPAP or considering extubation.

5.

Answer: A

Sepsis is a life-threatening organ dysfunction caused by a dysregulated host response to infection, with an increase in a SOFA score of 2 or more being associated with a more than 10% in-hospital mortality. This patient scores a minimum of 4 simply due to her noradrenaline requirement.

The overall mortality rate for STEMI is 8.1%.

SIRS criteria have been found to be unhelpful in definition of sepsis and have been superseded by the SOFA and qSOFA scores.

In 2016, the Third International Consensus Definitions for Sepsis and Septic Shock (Singer et al., JAMA) concluded that the term 'severe sepsis' is redundant.

A full septic screen should always be performed and empirical antimicrobial therapy commenced. In cases of urosepsis, a pathogen is often identified from urine or blood cultures (up to 78% in some studies).

6.

Answer: B

The Mental Capacity Act in the UK requires an IMCA to be appointed for serious medical treatment decisions where the patient lacks capacity, where there is no next of kin with whom to 'consult', and where the repercussions would have major consequences for the patient.

The hospital's learning disabilities team should be involved but they are unlikely to be able to help with the decision-making process at this point.

Unless the care home manager has been named as next of kin, you are not obliged to discuss the decision with them. However, often patients live in a care home for many years and the staff become close to the residents. It may be valuable to try and find out whether the patient was ever able to discuss end-of-life issues previously. The IMCA may wish to speak to staff at the care home for this reason.

Although it is the doctor's decision and responsibility to sign a DNAR or to withdraw life-sustaining treatment, this is done in close consultation with the patient and/or their next of kin. Occasionally, there can be significant disagreements between doctors and relatives and a decision may need to be escalated to the court of protection. At this stage, there is no disagreement and so there is no indication to discuss the case with the hospital legal team.

The most important priority is to appoint an IMCA.

7.

Answer: C

The only action which trumps the primary survey in a trauma call is to manage catastrophic bleeding (see NICE Guidance 39). If active pelvic bleeding is suspected then it would be reasonable to apply a pelvic binder as part of managing catastrophic bleeding, but that is not a strong suspicion from the information given here. Splinting the fractured leg at this point would not take priority over the primary survey.

Some major trauma centres may choose to perform full-body CT prior to performing the primary survey in specific patients. However, this is not standard practice.

8.

Answer: D

The patient has developed a left-sided pneumothorax, most probably as a complication of mechanical ventilation due to COVID pneumonia. Using lung ultrasound, the presence of a lung point has 100% specificity for the diagnosis of pneumothorax. However, a lung point cannot be visualised in totally collapsed lungs.

The absence of lung sliding, lung pulses and B-lines can also be associated with a pneumothorax, but they are not specific to its diagnosis. However, these findings have high negative predictive values. That is, if they are observed then they effectively rule out a pneumothorax at the point on the chest wall at which the probe is being applied. A-lines are present in patients with and without a pneumothorax. However, if A-lines are present in the absence of lung sliding, the reported sensitivity and specificity are approximately 95% and 94% respectively for pneumothorax.

9.

Answer: A

The patient is presenting with a symptomatic pericardial effusion. Pericardial effusions can be caused by any disease that can cause an acute pericarditis. Studies have shown that in patients undergoing pericardiocentesis, the most common aetiology was malignancy. Up to one-fifth of patients had an undiagnosed malignancy at time of pericardiocentesis. After malignancy, the remaining causes in order of frequency were idiopathic, acute pericarditis, trauma, other (which included cardiac failure) and uraemia.

10.

Answer: C

Current European Society of Intensive Care Medicine (ESICM) 2021 guidelines on sepsis suggest adding vasopressin if MAP remains inadequate despite low to moderate dose noradrenaline (e.g. 0.25–0.5 mcg/kg/min), rather than escalating the dose of noradrenaline. If vasopressin fails to maintain the required MAP, then adrenaline should be considered. Giving further fluid is immediately ruled out as the most appropriate next step, as the SVV is 5%, which suggests this patient is unlikely to be fluid responsive. It is suggested that corticosteroids are added at a dose of noradrenaline or adrenaline ≥0.25 mcg/kg/min at least 4 hours after initiation. Dobutamine is recommended in the presence of cardiac dysfunction with persistent hypoperfusion despite adequate volume status and arterial pressure.

11.

Answer: C

There are three types of necrotising fasciitis:

- Type I – polymicrobial, may be gas forming, usually occurs either following surgery/injury or abdomen/head/genitals (Fournier's gangrene), patients usually have co-morbidities, commonly develop septic shock
- Type II – monomicrobial with Group A *Streptococcus*, non-gas forming, often occurs at the extremities, can affect anyone including young fit patients, associated with toxic shock syndrome
- Type III – monomicrobial infection with *Clostridium perfringens* or *septicum*, often gas forming, usually with penetrating trauma, surgery or intravenous drug use, may be deeply invasive and associated with intravascular haemolytic anaemia

Mortality is usually around 20–40%. If toxic shock develops then mortality can be more than 60%. Noradrenaline 0.05 mcg/kg/min in a sedated patient does not suggest the presence of toxic shock, though this may develop later.

12.

Answer: B

When peripheral access is used for vasopressors, patients are more likely to have vasopressors started to achieve a MAP >65 mmHg within one hour. Delay in achieving a MAP >65 mmHg using vasopressors is associated with increased mortality. She has already received 40 mL/kg of fluid resuscitation, and though further fluids may be indicated, her MAP will need to be increased sooner rather than later. A central line and arterial line will be required in this patient in due course, especially as peripheral vasopressors should only be used for a short period of time. So central access will be needed for longer term vasopressor use. The use of albumin is suggested in patients who have received large volumes of crystalloids but may not immediately improve the MAP at this point.

13.

Answer: D

British Thoracic Society (2019) guidelines for the management of acute asthma in adults advise that in most cases beta-2 agonists (e.g. salbutamol and terbutaline) in high doses act quickly to relieve bronchospasm with few side-effects. They should be administered as early as possible, preferably in an oxygen-driven nebulised form. There appears to be no difference between salbutamol and terbutaline in terms of efficacy, so either can be used. Nebulised adrenaline does not have any significant benefit over terbutaline or salbutamol. Intravenous salbutamol should be used in patients where inhaled therapy cannot be used reliably. Steroids should be given to all patients with an acute asthma exacerbation and continued until recovery (minimum five days). Intravenous magnesium is recommended in patients who have not had a good initial response to inhaled bronchodilator therapy.

14.

Answer: D

The Society of Critical Care Medicine (SCCM) recommends the use of viscoelastic testing in critically ill patients undergoing procedures with acute-on-chronic liver failure. Other measures, aside from viscoelastic testing, consistently fail to provide reliable assessments of overall haemostatic function and risk of bleeding. Global coagulation status can be assessed using viscoelastic testing and allows for real-time global and functional evaluation of any changes in the pro- and anticoagulant pathways.

15.

Answer: B

It is likely that this woman has either suffered massive pulmonary embolism (thrombotic or amniotic) or that she has had some other major cardiac event leading to cardiogenic shock. There are many other possible diagnoses (including sepsis, ischaemic gut, etc.) but these are the most likely.

CTPA would be useful to demonstrate filling defect and confirm the diagnosis, but she is arguably too unstable for transfer to CT scan and CT will not give you information to guide your cardiovascular support.

There should be extreme caution if considering administering thrombolysis since she is post-op.

If her presentation is secondary to PE, focused echocardiography will be able to demonstrate a dilated right ventricle and systolic impairment.

16.

Answer: D

Daily surgical review should happen routinely but there does not appear to be a need to call for urgent review – her surgery was yesterday so postoperative pain is not unexpected. This appears to be a pain management problem.

It is not impossible that there is cord compression but her lower motor weakness is more likely secondary to the epidural which she has in situ.

From the information you have, it sounds as if the epidural is in the correct space – there are signs of sympathetic and motor blockade. However, the block is too low to manage her pain symptoms. Ideally, it would be better to get the epidural block to the right level, rather than remove the epidural and replace it with a morphine PCA which could result in nausea, constipation and respiratory depression.

Increasing the rate from 6 mL/h to 8–10mL/h might make some difference but it will be slow to take effect. If you give a bolus dose down the epidural, you can test to be assured that the catheter is in the right space and you can raise the level of the block, hopefully reducing her pain. After that you may need to increase the rate or remove the catheter, depending on whether the epidural block is good enough.

17.

Answer: D

The RSBI is the ratio of respiratory frequency to tidal volume (f/V_T). Following a systematic review of 20 RSBI studies (2001), it was concluded that a negative RSBI (i.e. ≥ 105 breaths/min/L) was associated with a large increase in the probability of weaning failure. Conversely, a positive RSBI (i.e. <105 breaths/min/L) is associated with only a small increase in the probability of weaning success. These findings suggest that greater emphasis should be placed on identifying patients with a negative RSBI. The RSBI has positive and negative predictive values of 78% and 95% respectively.

None of the other indices listed are considered superior to the RSBI in predicting success from weaning. For example, the positive and negative predictive values of the dynamic CROP index are 71% and 70% respectively.

18.

Answer: C

This history could be consistent with several diagnoses.

- Pregnancy-associated cardiac failure. This could be cardiomyopathy but the history of infection as a child (rheumatic fever is endemic in India) makes you consider decompensation of mitral stenosis due to the physiological changes of pregnancy.
- Pulmonary embolism. She is high risk for DVT and PE.
- It is possible that she could have chest sepsis or sepsis of another source, or indeed tuberculosis, but her temperature is normal, so you are more concerned that this is cardiac in origin.

You would certainly perform blood cultures, but an echocardiogram would be most useful to look for cardiomyopathy and mitral stenosis, and would also suggest PE if there is right ventricle dilation, systolic impairment and raised pulmonary artery systolic pressures. You would rather avoid CTPA if possible due to ionising radiation. D-dimer is not a discriminatory investigation and you will need to wait for the result.

Index

Notes:
Abbreviations used in the index are listed on pages 13–14.
Page numbers in *italics* indicate figures and those in **bold** denote tables.

'60/60' sign, 123

A

Abbreviated Injury Score (AIS), 288, 290
ABCDE approach/assessment
  COVID-19, 316
  drug overdose, 240–241
  fire/burns injury, 280–281
  haematemesis, 94
  maternal haemorrhage, 261
  polymorphic ventricular tachycardia, 225–226
  road traffic collision, 71
  seizures, 157
ABCDEF bundle (acronym), 153
ABCS (Alignment, Bony Structures, Cartilage and
    Soft tissues), 282
abdominal pain
  biliary colic, 65
  pancreatitis *see* pancreatitis, acute
  severe, causes, 65–66
  vomiting with, 60–70
    diagnostic imaging, 67
    see also diabetic ketoacidosis (DKA)
abducens nerve (VI), 190, 207
ABO blood groups, 75, 76
abscesses, intracranial, 188
acetylcholinesterase inhibitors, 53
N-acetylcysteine (NAC), 241, 242–243, 245
aciclovir, 159, 162, 164
acidaemia, metabolic
  in diabetic ketoacidosis, 61, 62, 63
  in haematemesis, 95
acidosis
  metabolic *see* metabolic acidosis
  mixed respiratory and metabolic, 133, 157
acid suppression therapy, 95
Acinetobacter, 10
acquired immunodeficiency syndrome
    (AIDS) *see* AIDS
acrodermatitis enteropathica, 235

acronyms *see* mnemonics and acronyms
activated charcoal, 242, 243
activated coagulation time (ACT), 269
ACURASYS trial, 111
acute cardiac event
  chordae tendinae rupture, 39, 266
  respiratory distress I in, 39
  see also cardiac arrest; myocardial infarction (MI)
acute heart failure, 184–186
  definition and types, 184
  treatment principles, 184–185
acute inflammatory demyelinating
    polyradiculoneuropathy (AIDP), 48
acute kidney injury (AKI)
  after cardiopulmonary bypass, 269
  CRRT in *see* continuous renal replacement
    therapy (CRRT)
  'early' *vs* 'late' renal replacement therapy, 113
  hepatorenal syndrome, 250
  in obstetric patient, 256, 258
  pre-renal, in diabetic ketoacidosis, 64
  in rhabdomyolysis, 87
    mechanism, 87–88
  in sepsis and critical illness, 113, 214
  severity
    creatinine and urea use, 89
    KDIGO classification, 87, **88**
  troponin levels, 215
acute liver failure *see* liver failure, acute
acute medical care unit (AMU), 293
acute motor axonal neuropathy (AMAN), 49
acute motor sensory axonal neuropathy
    (AMSAN), 49
acute respiratory distress syndrome (ARDS),
    69, 79, 111
  in acute pancreatitis, 69
  after blast injury and fire, 280, 285, 286, 289
  CABP complication, 268
  chest radiography, 110, *110*
  in chest sepsis, 110, *110*, 112, 114, 264
  in COVID-19, 308, 310, 314